Introductory Mental Health Nursing

THIRD EDITION

Donna M. Womble, RN, BS, MEd

Program Coordinator,
Assistant Professor of Nursing (Retired)
Health Occupations—Vocational Nursing
South Plains College
Plainview, Texas

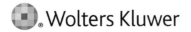
Wolters Kluwer

Philadelphia • Baltimore • New York • London
Buenos Aires • Hong Kong • Sydney • Tokyo

Acquisitions Editor: Christopher Richardson
Product Development Editor: Shana Murph
Editorial Assistant: Zachary Shapiro
Production Project Manager: Priscilla Crater
Design Coordinator: Terry Mallon
Manufacturing Coordinator: Karin Duffield
Marketing Manager: Dean Karampelas
Prepress Vendor: Aptara, Inc.

9 8 7 6 5 4 3 2

Printed in China

Library of Congress Cataloging-in-Publication Data
Available upon request
ISBN: 978-1-4511-4714-8

DEDICATION

To my wonderful family,
Tanya, Julie, Jimmy, and Hagen

Reviewers

Adrienne Blanks, MSN
Program Head, Nursing Education
Southside Virginia Community
    College
Keysville, Virginia

Anu Chiarelli, RN, BA, MA
Instructor, School of Health,
    Justice, and Human Services
Bow Valley College
Alberta, Canada

Sherri Comfort
Practical Nursing Faculty/
    Department Chair
Holmes Community College
Goodman, Mississippi

Ruth Gladen, MS, RN
Associate Professor
North Dakota State College
Wahpeton, North Dakota

Eula Jackson, MSN, PhD
Nursing Instructor
Reid State Technical College
Evergreen, Alabama

Nora James, MSN
VN Coordinator
Lee College
Baytown, Texas

Mary Lynn Kosinski, RN, BSN
Instructor, Practical Nursing
    Program
Flint Hills Technical College
Emporia, Kansas

Esther Labro-Aguilar, RN, BSN
Practical Nursing Coordinator
Sprott Shaw College
British Columbia, Canada

Annitta Love, MSN, RN
Program Coordinator/Director
    Practical Nursing
H. Councill Trenholm State
    Technical College
Montgomery, Alabama

Ruth Malone, MSN, RN
Director of Clinical Education
Galen College of Nursing
Louisville, Kentucky

Renee Moss, BSN, RN
Nursing Instructor
Phillips Community College of the
    University of Arkansas
DeWitt, Arkansas

Lauren Mullen, RN, MSN
Nursing Instructor
James Madison University
Harrisonburg, Virginia

Noel Nesbitt, RN, PhD
Practical Nurse Program
    Coordinator
Delta College
Covington, Louisiana

Sharon Nowak, RN, MSN, EdD
Professor of Nursing
Jackson College
Jackson, Michigan

Mary Olson, BSN, MSN
Practical Nursing Program Director
St. Paul College
St. Paul, Minnesota

JoAnne Pearce, MS, RN
Director of Nursing Programs
Idaho State University
Pocatello, Idaho

**Cheryl Pratt, EdD, MA, RN,
PHN, NEA-BC**
Nursing Dean
Rasmussen College
Mankato, Minnesota

Carol Price, APRN, PMHNP-BC
Assistant Professor of Nursing
Somerset Community College
Somerset, Kentucky

**Martha Sanderford-Smith,
MA, MSN, RN**
Adjunct Faculty
St. Louis College of Health Careers
Fenton, Missouri

Linda Sheets, MSN, RN
LPN Instructor
Lake Technical College
Eustis, Florida

**Rox Ann Sparks, RN, MSN,
MICN, LNC**
Assistant Director of Vocational
    Nursing
Merced College
Merced, California

Arlene Spinner, MSN
Assistant Professor
LaGuardia Community College
Long Island City, New York

Barbara Taylor, MSN, RN
LPN Instructor
Walton Career Development Center
DeFuniak Springs, Florida

Laura Travis, MSN, BSN
Health Careers Coordinator
Tennessee Technology Center at
    Dickson
Dickson, Tennessee

Preface

After using the first edition of this textbook in teaching Mental Health and Illness, I am excited to continue to improve the content to provide the preparation students need as they learn the basic principles and foundation for the mental health issues that are present in every aspect of the health care industry. I have observed the result as students apply the nursing process working with clients in their clinical rotations. Students consistently cite the readability and format as strengths of the book. Although this level of student nurse does not always have the opportunity for inpatient psychiatric unit experience, the majority of LPN/LVN graduates will encounter the mental issues in a variety of health care settings. I attempted to integrate these demographics of employment and functional roles into the text of this book. Regardless of the level of nursing credentials, it is essential for every nurse to have a basic understanding of how the mind and body work and influence the way we function as human beings.

It is often difficult for us to understand our present behavior and situation unless we have some conception of how we got to this point. Most of us do not realize that our perception of the world around us is influenced by all of our previous life experiences. Each experience is incorporated into our memory forming a screen through which new experiences are filtered. It is this predisposed view created in our mind that influences our insight and awareness of the present. Because students in the LPN/LVN programs do not typically have a theoretical foundation in psychology, it is difficult for them to conceptualize these basic concepts. Yet, they are the basis for current psychotherapeutic treatment methods. It is the aim of this text to provide a summarized overview of the theories integral in current treatment modalities. The presentation of human dynamics and the balance between adaptive and maladaptive responses to both internal and external stressors sets the climate for the presentation of the disorders.

This book presents the subject of mental health and illness by first establishing the essential groundwork. Unit I presents a picture of mental health and mental illness including an expanded section on the cultural, ethnic, and religious influences. A basic understanding of how mental issues are viewed or approached is needed for the multicultural diversity of our current population. Factors that affect our mental health are also discussed in this unit. Human emotions, stress, anxiety, grief, and loss are discussed along with the variables of human response to these factors. A new chapter has been added to address the role of anger, violence, and abuse as contributing factors. The impact of domestic violence, abuse, and bullying on the victims and on our society as a whole is discussed. Assessment of the induced trauma along with the subjects of crisis and suicide prevention are presented in a context of intervention and treatment. Chapter 3 presents various theories of personality and psychological development and how this shapes the holistic nature of who we are and our behavior as human beings.

Building on these concepts, Unit II discusses the delivery of mental health care, beginning with early views up to the present issues. The section on outpatient mental health settings and community mental health services is expanded to include more information on services offered in promoting wellness and quality of life for those with mental illness. Legal and ethical considerations, including client rights and accountability are addressed. The various practice settings for mental health care, both conventional and unconventional are included to provide a broad picture of how mental health is a common encounter in every health care setting. Initiation of the treatment process beginning with an introduction to the treatment team, the functions of a holistic approach, and the client's role in recovery are discussed.

In Unit III we will look at the nursing process as it applies to mental health nursing. This will include the art of therapeutic communication, techniques to facilitate communication, and things that hinder interaction with the client in a mental health setting. In addition, the components of a therapeutic relationship and ways to establish nurse–client interaction in potentially difficult situations are integrated.

Unit IV deals with the specific psychiatric disorders and includes updated information and changes initiated in the newly published DSM-5. The classification of psychotropic drugs, their action and therapeutic use are incorporated into the discussion of treatment methods associated with each group of disorders. Information sources on the disorders are an additional inclusion. The latter section of this unit addresses the mental health disorders of the child and adolescent. A new discussion of the intellectually disabled child and adult is included in the information. Chapter 9 will address the issues and types of mental disorders in the older adult.

Chapter objectives are written concisely and purposefully to anticipate learning outcomes. Specifically, they are intended to provide a mindset for the student to incorporate knowledge into application. Key terms are bold-faced in the manuscript to provide easy access to their meaning. Thought-provoking questions are posed throughout each chapter as Mind Joggers to encourage critical thinking. Important information is summarized or added in the form of Just the Facts margin supplements. Boxes and tables are located throughout the book to give the student resource information in an easily viewed and compressed arrangement. Case applications are integrated into the text to provide opportunities for reflective thinking and content application. Questions will lead the student to utilize the nursing process in resolving identified problems.

Each chapter is followed by an integrated study guide, or worksheet, with various methods of assessing the subject content. This component is designed to stimulate deductive thinking and reasoning. Questions are written so that the answers are easily discernible after reading chapter content. Terminology and key terms are reinforced through completion and matching exercises. Multiple-choice questions are written using an NCLEX item-writing format to help prepare students for entry-level testing. An answer key is provided for all worksheets at the back of the textbook. A support bibliography for content is provided at the end of each chapter.

It is my mission and hope that the third edition of this textbook will continue to help students better understand the mental processes and how they are affected by factors in our everyday lives. It is my anticipated challenge that students will experience self-awareness and personal growth as they learn with a realization that to experience this energizes them to help others. Helping ourselves and recognizing how and why we think and act as we do is often the most beneficial side effect of this subject. By being willing to confront and change those things that can be changed and accept the unchangeable in our own life, we can open doors that allow us to role model this for our clients.

Acknowledgments

As I contemplated a third edition of this textbook, my focus centered on what makes this information most useful for students and future nurses in the workplace. The application of knowledge to the actual clinical situation is the essence of its value. The feedback from students and faculty has proven most beneficial in putting together a revision of this textbook that will provide current information that can be applied in various health-care settings. Positive comments from students have cited the readability and presentation of material as beneficial to their overall experience in mental health nursing. This response and that of reviewers have been the driving force behind my dedication in writing this revision.

One comes to appreciate the entire process of publication throughout the many hours that are required in the development of the finished product. I would like to extend my sincere thanks to Christopher Richardson, Executive Editor, for his support of my textbook revision, and to Zachary Shapiro, Editorial Assistant, at Lippincott Williams & Wilkins for his assistance with details of the editorial process. My Product Development Editor, Shana Murph, has been very helpful and encouraging throughout the revision. It is this positive reinforcement that drives the energy necessary to stay fixed on completion of the project. My thanks also to the entire Production team at Lippincott Williams & Wilkins for all of your expertise and creativity that crafts the product to publication. I sincerely appreciate each and every one of you!

The incredible love and support I have received from my wonderful family have lifted me through the long dedicated hours that are invested in a manuscript. To my priceless family, Tanya, Julie, Jimmy, and Hagen, you are my most precious gifts and blessings. Words cannot express my deep love and respect for each of you and the incredible gifted individuals you are. Thank you for believing in me and encouraging me forward during the months of this revision. Although illness has claimed the life of my husband Grady, my heartfelt thanks to his family for their continued support as I have worked on this revision.

I want to extend my sincere gratitude to the families of the two young men who have so willingly shared their story and struggles in living with a mental illness. Thank you also, to my support system of coworkers and friends who have been my cheering section over the past months. A special thanks to my dear friend, Dr. Corky Terrell, for her encouragement and friendship that kept driving me with the passion and motivation I needed to see this project to the finish line.

As I complete another edition of this book, I want to continue to acknowledge the major motivation for the original manuscript. My late husband, Charlie, who died in 1999 from complications related to early-onset Alzheimer's disease, was perhaps the single-most driving reason I tackled the challenge to author a textbook. Throughout my nursing career, I have been devoted to the care-giving of many clients with this devastating disease and other mental disorders. I have had the privilege of teaching and mentoring many nursing students in the skills and application of mental health nursing. In spite of all the experience, I was still ill-prepared for the role of care-giver throughout the long journey of loss during the extent of his illness. He wanted others to know what he was experiencing, and for the opportunity to be his voice and fulfill those wishes has been a labor of love.

I am thankful most of all to my Heavenly Father for blessing me with the ability to give back to others what experience has taught me. My hope and prayer is that the students who read and study this textbook will continue to offer knowledgeable and compassionate care to those who search for the balance of mental health and those who encounter the challenges of mental illness along life's path.

Contents

Mental Health and Mental Illness

⊙ Learning Objectives

After learning the content in this chapter, the student will be able to:

1. Describe the nature of mental health and mental illness.
2. Define mental health nursing as it relates to human behavior.
3. Describe how culture, ethnicity, and religion influence the perception of mental health and mental illness.
4. Define stress and its relationship to anxiety.
5. Identify factors that contribute to stress and anxiety.
6. Differentiate between adaptive and maladaptive coping strategies.
7. Define grief as a process.
8. Identify factors that may contribute to dysfunctional grief.
9. Discuss ways to assist individuals to cope with the grieving process.

⊙ Key Terms

acceptance
adaptation
adaptive coping
anticipatory grief
anxiety
bargaining
bereavement
burnout
chronic sorrow
conventional grief
cultural identity
denial
depression
distress
dysfunctional grief

eustress
external stressors
"fight or flight" response
grief
internal stressors
loss
maladaptive coping
mental health
mental illness
palliative coping
reframing
stress
stress reaction
unresolved grief

Defining Mental Health and Mental Illness

As human beings, we exist in a society composed of many different types of people. Although genetics provides a blueprint for our physical body, the human mind is unique in that it contains a combination of our thoughts, perceptions, memories, emotions, will, and our reasoning. Each of these is developed as we think, feel, and react to the world around us. We interact with our own thoughts in a private way with the ability to communicate them to others as we choose. The well-being of this aspect of our body may be referred to as the state of or health of the mind.

Mental Health

According to the World Health Organization, **mental health** can be viewed as a "state of well-being in which the individual realizes his or her own abilities, can cope with the normal stresses of life, can work productively and fruitfully, and is able to make a contribution to his or her community". It can be said that a person is only in a complete state of health when physical, mental, and social well-being are intact. Mental health encompasses a balance between all these aspects of life. It impacts the way we see our surroundings, how we think, and the decisions we make. How we feel about ourselves and those around us has an influence on how we cope with life and meet the expectations it creates. Our ability to act independently directed by inner values and strengths, to face life with assurance and hope, and seek a meaningful balance between work, play, and love produces satisfying relationships with others. Further evidence of mental health is seen in our ability to function well alone or with others, to make sound judgments and accept responsibility for the outcomes, to love and be loved, and to respond with humor when life gets tough.

Mental Illness

Defining mental illness or disorders is complicated because there are various views and interpretation. For the purposes of this textbook, **mental illness** or a mental disorder can best be understood according to the DSM-5 definition as a "clinically significant disturbance in an individual's cognition, emotion regulation, or behavior that reflects a dysfunction in the psychological, biological, or developmental processes underlying mental functioning." Whatever the cause, the disorder is usually associated with a "significant impact on the social, occupational, or other activities" in the life of the individual. Based on the 2010 census report by the National Institute of Mental Health, an estimated 26.2% or one in four adult Americans has a diagnosable mental disorder. While less in number, those with a serious mental illness average about 6% and are a leading cause of disability in this country. Approximately 36% of these are receiving treatment. According to the World Health Organization Mental Health Atlas in 2011, mental illness accounts for approximately 13% of the economic load imposed on the economy worldwide. However, most countries invest less than 3% of their budget in mental health care.

Causes and descriptions of mental disorders are many and varied. However, by comparison with the indicators of mental health, a state of mental illness might be characterized by disarray in these same areas of the persona. For example, in mental illness, there is a general dissatisfaction with oneself and one's ability to meet the challenges of the environment. Interpersonal relationships are ineffective and unsuccessful as mental distress impacts the emotional stability and coping efforts of the individual. Thinking is often distorted as misconceptions and thinking errors take the place of rational and realistic processing. The discomfort experienced in the mind sets in motion the behavioral patterns characteristic of the various mental disorders.

Cultural, Ethnic, and Religious Influences

Racial and ethnic minority groups make up a significant portion of the American population, providing a wealth of strength, traditions, and cultural contributions to society in general. According to the U.S. Census Bureau projections, it is estimated that by the year 2060, the U.S. population will be older and more diverse racially and ethnically with the white non-Hispanic population peaking by 2024. The Hispanic population is predicted to more than double between the years 2012 and 2060. Among the ethnic and racial populations recognized by the federal government in

TABLE 1.1	U.S. Demographics 2012 (Projections based on 2010 Census)
ETHNIC ORIGIN	**POPULATION**
Total population, 2012 estimate	313,914,040
White only	197.8 million
Black or African American	41.2 million
American Indian/Alaska Native	3.9 million
Asian	15.9 million
Native Hawaiian/other Pacific Islander	706,000
Hispanic or Latino	53.3 million
Two or more races	7.5 million

Data from U.S. Census Bureau Projections 2012 (http://www.census.gov/newsroom/releases/archives/population/cb12–243.html). Accessed November 22, 2013.

the United States are White alone, Black or African American alone, Hispanic or Latino, Asian alone, American Indian and Alaskan Native alone, Native Hawaiian and Other Pacific Islander alone, and Two or More Races. There are many mixed groups in addition to those listed above, who have immigrated and become integral in the multicultural make-up of America (Table 1.1). Each group differs from one another and from society with respect to their own culture and traditions.

Cultural Heritage—Beliefs, Norms, and Values

Culture is a term that describes a common heritage and a set of beliefs, norms, values, and behaviors that are unique to each. This binding force between members of each group is often referred to as **cultural identity**. Cultural identity may include a common language, family customs, country of origin, religious and political beliefs, sexual orientation, gender, and an established culture within the geographic locale where the group resides. Factors related to the group to which one belongs also affect how people relate to one another. Behavior often mirrors that of the group and may be altered as cultural changes occur within the group.

With all of these differences among cultures, it is not surprising that variances can be seen among them in the manner in which they perceive, cope with, and manage mental health issues. Although many families meet the challenge of a

member's mental illness by seeking professional care, the stigma and shame created by a mental illness can lead some families to hide and deal with the affected person in their own ways. While some may respond outwardly to life situations, others may be discouraged from visibly showing emotional and mental problems. The tendency to seek help from religious or faith healers within the cultural group rather than professional providers is common. In response to atypical mental behaviors exhibited by a family member, families may simply deny that a problem exists. Others may see the symptoms as a punishment or judgment for wrongdoing. Some cultural beliefs conclude that mental symptoms are related to witchcraft, demon possession, or substance abuse and can be eliminated by remedies such as folk customs of healing arts, forms of magic, traditional medicines and herbs. Religious rituals using prayer, touch, candles, eggs or pollen, weed roots, pictures, and medals are common healing practices provided by those seen as healers within the group. Other patterns of religious coping may include prayer, religious music, talking to God, or meditation.

Despite the availability of mental health services, engrained and endeared cultural patterns of resolution remain the customary choice for certain individuals when managing mental illness. Regardless of educational preparation, the beliefs and traditions that are handed down from generation to generation are strong and viable within the cultural or ethnic community (Table 1.2).

Factors That Affect Mental Health

Mental health is achieved as we forage a balance between the ups and downs of everyday life. In the course of our lifetime, we encounter enumerable issues that require us to adapt both physically and emotionally. Stress and anxiety are unavoidable issues that confront us daily making it necessary for us to be flexible and adaptive. The events that cause grief and loss are difficult to accept as the reality of the situation is imposed. Faced with these challenges, our mental equilibrium may become temporarily disrupted, during which time our ability to reestablish a stable state depends on our adaptive resources at that particular time. Each individual will respond in different ways based on conditioning, cultural influence, and the mental resources available at the time. It is our

TABLE 1.2   Select Culture-Bound Terminology

TERM (IDIOMS)	CULTURE	BEHAVIOR OR SIGNIFICANCE

Amok
Cafard or cathard
  ideation
Mal de pelia
lich'aa
	Malasia, Laos,
	  Philippines
	Polynesia
	Puerto Rico
	Navajo
		Brooding followed by violent or aggressive behavior with persecutory ideation, amnesia, exhaustion, and automatism (psychotic episode)

Ataque de nervios	Latinos, Haitians,
	  or other Pacific
	  Islanders
		Attacks of crying, shouting, trembling, heat in chest rising to head, verbal or physical aggression—sense of being out of control. Most common following a stressful event relating to a family member. May be associated with suicidal ideation, disability, or acute distress (anxiety, mood, somatoform, or dissociative disorders)

Bilis, colera, muina	Latinos	Inner core body imbalance (hot and cold variances in body and between material and spiritual aspects of body). Acute nervous tension, headache, trembling, screaming, stomach disturbances, and possible fainting are common (anxiety, chronic fatigue)
Boufee delirante	West Africa/Haiti	Sudden outburst of agitated and aggressive behavior, confusion, and psychomotor agitation. May have paranoid ideation or hallucinations (brief psychotic disorder)
Brain fag	West Africa	Difficulty in concentrating, thinking, memory; pain pressure or tightness around head and neck, blurred vision (anxiety, mood, somatoform disorders)
Dhat syndrome Jiryan Sukra prameha Shen-k'-uei	India Sri Lanka China	Severe anxiety and hypochondrial concerns associated with seminal secretions, whitish discoloration of urine, feelings of weakness/fatigue (anxiety and somatoform disorder, erectile dysfunction)
Ghost sickness	American Indian	Preoccupation with death and the deceased sometimes associated with witchcraft. Bad dreams, weakness, feelings of danger, anorexia, fainting, fear, anxiety, hallucinations, feelings of doom

Khyal cap or "wind
  attacks"
	Cambodians,
	  Sri Lanka, Korean
		Panic attacks, dizziness, palpitations, shortness of breath, anxiety. Attacks include concern that a windlike substance will rise in the body causing serious effects (panic attacks, generalized anxiety disorder, agoraphobia, PTSD)

Koro Suo yang Rok-joo	Malaysian origin China Thailand	Episode of sudden and intense anxiety that the penis (or vulva/nipples in female) will recede into the body possibly causing death
Latah	Malaysian, Indonesian	Hypersensitivity to sudden fright with echopraxia, echolalia, dissociative or trancelike behavior

Amurakh, irkunii, ikota,
  olan, myriachit,
  mnekeiti, bahtschi
  imu, mali-mali, silok
	Siberian, Thailand
	Japan, Philippines	

Locura	Latino	Severe chronic psychosis attributed to inheritance, effects of life difficulties. Incoherence, agitation, auditory/visual hallucinations, inability to follow societal rules of interaction, possible violence and unpredictable behaviors
Nervios	Latinos	General state of vulnerability, emotional distress, somatic symptoms, and inability to function. (Major depressive disorder, generalized anxiety disorder, somatoform disorder, schizophrenia)
Rootwork Mal puesto or brujeria	African American European Latino	Illness ascribed to hexing, witchcraft, sorcery, or evil influence of another person. Symptoms of anxiety, gastrointestinal complaints, weakness, dizziness, fear of being poisoned or killed (voodoo death). "Roots, spells, hexes" can be "put" on other persons causing emotional and psychological problems. Can be "taken off" by a "root doctor" (healer in this tradition) or "curandera" in Latinos

Susto, espanto, pasmo,
  tripa ida, perdida del
  alma, or chibih
	Latinos, Mexico,
	  Central and South
	  America
		"Fright" or "soul loss" attributed to a frightening event that causes soul to leave the body resulting in unhappiness and sickness. Symptoms of depression, sadness, lack of motivation; somatic symptoms of headache, stomachache, diarrhea. Ritual healings to restore balance between body and soul (major depressive disorder; PTSD, somatoform disorders)

Data adapted and used with permission from American Psychological Association: *Diagnostic and statistical manual of mental disorders, Appendix I,* (4th ed.). Washington, DC: 2000; American Psychological Association, and DSM-5, *Glossary of Cultural Concepts of Distress, Appendix,* pp. 833–883, Washington, DC: 2013, American Psychological Association.

challenge as human beings to learn to deal with these issues in constructive ways.

Stress and Anxiety

Stress and anxiety can arise from any thought or issue that creates frustration or a feeling of uneasiness. Situations are seen differently by everyone with some things being stressful to one and not to another. What causes the uneasy feeling is not necessarily apparent and adds to the tension experienced.

Defining Stress

Stress is defined as the condition that results when a threat or challenge to one's well-being requires the person to adjust or adapt to the environment. According to the well-known stress researcher Hans Selye, there are two kinds of stress. **Distress** in response to a threat or challenge is actually harmful to one's health. This is a negative stress and demands an exhausting type of energy. **Eustress**, on the other hand, is positive and motivating, as shown by one's confidence in the ability to master a challenge or stressor. This type of stress may actually enhance the feeling of well-being. For example, eustress is demonstrated in a football player whose stress about an upcoming football game challenges him to play better. Distress, on the other hand, might be seen in the student who is disqualified from the football team because of poor grades, resulting in a feeling of low self-worth.

Stress is further defined in terms of acute or chronic stress. Acute stress constitutes the reaction to an immediate threat, commonly called the **"fight or flight" response** when there is a surge of the adrenal hormone epinephrine or adrenalin into the bloodstream. It is referred to in this way because it provides the energy or instant strength to either fight or run away from a danger or threat. This type of response can occur in situations where there is a sense of imminent danger, such as when walking in a darkened parking lot or upon losing track of a child in a crowd. The response is usually reversed to a relaxation mode once the danger is past. Chronic stress occurs when the situation is ongoing of continuous, such as chronic illness of a family member or job-related responsibilities. It is important to recognize that most of us have experienced both acute and chronic stress situations, ones that we as health care workers share with our clients (Fig. 1.1).

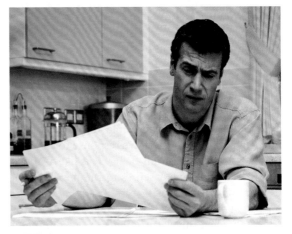

FIGURE 1.1

Stress is a common experience. Common sources of stress include work, family, money problems, and world events.

Common symptoms of stress generally fall into four categories: physical, mental, emotional, and behavioral (Box 1.1). The physical response to the stressor, or the **stress reaction**, is triggered by the arousal of the autonomic nervous system.

Just the Facts

When the perception of a stressful situation changes, the stimulation to the autonomic nervous system decreases.

BOX 1.1

Common Signs and Symptoms of Stress

- Increased heart rate and blood pressure
- Heart palpitations
- Increased respirations
- Abdominal cramping, nausea, diarrhea
- Headaches
- Insomnia
- Lack of concentration and memory
- Inability to make decisions
- Forgetfulness
- Confusion
- Anxiety
- Nervousness
- Irritability
- Frustration and worry
- Fidgety movements
- Nail-biting
- Smoking and drinking
- Yelling, throwing things

Defining Anxiety

Anxiety is defined as a feeling of apprehension, uneasiness, or uncertainty that occurs in response to a real or perceived threat whose source is not known. It is an automatic and unconscious biological response to a stressor that cannot be controlled by our conscious minds. Anxiety is such a natural occurrence that it is impossible to avoid. It is a build-in part of our instinctive response to an event that is a threat to our well-being. It is like a smoke detector that alerts our senses to the possibility of danger and prepares us to respond by either running or fighting. Anxiety is the mechanism that is triggered when the alarm sounds in our brain and actually prevents us from thinking logically about the situation. Therefore, anxiety may be present whether or not an actual danger exists. It can cause us to act impulsively not only when there is actual danger but also when we perceive the possibility of a threat. We cannot ignore the feeling of anxiety, but we often allow it to overshadow our logical and realistic thought processes.

Anxiety is the most basic of emotions seen in the statement that all behavior has meaning and purpose. Behavior is the result of our perceptions and thought processes and provides a clue to the underlying motive for action. It occurs at a deeper level than fear, which is a reaction to a specific, defined danger. Normal anxiety is necessary for survival and provides the energy needed to manage daily life and pursue life goals. Acute anxiety may be experienced by a person who faces a short-term stressor, such as undergoing surgery or a series of diagnostic testing. When anxiety persists over a long period, such as when a person faces a chronic illness, the chronic feeling is demonstrated by a sense of apprehension and overreaction to all unanticipated environmental stimuli. This state may be shown through chronic fatigue, insomnia, poor concentration, or impairment in work and social functioning. If the feelings of anxiety become too overwhelming, they may be repressed out of conscious awareness and expressed through behavior.

Just the Facts

Our behavior is the result of our perceptions and thought processes related to a particular situation.

The severity of the anxiety is expressed through an individual's perception and reaction to the stressor. This is usually exhibited in the person's physical, emotional, and mental behaviors. There are four levels at which anxiety may occur (mild, moderate, severe, panic), each escalating to a level more severe than the previous one. As anxiety increases, the person experiences an internal need to try to relieve it as soon as possible.

Mild anxiety is natural and motivating toward productivity with an improved sense of well-being. Anxiety that increases to a moderate level becomes uncomfortable and difficult to tolerate for extended periods. If this level of anxiety is not relieved, it progresses to a severe state that is physically and emotionally exhausting. The individual is desperate for a way to relieve the mental and emotional turmoil. If steps are not taken to decrease a severe level of anxiety, the state of panic may develop, possibly leading to hysteria, suicide attempts, or violence. The physical and psychological symptoms for each level of anxiety are described in Table 1.3.

Contributing Factors to Stress and Anxiety

An individual can experience both external and internal stressors (Box 1.2). **External stressors** are those aspects of the environment that may be adverse, such as an abusive relationship or poverty-level living conditions. **Internal stressors** can be physical, such as a chronic illness or terminal condition, or psychological, as in continued worry about financial burdens or a disaster that may never happen. Research has also shown that heart disease tends to be more prevalent in people who are highly driven, competitive, ambitious, and success-oriented and have a chronic sense of time urgency and a chronic hostile personal style (referred to as type A personality) than in those who are more relaxed and easygoing (referred to as Type B personality).

Both positive and negative aspects of life may include a fair amount of stress. For example, if you were experiencing your first day on the job after a promotion, your heart might be pounding and your muscles tense as you adapt to the new position. By contrast, an environment of everyday stress such as marital discord or difficult work demands may eventually pose a threat to one's health. It is important to recognize that many times we view external circumstances as the cause of our stress, but in reality, we create most of our own stress by choosing to make ourselves miserable and upset. When we monitor our anxiety-producing thoughts, our irrational thinking tends to over generalize and exaggerate things.

TABLE 1.3 Common Signs and Symptoms of Anxiety

LEVEL OF ANXIETY	PHYSICAL SYMPTOMS	PSYCHOLOGICAL SYMPTOMS

Mild Level	Increased awareness
	Increased energy
	Slight discomfort
	Restlessness
	Irritability
	Mild tension-relieving behaviors
	   (fidgeting, nail-biting, foot-tapping,
	   lip-chewing)
		Sharp perception of reality
		Alert and aware of environment
		Able to identify things producing anxiety
		Motivated
		Preoccupied at times
		Good concentration
		Reasoning and logical thought processes
		Attentive

Moderate Level	Voice tremors Muscle tension Rapid speech—change in pitch Difficulty concentrating Shakiness Repetitive questioning Misperception of stimuli Inability to complete tasks Autonomic response Headaches, insomnia Pacing Decreased eye contact	Reduced perceptual ability Decreased attentiveness Needs things repeated to grasp Still functional but problem-solving ability decreased (requires guidance) Decreased motivation and confidence Increased irritability Feeling of being tied in knots Bouts of crying and outbursts of anger Inability to learn or problem-solve
Severe Level	Feelings of impending doom Confusion Purposeless activity Increased somatic complaints Hyperventilation Palpitations Loud and rapid speech Threats and demands Increased pacing Diaphoresis Poor or no eye contact Insomnia Rapid speech Eye twitching Tremors	Distorted perception of reality Attention to details—loses sight of whole picture Focused totally on self and anxiety Defensiveness Oversensitive to comments from others Verbal threats Lacks reasoning or logical thought processes Unable to problem-solve
Panic Level	Hysteria Incoherent Suicide attempts Violent behavior Unintelligible speech Feelings of terror, extreme fear Immobility Dilated pupils Withdrawal Out of touch with reality	Irrational and disorganized thought processes Absent perceptual ability Unaware of reality Unable to perceive environment Depersonalization Delusional thinking Disorientation

This tends to give our thoughts an "all or none" frame of thinking. This type of thinking also leads to anticipating the worst possible outcome for situations. This is illustrated by an individual who is hit by the car behind him while driving in traffic. Believing that if he drives a car again, he will have an accident, he no longer drives a vehicle.

Some events create more stress than others. A major factor in whether the stressor becomes a strain on the individual is the unpredictability of situations over which the person may have little or no control. A fireman, for example, faces uncertainty and ongoing threat of danger or injury with each call of duty, or the intermittent pressure experienced by policemen when responding to a 911 call. Emotional triggers for higher levels of stress are those that are uncontrollable, repetitive, unexpected, and intense in nature, such as is experienced by nurses in critical patient care situations. Stress is greater and damage more likely in these situations, and can lead to job-related burnout or mental, physical, and emotional exhaustion. Disorders related to anxiety are discussed in Chapter 9.

BOX 1.2

Internal and External Stressors

External Stressors

- Physical environment (noise, bright lights, weather, crowds)
- Major life events (death of a loved one, divorce, loss of a job, marriage)
- Work-related (rules, deadlines, production pressures, gossip)
- Social (bossy or aggressive persons, strained friendship, marital affairs)
- Everyday life (schedules, household duties, family conflict)

Internal Stressors

- Personality traits (perfectionist, workaholic, worrier, loner)
- Negative self-talk (pessimism, irrational thinking, self-criticism)
- Thinking snags (all or none approach, unrealistic and inflexible expectations)

Just the Facts

Job-related **burnout** is a condition of mental, physical, and emotional exhaustion with a reduced sense of personal accomplishment and apathy toward one's work.

Mind Jogger

What types of stress might be more damaging than others?

Coping with Stress and Anxiety

In most situations, the sense of control an individual feels over a particular stressor determines how he or she thinks about or perceives it. The first step in coping with a threatening situation is to assess if it really is what it seems to be. Once this has been determined, options can be reviewed to resolve the problem. The solution may be one of trying to deal with the situation itself, or one of controlling the emotional reaction that is felt in response to the stressor. A student who feels overwhelmed by requirements for taking a full semester course load with a fear of failing may decide to drop one or two classes to perform better in the remaining subjects. Another student with the same course load may decide to work out in the gym each day, along with budgeting time between the required subjects to deal with the stress.

Coping Strategies

Coping strategies are the methods we use to manage stress and anxiety. Coping strategies generally fall into four categories: adaptive, palliative, maladaptive, and dysfunctional. A person's successful management of stress or anxiety is referred to as **adaptation**. Therefore, when a person uses a rational and productive way of resolving a problem to reduce anxiety, it is said to be **adaptive coping**. If the solution temporarily relieves the anxiety but the problem still exists and must be dealt with again at a later time, the strategy is termed **palliative coping**. These two types of coping usually result in a positive outcome. For example, a drama student feels anxiety as time for a performance approaches and asks a classmate to review the script to refocus on the lines. A second student who feels anxious about the performance goes jogging with music to relieve the anxiety and increase his mental alertness to remember his lines.

On the other hand, maladaptive and dysfunctional strategies usually do not result in a positive outcome. If unsuccessful attempts are made to decrease the anxiety without attempting to solve the problem, the strategies are described as **maladaptive coping** and the anxiety remains. For example, the drama student might decide to ignore the anxiety and go to a movie the afternoon before the performance and rapidly look over the lines immediately before going on stage. During the performance, he forgets several of his lines and has to be prompted. The individual who does not attempt to reduce the anxiety or solve the problem is considered to have dysfunctional coping in response to the stressor and the emotional response. For example, another student decides to get drunk the night before the performance, fails to show up for the performance until the second act, and is replaced by his understudy.

Mind Jogger

Does avoidance of a conflict situation create or reduce anxiety?

Promoting Adaptive Coping Strategies

In managing and coping with the anxiety we experience in response to stress in our lives, it is important to accept the anxiety rather than fight it. Stress is a part of life. We have a choice to replace negative feelings with more positive ones. We can stand back and look realistically at the situation as we function along with the anxiety. We expect the best. The outcome is rarely as bad as what we fear the most. Our perception of the stress situation often involves thinking that expects the worst or is driven by negative thoughts. Coping strategies, whether adaptive or maladaptive, are learned by observation of those who model them in our family and social environment. We tend to use those skills that we know to deal with life stressors.

Nurses play a major role in helping clients with anxiety to cope more effectively. We must recognize that to help our clients deal with their level of stress, we must learn to handle our own. Two examples of effective coping strategies are reframing and visualization. **Reframing** is a way of restructuring our thinking about a stressful event into one that is less disturbing and over which we can have some control. Table 1.4 illustrates examples of how irrational beliefs can be reframed into rational thoughts. By changing our view to a more realistic expectation, we can pursue a solution more clearly. Taking a mental escape to a place of peaceful solitude is also an effective means of coping with stress. This form of visualization can momentarily allow a reprieve from the stress to a place of peaceful solitude (e.g., visualizing a vacation spot or pastime that brings relaxation, imagining oneself on the seashore listening to the sounds of water and sea gulls). The escape provides a temporary defense withdrawal from the anxiety, giving the individual renewed energy. Each time we are successful in dealing with an anxiety-producing situation, there is a better chance that we will manage to control the anxiety the next time.

Some other effective techniques for managing anxiety include Positive self-talk and reframing irrational thinking.

- Positive self-talk and reframing irrational thinking
- Assertiveness training
- Problem-solving skills—view problems as opportunities for growth
- Communication skills
- Conflict resolution
- Relaxation techniques
- Meditation
- Support systems
- Practical attitude
- Sense of humor
- Self-care (diet, exercise, sleep, leisure, avoiding things that increase stress such as caffeine and alcohol)
- Faith in spiritual power and in yourself

Mind Jogger

How might failure to achieve one's ambition be seen as a positive experience?

Grief and Loss

Grief is defined as the emotional process of coping with a loss. Instinctively, we associate this process with the death of a loved one, such as a spouse, parent, or child, or of any person who is important in our life. In a broader sense, the reality of loss can be applied to the absence of anything that is significant or meaningful to our existence. This can include a separation or divorce, loss of a body part, threat to one's health, loss of a job or source of income, and losses that result from a natural or imposed disaster. All of these events or circumstances may leave the person with a sense of emptiness, hopelessness, and detachment from the meaning that previously was found in life. The extent to which emotional energy was previously invested in these objects, persons, and relationships will determine the intensity with which an individual responds to the absence of that object. Although a person may experience sadness or sorrow in response to making a mistake or doing something that is hurtful to another, the grief felt as the person adjusts to the absence of the endeared person or object is a deeper and longer lasting emotion that involves time and emotional energy.

Loss can be an actual or perceived change in the status of one's relationship to a valued object or person. This concept is easily associated with

TABLE 1.4   Examples of Reframing Irrational Thoughts

IRRATIONAL BELIEF	RESTRUCTURED POSITIVE THOUGHT
I always mess things up	Even if things didn't turn out right this time I can do it different next time
He never does what I want him to do	If I want him to do something I need to communicate that to him
She never pays any attention to me	If I give her more attention, she might be more attentive to me
I should have done better on the exam	I can study harder and do better on the next one
I can't be happy unless I am loved by the person I really care about	If this person does not return my love, I can give my energy to finding someone better

Case Application 1.1

"Lost and Alone"

The clinic nurse is assessing Art, a 56-year-old farmer, whose wife died 6 months ago from ovarian cancer. He describes himself as "lost, forgetful, and unable to concentrate." He states that, "I seem to cry at the most inconvenient moments, so I just stay to myself." The nurse notes his expression is sad and he avoids eye contact. Art says he has no appetite and just "doesn't care anymore." When asked about his farming operation, he states he has lost interest in doing anything and has turned the farming over to his son.

What feelings might be responsible for Art's symptoms?

_____

_____

How should the nurse respond to Art?

_____

_____

What stage of the grief process is Art likely experiencing?

_____

_____

What referrals may be appropriate for Art?

_____

_____

the death of a valued person or pet. There is also a major loss when losing a home to fire or natural disaster with a lifetime of memories suddenly gone from view and reality. The loss may be seen as the lack of certainty that a goal or desired outcome will be achieved, such as not receiving a job promotion or an academic failure. The attachment bond that is seen as strong and secure is suddenly shattered, making a person vulnerable to an unstable emotional response. Grief is the emotion encountered when an individual is confronted with a loss. It is a feeling of sadness and despondency centered on the experience itself. These feelings may lead to behaviors such as forgetfulness and crying at unpredictable times. It is helpful for the person to be reassured that this is a common reaction to grief. Tears are accepted as a part of the healing that takes place in the months after the loss. How people mourn a loss is also influenced by their personal, familial, and cultural beliefs or customs. The amount of time allotted to the mourning period or how families may view sympathy and support during the time of sadness is often determined by these factors. For example, some people prefer to be alone as they mourn a loss, while others may do so openly for a specified time or with specific rituals and family gatherings.

Types of Grief

Anticipatory grief may be seen in individuals and families who are expecting a major loss in the near future. This concept is helpful to nurses in understanding the reaction of the terminally ill client and the family members who will be left to mourn the death of their loved one. In this case, death is inevitable and there is a time of preparation and closure that can ease the emotional pain at the actual time of death. This is the premise for hospice care, which provides palliative nursing and supportive interventions to assist the client and family members in coping with the imminent loss. The nurse can also apply this concept to those in the acute care setting who may be anticipating or facing the loss of a body part (e.g., amputation of a limb or a mastectomy) or change in body functioning (e.g., urinary or bowel diversion; chronic illness such as diabetes, emphysema, heart disease) that may inflict a major alteration in lifestyle.

Conventional grief is primarily associated with the grief that is experienced following a loss. This process of **bereavement** or adapting to loss may take days, weeks, or years, depending on the sense of loss for the person involved. Each person responds to loss in a personal and unique way and time. This response is based on the person's level of development, past experiences, and current coping strategies.

Children and adolescents respond according to the level at which they understand the concept of death or loss. Table 1.5 shows how the response reflects the age-related cognitive and psychological developments of the child. For example, a toddler may respond to separation from a parent or attachment figure with anxiety but has no concept of loss. Should that attachment figure not return, the child will usually adapt to another attachment figure who is nurturing. The preschool child reacts with magical thinking, such as in a 5-year-old child who says, "Grandpa is sleeping. Will he wake up in time to take me to the park?" The concept of death as a finality is not yet understood. Associated with the growing moral concept of right and wrong, the school-age child may feel a sense of guilt or responsibility for a loss, such as when a parent is absent following a divorce. Although adolescents understand the concept of death as finality, it is difficult for this age group to fit death or loss into their search for an identity.

 Mind Jogger

How might environmental factors during childhood affect a person's ability to cope with loss?

Adults may view loss as temporary or permanent, and most adults are able to accept their losses and grow from these situations. Acceptance often opens the door of opportunity for new and expanded life experiences. An example of this is seen when one experiences failure in a given situation such as divorce, job promotion, or academic challenges. Failure, if viewed realistically can allow the individual to try again more successfully. Learning what contributed to the loss can open the door for a new challenge. It is important to remember that regardless of age or circumstances, bereavement is a natural, healthy, and healing process that emerges in response to any significant loss.

Mind Jogger

What objective signs might indicate a person has reached acceptance?

Grief as a Process

The grieving process describes a series of occurrences in the resolution of loss. This process provides support as an individual works through the feelings of anger, hopelessness, and futility that accompany loss. It provides time to put things into perspective, to place into memory that which is gone, and to emerge with a newly developed embrace of life. Life is an evolving challenge of events that inevitably requires us to cope with disappointment and loss. Learning to deal with these situations in small increments better prepares us to deal effectively with a major loss. We can learn to accept loss as part of living, or we can choose to react with hostility, often suppressing the anger into hidden feelings that eventually may erupt in negative or maladaptive patterns of behavior such as substance abuse or suicide. Learning to cope or adapt to loss involves giving ourselves the right to grieve in whatever timeframe is needed to go through the process. It is important to recognize and accept the feelings, such as anger, fear, and guilt, that are normal and appropriate part of grieving (Box 1.3).

TABLE 1.5	Age-Related Concepts of Loss
AGE GROUP	**CONCEPTUAL UNDERSTANDING OF LOSS**
Toddler	Egocentric and concerned with themselves
	Do not understand concept of loss
Preschool	Use magical thinking and may feel shame or guilt when thinking is associated with loss (i.e., belief that behavior is reason a parent is gone such as in divorce)
	Primitive coping mechanisms result in more intense response
	Do not understand death or its permanence
School-age	Still feel guilt and responsibility in associating negative actions with loss
	Respond to concrete, simple and logical explanation of death such as in the death of a pet (ages 9–10)
	Understand permanence of death and that some losses may be temporary
Adolescent	Able to understand the concept of death, but have difficulty accepting loss
	Perceive loss as a threat to their identity

Growth occurs as the bereaved person comes to the point of letting go of the past. This does not reduce the importance of the loss but allows the person to continue living with new perspective. In time, the sadness and loneliness felt as a result of the void left by the cherished object are replaced with hopefulness as one is freed from the previous relationship. This acceptance indicates that the grief process is coming to a close.

Just the Facts

Grief is the process of working through the emotional response to loss, reorganizing one's life, and accomplishing some degree of resolution or closure.

Stages of Grief

Perhaps the best known theory of bereavement is that of Dr. Elisabeth Kubler-Ross, a German psychiatrist, who described the stages that a person who is facing his or her own death or that of a loved one encounters before coming to actual acceptance of death as a final stage of life. Dr. Kubler-Ross believed that the dying is a lifelong process in which we repeat the stages each time we are confronted by loss.

Dr. Kubler-Ross identified five stages that we go through each time we are confronted with a loss or death. The first step is shock, disbelief, and **denial** that the event is happening. We want to avoid the reality of the loss and may act as if nothing has occurred or as though the lost object or person is still present. Denial actually allows us an adjustment period in which to gather coping strategies for the grieving work ahead.

As we realize that the loss is real, the denial gives way to feelings of bitterness, anger, and turmoil. Anger is expressed in many ways, often demonstrated openly in behaviors such as crying or expressions of self-blame and guilt. Some may turn the anger inward, resulting in physical illness and/or psychological dysfunction.

Anger usually is followed by **bargaining** as we attempt to postpone acceptance of the loss. As is often seen with terminal illness, this is a time when deals with God are attempted as a way to prolong the inevitable. Frequent labile moods are common and are often intermingled with continued anger and unwillingness to accept the loss.

The bargaining period is gradually followed by a deep sense of loss as the reality of what has happened or is anticipated settles. At this point we may withdraw from social interaction, choosing to spend hours and days alone in the depth of loneliness for that which is gone. **Depression**, the persistent and prolonged mood of sadness that may extend beyond 2 weeks duration, is a normal response in this process as we adjust to life without the loved object and the full impact of the loss. However, according to the DSM-5, in grief, "the predominant affect is feelings of emptiness and loss" (p 161), rather than self-doubt and self-critical mood. In grief, these feelings of sadness and desolation may be intertwined with good days of positive emotions, rather than being persistent as in depressive disorder. Self-esteem is usually intact and thoughts are primarily focused on the deceased. For some people this period may be overwhelming and recovery from the depth of sorrow felt is unlikely without professional support and guidance.

The final stage is that of **acceptance** when the person begins to experience peace and serenity. This is the time of letting go and allowing life to provide new experiences and relationships (Box 1.4).

Mind Jogger

How might body language indicate a sense of guilt or self-blame for a death or loss?

There are several theories that have evolved concerning the grief process, and while not absolute, the stages of grief supply a basis for understanding this process. A person may experience all stages in rapid succession or rally back and forth between stages, remaining in some longer than others. When the process of grieving becomes prolonged it may be seen as abnormal or maladaptive with symptoms of a major depressive episode such as extreme sadness, insomnia, anorexia, and weight loss. The person may consider these symptoms normal but may seek professional help for the insomnia or appetite loss. According to *DSM-5* the diagnosis of major depressive disorder is not generally assigned unless the symptoms are still present for at least 2 weeks duration after the loss and involve clear-cut changes in emotional and psychological functioning.

Dysfunctional Grief

Dysfunctional grief is a failure to complete the grieving process and cope successfully with a loss. If the person experiences a prolonged and intensified reaction, life may become meaningless and a mere existence centered on longing for that which is lost. These extended feelings a person has while attempting to deal with the loss are described as **chronic sorrow**. **Unresolved grief** describes situations when the grief process is incomplete and life is burdened with maladaptive symptoms continuing months after the loss has occurred. Factors that may contribute to unresolved grief, which then leads to the dysfunction include the following:

- Socially unacceptable death such as suicide or homicide
- Missing person related to war, mysterious disappearance, or abduction
- Multiple losses or losses in close succession (loss of several family members in short period with financial loss or disaster loss)
- Ambivalent feelings toward the lost person or object
- Unresolved grieving from a previous loss
- Guilt with regard to circumstances at or near the time of death
- Feelings of the survivor that he or she should have died with or instead of the deceased
- Consuming feelings of worthlessness with suicidal tendencies
- Physiological response to the loss with marked decrease in functioning
- Delusional thinking or hallucinations of seeing the image or hearing the voice of the deceased

Coping with Grief and Loss

Because the intensity of feelings at this level is often desperate, it is essential that the person with prolonged bereavement receive clinical attention and treatment. To deal effectively with the client experiencing grief, the nurse must face the reality of his or her own mortality and concept of death. The nurse is conditioned by experience and by cultural and religious beliefs that develop a response pattern toward loss. Most people experiencing a crisis of major proportion require assistance and support to complete the grief process. The nurse needs to respect and attempt to understand the importance of grieving for oneself and for others. It is important to avoid reassuring clichés, such as, "I know how hard it is" or "It was for the best." They only serve to decrease the genuineness of the support effort.

Using open-ended statements (e.g., "tell me what you are feeling now" or "can you tell me about what has happened?"), the nurse can determine at what point the person is in the grieving process. The nurse should also determine what support systems are available through family and friends, and what coping strategies the person may have used in the past that could be used to deal with the present situation. Through the use of leading statements such as, "You seem to regret some things. Can you tell me about that…," the nurse can determine whether there are any ambivalent feelings, guilt issues, anger, or feelings of helplessness. Recognizing that the process of grieving is very individualized, it is important to remember that the client will progress in the stages of grieving at his or her own pace, with some clients taking longer than others.

Interventions that will assist individuals to cope in the grieving process should encourage clients to be open and honest about their feelings with reassurance they are acceptable and normal as the process follows its course. Having the client journal his or her feelings or write a letter to the deceased can help to bring closure to the past relationship. Referral to a grief support group can provide additional help for the individual or family members. Encouraging the client to utilize family, religious, or cultural groups may also provide meaningful support. Success is determined as the client moves to establish new relationships and put the loss in perspective. Expressions of hope for the future and reinvestment in personal interests will demonstrate a positive self-image that is separated from the past relationship.

In Chapter 2, we will discuss other issues that affect mental health such as anger, violence, abuse, crisis, and suicide. All of these factors have the ability to disrupt an individual's mental state temporarily with most people adapting and growing from the experience. In other situations, as we will see in the mental disorders, the individual may be unable to retrieve a mental balance.

Summary

- Mental health is seen as a state of well-being in which the individual has an awareness of his or her own abilities and weaknesses, copes with normal stressors of life, works productively, and makes a meaningful contribution to society.
- Mental illness denotes clinically significant behavioral or psychological patterns that occur in an individual that cause distress or disability in the person's life. Disorders manifest as inappropriate behavioral patterns that result from the distortions and discomfort experienced in the mind of the individual. Thinking errors and misconceptions often lead to irrational and unrealistic processing.
- Mental health is achieved as we forage a balance between the ups and downs of everyday life. Factors that require us to adapt both physically and emotionally and may affect mental health include stress, anxiety, psychological crisis, grief, loss, anger, violence, and abuse, to name a few.
- Stress and anxiety are considered a part of everyday living. Mild stress is motivating and propels us to function at optimum levels toward accomplishment and success.
- Acute stress is triggered by an overwhelming sense of danger or threat over which we feel a lack of control. Chronic stress relates to a situation that is experienced on a continuous basis.
- Stress triggers an autonomic nervous system response that results in an unconscious feeling over which our conscious mind has no control. Both internal and external stressors can cause the various responses. How one perceives a situation directly affects the sense of control felt over the stressor.
- Anxiety in response to stress can range from mild levels to those of panic. An individual response may be either adaptive or maladaptive based on this perception.
- Coping strategies are learned behaviors. Successful resolution of previous stressful situations will lead to more effective coping methods. Ineffective coping and emotional strategies lead to ineffective and unsuccessful interpersonal relationships.
- If a stressful situation is unresolved, a state of crisis or emotional disorganization can result. The ability to function is impaired and intervention by a support system is required to reestablish homeostasis and control.
- Grief is experienced in response to the anticipation of or the result of a loss. It is the process of mourning for and coming to terms with the reality of the loss and putting it into perspective as one moves forward. Reaction to loss changes with growth and maturation of individual cognitive ability.
- Elizabeth Kubler-Ross defined five stages of dying: denial, anger, bargaining, depression, and acceptance. Once the loss is accepted, a new period of growth beyond the esteemed object or person can emerge.
- Dysfunctional grief results from a failure to complete the grieving process in which the person experiences a prolonged and intensified sense of loss. Multiple factors may contribute to this unresolved grief often requiring professional intervention.
- Interventions that assist individuals with the grieving process should encourage openness and honesty about their feelings, while encouraging expressions of hope for the future and reinvestment in life interests.

Bibliography

American Psychiatric Association. (2013). *Diagnostic and statistical manual of mental disorders* (5th ed.). Washington, DC: American Psychiatric Publishing.

Bee, S., & Gibson, M. J. (1998). Mental health parity: An overview of recent legislation, AARP Research. Accessed November 13, 2013, from http://research.aarp.org

Bhui, K., King, M., Dein, S., & O'Connor, W. (2008). Ethnicity and religious coping with mental distress. *Journal of Mental Health, 17*(2), 141–151.

Daly, R. (2011). Reform-law mandate should boost MH screening in primary care. *Psychiatric News, 46*(1), 12–26. Government News. Retrieved November 20, 2013, from http://pn.psychiatryonline.org

Frisch, N. C., & Frisch, L. E. (2010). *Psychiatric Mental Health Nursing* (4th ed.). Albany, NY: Delmar Publishers.

Honeycutt, A., & Milliken, M. E. (2012). *Understanding Human Behavior* (8th ed.). Albany, NY: Delmar.

National Institute of Mental Health. (2013). Statistics – any disorder among adults. Accessed November 8,

2013, from http://www.nimh.nih.gov/statistics/1ANYDIS_ADULT.shtml

National Institute of Mental Health. (2013). FY 2013 Budget – Congressional Justification. Accessed November 8, 2013, from http://www.nimh.nih.gov/about/budget/fy-2013-budget-congressional-justification.shtml

Oscos-Sanchez, M. A., Lesser, J., Kelly, P. (2008). Cultural competence: a critical facilitator of success in community-based participatory action research. *Issues in Mental Health Nursing, 29*(2), 197–200.

Owen, S., & Khalil, E. (2007). Addressing diversity in mental health care: A review of guidance documents. *International Journal of Nursing Studies, 44*(3), 467–478. Retrieved November 13, 2013.

President's New Freedom Commission on Mental Health. (2004). Goal 3: Disparities in mental health services are eliminated. Retrieved November 12, 2013, from http://mentalhealth.about.com/library

Satcher, D. (1999). Overview of cultural diversity and mental health services. *Mental Health: A Report of the Surgeon General*, Chapter 2, Sections 7–8, National Institute of Mental Health. Retrieved November 13, 2013, from http://www.surgeongeneral.gov/library/mentalhealth//home.html

U.S. Census Bureau. (2012a). U.S. census bureau projections show a slower growing, older, more diverse nation a half century from now. Accessed November 9, 2013, from http://www.census.gov/newsroom/releases/archives/populatio/cb12-243.html

U.S. Census Bureau. (2012b). USA quick facts from the US Census Bureau. Accessed November 8, 2013, from http://quickfacts.census.gov/qfd/states/00000.html

World Health Organization. (2007). "What is mental health?" Accessed October 30, 2014, from http://www.who.int/features/qa/62/en/index.html

World Health Organization Fact Sheet N-220. (2007). Mental health: Strengthening mental health promotion, 1–2. Accessed November 9, 2013, from http://www.who.int/mediacentre/factsheets/fs220/en/

Student Worksheet

Fill in the Blank

Fill in the blank with the correct answer.

1. Mental health is achieved as forage a _____ between the ups and downs of everyday life.

2. Acute stress is a response to an immediate threat, commonly called the _____ or _____ response in which there is a surge of adrenalin into the blood.

3. When anxiety persists over a long period, its effect may be demonstrated by apprehension and _____ to all unexpected environmental stimuli.

4. A major factor in whether a stressor becomes a strain on an individual is the _____ of situations over which little or no control is possible.

5. Statements made to the person who is grieving that are seemingly appropriate but tend to be empty and show little support are termed _____.

Matching

Match the following terms to the most appropriate phrase.

1. _____ Anxiety
2. _____ Eustress
3. _____ Adaptation
4. _____ Denial
5. _____ Bargaining
6. _____ Cultural identity
7. _____ Reframing
8. _____ Burnout
9. _____ Distress

a. Positive restructuring of our thinking about a stressful event
b. Binding force between members of a cultural group
c. Feeling of apprehension, uneasiness, or uncertainty in response to a perceived threat
d. Adjustment period in which the reality of a loss is avoided
e. Positive and motivating stress
f. Condition of mental and emotional exhaustion with apathy toward one's work
g. Harmful response to a threat or challenge
h. Manner in which individuals manage their anxiety
i. Labile moods and attempts to make deals to postpone a loss

Multiple Choice

Select the best answer from the available choices.

1. Which of the following statements made by a client might indicate a possible problem with the individual's present state of mental health?
   a. "I am involved in many community activities."
   b. "My children don't care about me anymore."
   c. "I enjoy the solitude of living by myself."
   d. "I try not to let the little things upset me."

2. In general, a client diagnosed with a mental illness would demonstrate which of the following?
   a. Rational and realistic thought processing
   b. Ability to function alone or with others
   c. Disrupted interpersonal relationships
   d. Motivation by inner values and strengths

3. Amanda is an LPN/LVN who has worked in the dementia unit of a long-term care facility for the past 8 years. Recently, she has been calling in with various physical complaints and says she just doesn't care about the clients like she used to. It is most likely that Amanda is experiencing:

   a. Mental escape
   b. Crisis
   c. Burnout
   d. Dysfunctional stress

4. Which of the following statements reframes the irrational thought, "I will always be a failure," into a rational thought process?

   a. "I may fail at some things, but I am not always a failure."
   b. "I don't have to fail at anything."
   c. "I am my own worst enemy."
   d. "I usually fail because most things are just too difficult for me."

5. William owns a small business that has recently been experiencing reduced sales and profits. William obtained a bank loan to cover losses from the past few months and obtain merchandise for inventory. The bank loan will be due for repayment in 6 months. Which of the following describes William's solution to his anxiety over his financial situation?

   a. Adaptive coping strategy
   b. Palliative coping strategy
   c. Maladaptive coping method
   d. Dysfunctional management

6. A client is scheduled for a radical mastectomy. As the nurse enters the client's hospital room, the client ways, "It would be easier if I just didn't wake up from the surgery." The best response for the nurse to make at this time is:

   a. "You are just afraid now. Everything will look different tomorrow."
   b. "You feel it would be easier to die than to face the loss of your breast?"
   c. "Some people feel the way you do, but this does not mean the end of your life."
   d. "Why do you think it would be easier to die than to wake up after surgery?"

7. Maria has been in a comatose state for the past 8 months as a result of an automobile accident. Although doctors have told her husband, Reuben that there is no brain function, Reuben insists that she is showing purposeful response. Which of the following stages of grief is Reuben experiencing?

   a. Bargaining
   b. Anger
   c. Denial
   d. Depression

8. The nurse is caring for a client who has been told the radiation treatment of his cancer is not working. He is placed on hospice care and palliative relief of his pain. Which of the following will this client likely soon experience?

   a. Resolution
   b. Conventional grief
   c. Bereavement
   d. Anticipatory grief

9. The nurse is assessing a client whose wallet was stolen. The client is experiencing palpitations, hyperventilation, diaphoresis, and confusion. Although alert and talking, the client is unable to provide a name and address. The nurse would document this as the client experiencing which level of anxiety?

   a. Mild anxiety
   b. Moderate anxiety
   c. Severe anxiety
   d. Panic level

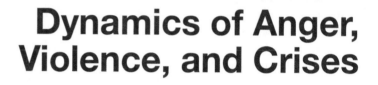

Dynamics of Anger, Violence, and Crises

⊙ Learning Objectives

After learning the content in this chapter, the student will be able to:

1. Define anger as a human emotion.
2. Describe what is meant by trait anger.
3. Identify ways that anger is outwardly expressed.
4. Define what is meant by aggression and violence.
5. Describe contributing factors that propel violent behavior.
6. Discuss the cycle of violence and its influence in situations of abuse.
7. Identify constructive ways of managing anger and aggression.
8. Describe the strategies of crisis intervention.
9. Describe components of a suicide risk assessment.
10. Identify approaches of intervention for prevention of suicide.

⊙ Key Terms

aggression
anger
batterer
bullying
developmental crisis
domestic violence
emotional abuse
hostility
physical abuse
psychological crisis

sexual abuse
situational crisis
stalking
suicidal erosion
suicidal gesture
suicidal ideation
suicidal threat
suicide attempt
trait anger
violence

Dynamics of Anger and Aggression

Negative human emotions tend to disrupt our feeling of internal comfort. They can range from a mild feeling of discontent to a volatile degree of hostile and potentially harmful outrage. Everyone has felt angry or upset at some point. Sometimes this emotion can have a short-term positive effect. However, not everyone is able to harness these feelings before they get out of control. The spiraling effects of this escalation in emotion are often at the root of abuse and the associated violence.

Defining Anger

Anger is an emotion triggered in response to threats, insulting situations, or anything that seriously hampers the intended actions of an individual. In one sense, anger is a natural adaptive response needed for survival in the face of a threat or danger. In most instances, however, the reaction may be directed at a specific person or, in a generalized sense, toward a group and even society itself. The anger builds into bitterness and becomes an unconscious hurt that breeds a desire to get even. These negative feelings are often expressed through hurtful words or actions toward another individual. The feelings can also be self-directed, resulting in varying degrees of guilt, anxiety, and depression. A mild form of anger may be described as annoyance that, if provoked, can escalate to a more volatile state. Anger can also be expressed aggressively, either verbally or non-verbally in the form of hostility, or can spiral to intense anger or rage that may result in violence toward the subject.

Trait Anger

Trait anger is often referred to as a general biological leaning toward a volatile personality that may be described by the person themselves as a "quick-temper," a feeling of becoming "hot" or feeling one's heart rate accelerate, or behavior that reflects a quick response of irritation and fury. The individual with this type of personality typically has a habitual response to frustrating circumstances that trigger a negative social outcome. The person may have difficulty interacting and encountering new relationships or social situations without preformed opinions or biases. This makes it more difficult to avoid conflict and tense atmospheres, while those with low trait anger may be able to compromise and develop longer solid relationships.

> ### Just the Facts
> People who are easily frustrated and angered usually have a history of being irritable, touchy, and quick-tempered from an early age.

Expressing Anger and Resentment

Both anger and resentment originate in our mental perception of a situation. This perception usually includes feelings of being wronged, ignored, cheated, or abused in some way. When we feel insulted, we form mental images that generate the need to fight back. This unconscious frustration becomes a person's private battle within the mind where emotions follow the thoughts. Getting angry is a way of using manipulation to cause an emotional reaction in another in order to get them to act in accordance with our thinking. This response is conveyed in our behavior. Many of these mental hurts are formed during the vulnerable defenseless years of childhood and the baggage is carried over a lifetime. Other situations such as cases of domestic violence, rape, and abuse can instill long-term emotional trauma and the desire for retribution. Suppressed over time, the hurt turns to resentment and often erupts in a destructive means of resolution. Anger blurs our vision, alters our focus, depletes our energy, creates painful emotions, and destroys teamwork. Concealed hurt is often turned inward as self-directed guilt resulting in depression or willingness to be the victim over and over again. This unexpressed anger can lead to both physical and psychological disorders.

In many instances, the outward reaction fueled by the emotions may be directed at a specific object or person, or in a generalized sense, toward a group and even the society itself. The indirect expression of resentment or chronic anger is often seen in the projection of the negative feelings toward another object or person. The anger builds into bitterness and becomes an unconscious hurt that breeds a desire to get even. These feelings can also be self-directed resulting in varying degrees of guilt, anxiety, and depression.

Mind Jogger

How might a person with embedded anger sabotage his or her own interpersonal relationships?

Unrestrained Anger and Violence

We all feel anger at some time and all tend to express our feelings in different ways. The person with high trait anger is more likely to respond with aggressive behavior or violence. Anger-based aggressive behavior is termed **hostility** or an intense feeling of animosity toward someone or something. This bottled-up resentment can preclude a confrontation of physical aggression and violent behavior. The term **aggression** can include behavior that may result in both physical and psychological harm to oneself or another that can occur both verbally and nonverbally. **Violence** is seen as a means to maintain power in a situation or relationship. This may be related to a misconstrued belief of entitlement, manipulation, rationalization, or indifference toward the feelings of another.

Rooted in a feeling of being wronged, the desire to retaliate or get even is a natural instinct. Given fuel, this bitterness and anger will send the individual into an aggressive overdrive. In this emotional state, the individual is physically capable of inflicting harm to another person or themselves. In other words, the anger is in control. Although inappropriate, violence and abusive behaviors are often learned responses in an environment where this is the norm. Growing up, the child learns to deal with frustration and disappointment by observing patterns modeled by the family members. Since the conditioned response may be reactive and automatic, actions may precede any effort to dissolve the intensity of the emotion, or to resolve the situation through problem-solving.

Along with family influence, the effect of peer relationships and the community where a child resides are major in the learned anger response. The child who is constantly subjected to a violent verbal or physical response to unleashed anger by adults in his or her living environment learns this behavior as a norm. The child may also be the object of the anger and receive both verbal and physical results of adult fury. Continued exposure to this negative world, the child is given few chances to develop trusting, positive relationships to counteract the cycle. When the child is confronted with his or her own feelings of anger, the immediate impulse is to utilize the defense that has been reinforced by a repeated pattern. The child will also gravitate toward friends or peer relationships that reinforce learned behaviors feeding the likelihood the child will continue a pattern of uninhibited response to anger and bitterness.

Influencing Factors for Violence

Although aggressive behavior may be seen as one way of expressing anger, it is not an acceptable outlet for these negative emotions. Acting out in a violent manner is never a positive way to handle the feelings associated with being frustrated or pent-up emotions. Violence has become a central theme to many of the shows on television, movies, and video games. Because these are seen as fictional and action packed, they are accepted as entertainment. The empirical evidence to support a link between violent video games and violent crimes is scarce. However, many feel the influence of the violent games may extend beyond the fictional moment and be seen in real-life events such as the infamous April 20, 1999 Columbine High School shooting in Littleton, Colorado, in which 18-year-old Eric Harris and 17-year-old Dylan Klebold killed 12 students and one teacher. They also wounded 23 people before turning their weapons on themselves. All these incidents of imposed violence on innocent children and adults involve an individual or individuals who respond with violence whether as a result of psychological imbalances (e.g., the Sandy Hook school tragedy in December, 2012 and the Aurora, CO theater massacre in July, 2012), or feelings of being wronged by someone or society in general (e.g., the Washington Navy Yard shooting in September, 2013).

Bullying

Another serious problem today is the issue of **bullying** defined as psychological harassment or physical confrontation used repeatedly to intentionally bring harm or humiliation to one seen as weak or different. This form of abuse gains strength because the abuser tries to seem stronger or cooler than the target victims. According to the National Education Association, it is estimated that 1 in 3 students in Grades 6 to 10 in the

---

BOX 2.1

Picture of Bullying

- Behavior is done repeatedly with intent to diminish or harm the victim
- Harassment is repeated daily
- Victim is one who is smaller or seen as weaker or different
- Bully usually has allies present who witness and encourage the behavior
- The bully enjoys the fear and trauma induced on the victim
- Harassment usually occurs during time when adult authority figure is not present

---

United States is either a bully or a victim of bullying. Bullying results in absenteeism, violence at schools, and adolescent suicide. It is a frightening experience for the victim that may be physical, verbal, or social. It can involve physically hitting, pushing, teasing, or destroying property belonging to the targeted individual. It can also be indirect such as texting, sexting, spreading rumors or excluding the victim from being part of the perceived group, or cyberbullying in which damaging entries may be posted on the Internet or social network that can cause serious and often irreparable harm. The person inflicting the bullying usually surrounds himself or herself with allies who enhance the bully's feeling of power. The bully continues to pick on the target daily while seeming to enjoy the obvious fright and fear of the victim. Timing of the harassment is usually during a time when an authority figure is not present. This pattern of repeated intent to diminish the victim and harm them distinguishes bullying from other types of conflict (Box 2.1). Problems extend beyond the children to the parents as children drop out of school and demonstrate symptoms of mental illness as a result of the psychological abuse. The problems experienced by these individuals may extend into adulthood with serious dysfunction in the individual's ability to function both in relationships and society in general.

The victims of bullying develop a feeling of low self-esteem and helplessness as a result of the repeated threats and taunting hurtful abuse. This sense of decreased self-worth can be devastating and lead to serious depression and emotional problems. Statistics show that children and adolescents who are bullied are more likely to think about or attempt suicide. According to a study at Yale University that examined bullying and suicide, bully victims are 2 to 9 times more likely to report suicidal thoughts than nonvictims. Suicide is the third leading cause of death among young people according to the Centers for Disease Control. Some instances of suicide occur after the victim has been encouraged to end his or her life or that the world would be better without them. Many acts of violence are also the result of bullying such as workplace shootings, robberies, and homicides. There is no Federal law against bullying although 49 states have legislation against this form of abuse. If a crime occurs as a result of the bullying, the crime can be prosecuted but at this point, the bullying is not illegal.

Domestic Violence and Abuse

According to the National Domestic Violence Organization statistics, "24 people per minute are victims of rape, physical violence or stalking by an intimate partner in the United States," and "nearly 3 in 10 women (29%) and 1 in 10 men (10%) in the US have experienced rape, physical violence and/or stalking by a partner and report a related impact on their functioning." Over 1,200 deaths were reported as the result of domestic violence in a recent study. An increasing number of research studies show that domestic violence and child abuse occur in the same families who also tend to have similar social and economic risk factors. Findings also show that children who grow up in families where abuse and violence are the norms demonstrate more likelihood of engaging in similar behaviors as youth and adults.

Domestic Violence Defined

Domestic violence is a pattern of behavior that is used by the perpetrator or **batterer** to gain power and control over another person through fear and intimidation that often includes threats or use of physical violence. This form of violence can take the form of emotional, physical, economic, and/or sexual abuse. The effects of domestic violence have no social or economic boundaries and can

---

Mind Jogger

With the increase in cyberbullying, what can be done by parents or the victims themselves to reduce the harmful effects?

---

affect anyone regardless of gender, ethnicity, race, religion, income, sexual orientation, or age. The effects leave the victim with a sense of fear and hopelessness that is often shrouded in secrecy by the individual induced by the intimidation of the abuser.

Physical abuse is an intentional injury to another person and can take the form of slapping, pinching, choking, scratching, stabbing, shooting, and homicide. **Emotional abuse** inflicts psychological trauma as words and nonverbal language are used to criticize, demean, or humiliate another person. Each incident further deteriorates the self-esteem of the victim as blaming by the abuser gives way to feelings of guilt in the abused. **Sexual abuse** and/or rape often accompanies other forms of abuse, and refers to any behavior using forced or unwanted sex that is inflicted on an unwilling participant. Any of these situations can also be accompanied by **stalking** which involves harassing or threatening phone calls, e-mails, texts, voice mails, mail, or unwanted appearances at the victim's place of employment, home, or other location. Stalking can also involve vandalism or forced entry of the victim's place of residence or vehicle. Abuse of a partner or parent also puts children in the home at risk for abuse and emotional and/or physical problems. There are also indications that as a result of the trauma, the child may be at greater risk for emotional problems or substance use and abuse.

> **Just the Facts**
>
> Domestic violence and abuse are patterns of behavior used by one person to control or have power over another through fear and intimidation with threats or acts of violence.

Risk Factors

There are factors that indicate the potential or warning signs for violence in people. These may include the following:

- A past history or family history of violence
- Are moody and over sensitive to criticism
- Are power-seeking or overly competitive
- Degrade or put down women
- Drug or alcohol abuse
- Always blame others for their problems or feelings
- Rationalize the use of violent behavior as needed to resolve a situation

- Expect others to meet their needs or wait on them
- Frequent arguing, cursing, or physical fighting
- Verbal threats against others
- Vandalism or harming animals

Recognizing these characteristics and their potential to trigger destructive behavior can contribute to the efforts to avert the continued escalating incidence of violence-related events. The problem does not belong to one segment of society but to society as a whole.

Cycle of Violence and Abuse

Violence toward an individual starts with verbal or physical threats and assaults that quickly victimize the person into going along with the abuse. There may be blaming, insults, name-calling, or accusations of infidelity. Often the abuser will be extreme in controlling the family money, stop the partner from getting a job or furthering their education, and isolating the family from relatives and friends. Stalking, threats of divorce, taking the children, and killing or harming the victim are mind games in the manipulation for power. During these violent episodes, the abuser may punch walls or doors, throw objects, break mirrors or windows, tear clothing or furniture, block driveways or take keys, and take money or means for independence of the victim. The abused individual may attempt to protect him or herself as the intensity of the attacks increases.

The emotional or verbal abuse often appears before the physical harm occurs. The contact level may include pushing, shoving, twisting limbs, slapping, punching, choking, hair pulling, forced sex, or threats with a weapon. Once major physical and emotional harm or battering has been done to the victim, the batterer or abusive partner usually tries to offer some type of gift or loving gestures of remorse and promises it will not happen again. Ironically, this presumed sorrow sets the victim up for the next step of abuse in which the perpetrator justifies the behavior by projecting the blame to the victim. The victim feels guilt and accepts the blame. Each incident of this violence cycle further depletes the victim's self-esteem and sense of worth as they feel trapped and powerless to end the cycle. Many women report that their partner has physically hit them at some point in their marriage or relationship. As many as 70% of women who are murdered are killed by their mate or partner, a male family member, or another male acquaintance.

Just the Facts

Explaining anger in a logical way to oneself defeats the fury of the emotion. Anger, even if justified, is an irrational means to an end.

There are many mistaken beliefs about the perpetrator and the victims of domestic abuse. As stated earlier, violence is a character trait and not the result of the relationship. It is not the partner who does something to trigger the abuse. Ownership of the subsequent violent response solely belongs to the abuser. Women often separate from an abusive partner only to return to the situation. This may be the result of fear of the abuser or because they are encouraged to "try again" to make the relationship work. Sometimes the woman feels a dependency on the partner for an income or because it would be detrimental to the children to break up the home. It is important to point out that mental health issues of depression, low self-esteem, anxiety, and fear are the result of battering and not the cause. The abuser will continue the cycle of abuse and violence until they get help. It is necessary for the abuser to recognize and take responsibility for his or her actions. It is also important that intervention in this situation involves providing a safe environment and counseling to help build a sense of power, self-worth, and support for the abused victim. The victim is usually in greatest danger right after the separation occurs as the batterer is flooded with a surge of anger and blame. The possibility of a tragic ending to this scenario is all too common in our society. Some available links and hotlines are listed in Box 2.2.

Mind Jogger

How can we as nurses help to prevent or advocate for the victim of domestic violence?

Managing Anger

Even as we recognize the instinctive reaction to anger is aggression, we can also be aware that we have the ability to be in control of our behavior. Just as we can choose a negative response, we can elect to develop steps toward managing or redirecting the anger in a constructive way. We might ask ourselves, what is it that sets me off or gets

---

BOX 2.2

Help for Domestic Violence and Abuse

- National Domestic Violence Hotline
  1-800-799-SAFE (7233)
  1-800-787-3224 (TTY)
- Safe Horizon Domestic Violence Hotline
  1-800-621-HOPE (4673)
- American Domestic Violence Crisis Line
  3300 NW 185th Street, Suite 133
  Portland, OR 97229
  Phone: 503-846-8748
  Toll-free: 1-866-USWOMEN (International Crisis
      Line)
  http://www.866uswomen.org
- National Resource Center on Domestic Violence
  6400 Flank Drive, Suite 1300
  Harrisburg, PA 17112
  1-800-537-2238 ext. 5
  TTY: 1-800-553-2508
  Fax: 717-545-9456
- Rape, Abuse & Incest National Network (RAINN)
  Hotline
  1-800-656-HOPE
- National Coalition Against Domestic Violence
  1120 Lincoln Street, Suite 1603
  Denver, CO 80203
  Phone: 303-839-1852
  TTY: (303) 839-8459
  E-mail: mainoffice@ncadv.org
- Individual State Information available at
  http://feminist.org/911/crisis_state.html

me riled? Recognizing the origin of the emotional response can identify triggers that allow us to be in touch with why we respond as we do. This awareness gives us the opportunity to assume control of the anger before we succumb to its fury.

Constructive Methods

Putting the situation in perspective with restructured thinking can help the person from overdramatizing the facts. Sensible reasoning can diffuse the anger, which left unchecked, will accelerate and can lead to negative and harmful consequences. The feelings created do not resolve the situation underlying the emotion, but rethinking the worst possible scenario can make it more palatable. For instance, if one feels like other people in the workplace are "always saying things behind my back," replace it with "maybe I can turn this around by saying nice things to them." This approach requires self-control to check one's volatile feelings before they lead to actions that are later regretted.

When the emotion of anger is elicited in a person, the result is both an emotional and an internal physiological combustion that stimulates and accelerates the system. In order to control the emotion, one must also take steps to decrease the body response. One way to manage the anger is to engage in some form of physical activity such as walking, jogging, playing tennis or a game of volleyball. The activity utilizes energy for a constructive purpose rather than an emotional outburst. People who know their temperament is easily irritated may want to plan a "time-out" period each day for exercise and meditation. Separating oneself from the situation allows the mind time to reflect and think about the cause of the feelings. Sometimes changing the timing surrounding the conflict (e.g., parental confrontation after school or at meal-time, arguing with a spouse after both mates are tired) and allowing a cool-down period before discussing issues can allow time to think about the emotions before the interaction and separate reaction from an impulsive action in words or deeds.

Another way to manage anger is through assertion. Assertion is standing up for one's rights, beliefs, or values in such a way that it does not hurt others in the process. This demonstrates a form of respect for oneself and for those with whom we interact. Thinking about the situation usually precedes assertive behavior. By this we mean that negative thoughts can be restructured and replaced with more rational ones. For example, a young couple is arguing over their vacation plans. The young woman says, "You never want to do what I want. I'm going to my mother's and you can go by yourself!" Restructured into a more rational approach, she might say, "I really want to see my mother on this trip. Could we work that in to your plan?" Reminding oneself that anger will not solve a problem can set the tone for facing the issue and finding a solution. Using "I" statements allow us to own our feelings and express our thoughts in a way that avoids attacking the other person. Volatile emotions can often be diffused when there is a mutual willingness to view a situation from more than one perspective. This approach of conflict resolution and improved communication can rechannel the negative feelings into a win–win situation where everyone benefits.

Mind Jogger

How can self-evaluation contribute to successful conflict resolution?

Talking with someone who will listen is also a positive means of reducing the intensity of emotions. If another person is not available, the individual can use a tape recorder to provide the listening ear. Sometimes writing or typing a letter but never sending it will allow the expression of thoughts and feelings without hurting the other person. Feelings are brought outward and mellowed by acknowledging them in print. This prevents the buildup of resentment or animosity over time that results in hostile feelings. Sometimes in talking with someone else, humor can add a dimension that lightens the impact of the feelings. An objective view from another person can sometimes help us to see the situation from another angle making it actually seem silly to be so angry. Counseling in anger management allows time to reflect and discover reasons behind the anger and learn new ways of coping with the feelings. Anger management groups also allow a person not only to see that other people also struggle with similar feelings and problems, but how they cope and control their anger. Anger management classes for perpetrators in domestic violence situations also address issues of power and control which are central to the abuse.

Perhaps the most effective means of dealing with the negative feelings of anger is forgiveness, both of someone else or oneself. Carrying anger or bitterness within us is like a chronic disease that is harmful to us both physically and psychologically. True joy and happiness are colored by the nagging negativity and animosity of our grudges and inability to rid our hearts of the need to get even. Forgiveness can permit us to let go of the hurt and allow ourselves to heal the bruises of emotional pain and bitterness. True forgiveness is cleansing and brings peace within. To forgive ourselves often involves an apology or confession to another person for something we may have done or didn't do. Learning to forgive is a difficult task, but once done will lift the negative burdens we have been carrying.

Crisis and Intervention

A **psychological crisis** differs from stress and anxiety in that a state of disorganization and disarray occurs in the individual as usual coping strategies fail or are not available. The total inability to control the situation and to function in daily activities leads the person to seek a way out. The

"Reactive Anger"

Since an early age, Kendall has had what most people called a "short fuse." Because he would always argue and start fights, it became difficult for him to make friends during his school years. In addition, nothing seemed to curb the angry response Kendall displayed when his parents tried to discipline him. Aside from his inability to control his temper, Kendall was intelligent and athletic. He made good grades and engaged in competitive sports. Social relationships remained an issue as he was controlling and impulsive.

After graduating from college, Kendall works in a pharmaceutical laboratory. Co-workers describe him as "touchy" and "easily ticked off," but very brilliant and efficient at what he does. On one particular day, Kendall is unable to contain his anger over an incident in which a lab technician makes an error in a chemical formula. Kendall becomes so irate and angry, he throws the flask across the room narrowly missing the young technician's head. The technician runs out of the lab screaming that "Ken has lost it this time." Kendall is put on leave from the company and is required to enter treatment for anger management.

How are anger and aggression evident in Kendall's situation?

_____

_____

In what ways might Kendall's behavior be a conditioned response?

_____

_____

What methods might be used to help him diffuse some of his anger before it controls him?

_____

_____

Case Application 2.1

level of anxiety increases to a severe or panic level during which the individual feels helpless and lost. Attempts to cope may meet with little success. The state of dysfunction is usually receptive to the right intervention that can help the person stabilize and regain a sense of power and control over his or her being.

Types of Crises

A model for crisis intervention developed in the early 1960s by Linder Mann and Gerald Caplan identifies two primary types of crisis situations. A **developmental crisis** may occur at a predictable time period in an individual's life related to maturational stages (e.g., teenage, mid-life, or old-age crises) and changes. The other type, a **situational crisis**, is unpredictable and sudden without warning such as a fatal illness diagnosis, plane crash, natural disaster, or sudden death. Thoughts are dismantled and behavior changes in response to these crisis situations. People become confused, feel helpless and lost, and are easily angered and agitated.

It is important to note that intervention is not to the actual event or situation but to deal with the individual response to that situation. Intervention is an attempt to offer help to the client in the way of support, resources, and short-term stabilization.

Just the Facts

Disorganization may result from an unrealistic perception of a threatening event, lack of a support system, or inadequate coping ability.

Crisis Intervention

A state of psychological crisis is intolerable for more than a few weeks if help is not received. Resolution will usually allow the person to either emerge at a higher and more productive level of functioning, at the same level, or at a lower level of coping ability. The outcome depends on the actions taken by the individual to cope with the crisis and those taken by others to intervene. During a crisis, an individual is often more receptive to support from others and can learn adaptive coping strategies to assist in the resolution. Reassuring the person that he or she is mentally healthy and has coped with a crisis in the past often helps the person to reinvest in his or her ability to face the current state of chaos.

Intervention deals with the present situation and resolution of the immediate issue. It is important to assess the events that led up to the crisis. Listening to what the client says both verbally and nonverbally gives insight into the event or problem from the client's perspective. It is important that the intervention offers hope to the individual and a plan for resolution of the crisis with specific steps. Focusing on the present situation and keeping a reality-based approach helps the person to concentrate on a specific task. At this point, the person may be able to make a temporary form of resolution that allows him or her to function and move on with daily activities.

Early intervention in assisting the individual to manage the current situation promotes the best chance for a positive outcome. Once the anxiety level is reduced to a tolerable level, the individual can be assisted in defining the problem, determining available support, and setting realistic goals for resolution of the issue. The nurse is

integral in providing support and returning control to the client. This allows the nurse to help the client identify alternative ways of reducing the anxiety and feelings of powerlessness. It is important for the nurse to remain nonjudgmental and to resist letting personal feelings interfere with an objective view of the client's problem. Establishing a sense of trust and respect will help the client focus on his or her feelings. Allow the client time to sort through his or her thoughts as you begin questioning. Using open-ended statements (e.g., "Can you tell me what happened right before you started feeling this way?"), will also help the client work through the details that led up to the current crisis. Listen for meaning behind statements that help to define the situational trauma the client is experiencing. If the person is suicidal, protective measures must be initiated to provide a feeling of safety and security. This feeling will allow the individual a temporary sanctuary in which the inner resources can be stabilized. Outcomes are aimed at promoting optimum psychological and physiological functioning. Therapeutic strategies are designed to assist in mobilizing the client's currently available coping mechanisms and developing new

Case Application 2.2

"Nathan in Trouble"

Nathan feels that his world is coming to an end. Seventeen years ago, his fiancé was badly beaten by an intruder and left with multiple scars and a loss of vision in one eye. Last week, Nathan learned that the intruder was due to be released from prison and would be returning to the community. Nathan is so worried about further danger to the girl who is now his wife that he cannot sleep, eat, or function. Nathan feels that he will not be able to control his impulse to kill the man if he sees him.

How does Nathan's problem demonstrate a crisis situation?

_____

_____

What is the first step of the intervention to help Nathan?

_____

_____

Why is it so important to listen to what Nathan says both verbally and nonverbally?

_____

_____

strategies to assist in preventing future emotional states of dysfunction.

Mind Jogger

How would the need for intervention increases for someone experiencing several potential crisis situations at one time?

Suicide

Each year, there are many people who contemplate or complete suicide, or self-inflicted death. Although some people are at a greater risk, people of all ages, races, and socioeconomic status commit suicide. According to the National Institute of Mental Health (NIMH), in 2007, suicide was the 10th leading cause of death in the adult population of the United States. Approximately 11 attempted suicides occur for every suicide that ends in death. Males and the elderly are more likely to have attempts that end in death than females and youth. Among children and young people ages 15 to 24 years, suicide ranks as the third ranked cause of death. Statistics show that about four times as many males die by suicide as females. Firearms, suffocation, and poisoning tend to be the most common methods used. A familial history of mental disorders is shown to increase the risk for suicidal behaviors. Research also demonstrates that the risk increases when depression, other mental disorders, or substance-related disorders are involved. It is estimated that more than 90% of those who succeed in ending their life by suicide have one of these problems. In addition, research also shows the risk is associated with decreased levels of the neurotransmitter serotonin in the brain. This has been found in persons with depression, impulsive disorders, and those having a history of attempted or fatal suicide (NIMH).

Risk Factors

Some identifiable factors can put a person in a mindset leading to the actual decision to end his or her life. For example, a person may distance himself or herself from others with a feeling of hopelessness and worthlessness. This despondency may be related to loss of a love object, loss of health, or an escape from the realities of life. Other factors may include substance abuse or loss of control over situations that seem hopeless. Any kind of loss has the potential to precipitate depressive symptoms. In a person who is depressed, the symptoms may go undetected by family members or friends. **Suicidal erosion**, or the long-term accumulation of negative experiences throughout a person's lifetime can lead to suicidal thoughts, occurs not as a result of a single factor that leads to suicidal thoughts, but because of a combination of situations over time. In addition, risk factors for adolescents and youth include depression, alcohol and drugs, bullying, physical or sexual abuse, and behavior disorders. Most suicide attempts are expressions of severe internal and mental distress. Box 2.3 provides a list of warning signs or "flashing lights" that indicate the person may be considering suicide as a way out.

There are four levels of risk that apply to the person who may be contemplating suicide. A verbalized thought or idea that indicates the person's desire to do self-harm or destruction is **suicidal ideation**. This person may have recurrent thought processes that center on death as a means of ending mental and physical anguish. A further step is taken if the person has devised a plan for ending his or her life. A statement of intent is considered a **suicidal threat** and is usually accompanied by behavior changes that indicate the person has defined their plan. Action that indicates the person may be about ready to carry out the plan is considered a **suicidal gesture**. If the person actually carries out a **suicide attempt**, the possibility of success is a reality. This is often the last desperate cry for help by

---

BOX 2.3

Suicide Warning Signs

- Talks about suicide
- Difficulty eating and sleeping
- Increased substance use
- Social withdrawal
- Loss of interest in school, work, or pleasure activities
- Giving away possessions
- Previous suicide attempt
- Unnecessary risk-taking
- Recent major loss
- Preoccupation with death and dying
- Lack of attention to personal hygiene

a person who sees no other alternative. To the person who is unable to see any other way of improving the present situation, suicide seems to be a logical and rational solution. It is important that any person who appears to be suicidal is not left alone and assisted in securing immediate mental health treatment.

Risk Assessment and Intervention

A risk assessment should be done on the first contact with the person. It is important that this assessment determines the lethality and immediacy of the crisis. Is the person thinking about suicide now or has he or she thought about it in the past few months? If the answer is yes, was it a passing thought or a continuing thought (suicidal ideation)? Does the person have a plan (suicidal threat) and do they have the means available to carry out their plan (suicidal gesture)? Has the individual actually attempted to carry out the plan (suicide attempt)? The assessment should address the suicidal desire, suicidal capability, suicidal intent, available support system, and the individual's sense of purpose. Once a crisis intervention assessment has been made, the risk designation can be assigned and a plan for treatment can be initiated.

Just the Facts

To the person who is unable to see any other way of improving his or her present situation, suicide may seem to be a logical and rational solution.

Other signs to consider are reports from family or friends that the individual may have recently expressed a desire to die or wanting to kill him/herself, or about being a burden to family. The person may feel trapped in a presumably inescapable situation, such as an individual who is caught stealing money from the company they work for and faces litigation and an uncertain future. The person may also have exhibited reckless behavior or an increased use of alcohol or drugs. Withdrawal from friends and family events or giving away items that previously had significant meaning to the individual can also indicate a loss of the will to live.

BOX 2.4

If You Think Someone Might be Suicidal

- Do not leave the person alone
- Try to get the person immediate medical help
- Call 911
- Eliminate access to firearms or other potential suicide tools
- Remove any unsupervised access to prescription or OTC drugs

(NIMH, 2013)

Steps for Prevention

Individuals who indicate that they are thinking about or wanting to kill themselves need help. It is imperative to listen and find support for the person. Box 2.4 provides steps that anyone can take if he or she feels that another person is suicidal. Suicide crisis centers have hot lines that can provide assistance from medical and mental health professionals. Talking to someone who is trained to lend a listening ear is often a lifesaving intervention. Client Teaching Note 2.1 provides information for the National Suicide Prevention Lifeline and Veteran's Crisis Line.

It is important that interventions focus on the immediate danger to and safety of the individual. The person in an acute crisis situation should never be left alone. A rapport should be established that conveys a calm and caring attitude or genuine concern for the life and story. If the individual has called the crisis line, the person is asking for help—the help-seeking should be validated as the first step in a solution to his or her problems and treatment can be initiated.

CLIENT TEACHING NOTE 2.1

SUICIDE PREVENTION LIFELINE

If you are in a crisis and need immediate help:

Call this toll-free number, available 7 days a week, 24 hours a day: Lifeline at 1-800-273-TALK (8255). This will put you in touch with the National Suicide Prevention Lifeline. You may call or anyone else may call for you. All calls are confidential and answered immediately.

Veteran's Crisis Line: 1-800-273-8255 or text to 838255.

(NIMH, 2013)

Summary

- Anger describes the emotion elicited in response to a threat, insult, or circumstance that prevents us from following through with intended actions or desires. Anger drives the response of aggression and bitterness that can lead to hostility and outward attacks toward another person or object.

- Bullying is a form of psychological harassment or physical confrontation used to intentionally bring harm or humiliation to one who is seen as weak or different. This form of abuse is done both directly and indirectly as in cyberbullying which can cause irreparable damage to the individual. Both the victim and family members may be affected in some way by the destructive attacks of degradation.

- Domestic violence is a pattern of behavior that is used by the abuser to gain power and control over another person through fear and intimidation that often includes threats or use of physical violence. This form of violence can take the form of emotional, physical, economic, and/or sexual abuse.

- The cycle of abuse is seen in domestic violence, physical, emotional, and sexual abuse. Beginning as put-downs and verbal accusations of control escalates to physical attacks that can endanger the victim and cause serious bodily harm. Seeming remorse and gift giving are soon replaced with a repeat of blaming and further abuse that repeats the cycle. Fear of the abuser and the unknown holds the victim captive in the repetitious sequence.

- Our mental perception of a situation in which we feel wronged or cheated leads to an unconscious battle that grows to internal guilt and pain.

- Anger and resentment can be channeled constructively into physical activity, assertive "I" statements to own feelings, talking to one who will listen, and learning to forgive. We have the ability to think before we act and take control of our negative emotions in a manageable way toward a positive outcome.

- Anger, depression, and guilt are among factors that can cause an individual to attempt or actually be successful at ending his or her own life. Assess the content of suicidal thoughts or ideations, and if the person has a plan and/or means to carry out the plan, to determine the lethality of the method of attempt.

- A developmental crisis can occur at a predictable period of a person's life such as mid-life or old-age crisis, whereas a situational crisis is unpredictable and happens suddenly such as an automobile crash, natural disaster, fire, explosion, or sudden death. Thoughts are dismantled and behavior changes in response to these crisis situations.

- The goal of crisis intervention is to reduce the anxiety to a level that will allow the client to look at the situation more realistically toward a resolution.

Bibliography

Abrams, M. (2013). Learn the difference between anger, aggression, and violence, Excerpt from Anger Management in Sport. Retrieved November 22, 2013, from http://www.humankinetics.com/excerpts/learn-the-difference-between-anger-aggression

American Psychological Association. (2008). Controlling anger – before it controls you. Retrieved October 13, 2013, from http://www.apa.org/topics/controlanger.html

Bruehl, S., Liu, X., Burns, J. W., Chont, M., & Jamison, R. N. (2012). Associations between daily chronic pain intensity, daily anger expression, and trait anger expressiveness: An ecological momentary assessment study. *Pain, 153*(12), 2352–2358. Retrieved October 13, 2013.

Edwards, R. D., & Stoppler, M. C. (2010). Domestic violence. Retrieved December 7, 2013, from http://www.medicinenet.com/domestic_violence/article.htm

Honeycutt, A., & Milliken, M. E. (2012). *Understanding human behavior* (8th ed.). Albany, NY: Delmar.

Kassinove, H. (2013). *How to recognize and deal with anger.* American Psychological Association. Retrieved October 13, 2013, from http://www.apa.org/helpcenter/recognize-anger.aspx

Kim, Y. S., & Leventhal, B. (2008). Bullying and suicide. A review. *International Journal of Adolescent Medicine and Health, 20*(2), 133–154. Retrieved December 6, 2013.

Lee, R., Walters, M., Hall, J., & Basile, K. (2013). The behavioral and attitudinal factors differentiating male intimate partner violence perpetrators with and without a history of childhood family violence. *Journal of Family Violence, 28*(1), 85–94. Retrieved November 13, 2013.

Lobbestael, J., Arntz, A., & Wiers, R. W. (2008). How to push someone's buttons: A comparison of four anger-induction methods. *Cognition and Emotion, 22*(2), 353–373. Retrieved November 24, 2013.

Mahon, N. E., Yarcheski, A., Yarcheski, T. J., & Hanks, M. M. (2010). A meta-analytic study of predictors of anger in adolescents. *Nursing Research, 59*(3), 178–184. Retrieved October 30, 2013.

Mendoza, D. W. (1993). A review of Gerald Caplan's theory and practice of mental health consultation. *Journal of Counseling and Development, 71*(6), 629.

Michalopoulos, H., & Michalopoulos, A. (2009). Crisis counseling: Be prepared to intervene. *Nursing, 39*(9), 47–50. Retrieved November 30, 2013.

National Domestic Violence Hotline/Statistics. (2012). Retrieved December 7, 2013, from http://www.thehotline.org/is-this-abuse/statistics/

National Education Association. (2012). Our position and actions on school safety, bullying and harassment. Retrieved November 17, 2013, from http://www.nea.org/home/19535.htm

National Education Association. (2013). How to identify bullying. Retrieved November 17, 2013, from http://www.nea.org/home/533359.htm

National Institute of Mental Health. (2013). Suicide in the U.S.: Statistics and Prevention. Accessed October 19, 2014, from http://www.nimh.nih.gov/health/publications/suicide-in-the-us-statistics-and-prevention/index.shtml

Powley, D. (2013). Reducing violence and aggression in the emergency department. *Emergency Nurse, 21*(4), 26–29. Retrieved November 16, 2013.

Sadeh, N., & McNiel, D. E. (2013). Facets of anger, childhood sexual victimization, and gender as predictors of suicide attempts by psychiatric patients after hospital discharge. *Journal of Abnormal Psychology, 122*(3), 879–890.

Shorey, R. C., Brasfield, H., Febres, J., & Stuart, G. L. (2011). The association between impulsivity, trait anger, and the perpetration of intimate partner and general violence among women arrested for domestic violence. *Journal of Interpersonal Violence, 26*(13), 2681–2697. Retrieved November 13, 2013.

Sturrock, A. (2012). Assessing the risk of aggression and violence among service users. *Mental Health Practice, 15*(5), 26–29. Retrieved November 24, 2013.

Wilson, D. R., Vical, B., Wilson, W. A., & Salyer, S. L. (2012). Overcoming sequelae of childhood sexual abuse with stress management. *Journal of Psychiatric & Mental Health Nursing, 19*(7), 587–593. Retrieved November 14, 2013.

Wright, M. F., & Li, Y. (2013). Normative beliefs about aggression and cyber aggression among young adults: A longitudinal investigation. *Aggressive Behavior, 39*(3), 161–170. Retrieved November 14, 2013.

Student Worksheet

Fill in the Blank

Fill in the blank with the correct answer.

1. _____ is often turned inward as self-directed guilt resulting in depression or willingness to be a perpetual victim.

2. Both anger and resentment originate in our _____ of a situation.

3. _____ is used repeatedly to intentionally bring harm or humiliation to another who is seen as weak or different.

4. _____ _____ can take the form of physical, emotional, economic, and/or sexual abuse.

5. Violence toward an individual starts with _____ or _____ threats and assaults that quickly victimize the person into going along with the abuse.

6. _____ is standing up for one's rights, beliefs, or values in such a way that it does not hurt others in the process.

Matching

Match the following terms to the most appropriate phrase.

1. _____ Crisis
2. _____ Hostility
3. _____ Stalking
4. _____ Suicidal erosion
5. _____ Trait anger
6. _____ Aggression
7. _____ Suicidal gesture

a. Action that indicates that self-harm may be imminent
b. Verbal or nonverbal behavior that can result in harm to oneself or another
c. General biological leaning toward a volatile personality
d. State of emotional disorganization and loss of control
e. Abuse that involves harassment or threatening behaviors
f. Intense feeling of animosity toward someone or something
g. Long-term accumulation of negative experiences throughout a person's lifetime

Multiple Choice

Select the best answer from the available choices.

1. A client is brought to the emergency room in a state of crisis following a motor vehicle accident in which her mother was killed. Which of the following statements by the nurse would be most appropriate to determine the client's perception of the situation?
   a. "What family members are available to be here with you?"
   b. "Can you tell me what brought you to the hospital today?"
   c. "How have you handled things like this in the past?"
   d. "It will take time to realize what has happened."

2. A call is received by the crisis hotline with the person stating, "I have a gun and I am going to shoot myself." Which level of lethality is demonstrated by this individual?
   a. Suicidal erosion
   b. Suicidal ideation
   c. Suicidal gesture
   d. Suicidal attempt

3. Matthew is 24 years of age and having severe symptoms of headaches, crying episodes, and anorexia. He states his girl-friend left him, he lost his job because of excess absences, and now his landlord has evicted him from his apartment. The nurse would recognize this client may be having symptoms of a/an:

   a. Situational crisis
   b. Maturational crisis
   c. Developmental crisis
   d. Identity crisis

4. Which statement would be correct in describing the perpetrator in a situation of domestic abuse? (Choose all that apply).

   a. History of degrading or putting down women
   b. Family history of alcohol abuse and violence
   c. Likes to watch action-packed movies on television
   d. Frequently involved in fights and vandalism
   e. Has had numerous intimate relationships

5. A 16-year-old girl tells her mother she is being bullied by other kids at school. She is distraught and doesn't want to go to school. Which statement by the girl would separate this situation from other reasons for not wanting to attend classes?

   a. "The girls were teasing me all day yesterday about my hair cut!"
   b. "I can't do what the gym teacher wants and they make fun of me."
   c. "They wait for me in the hall every day and make fun of me in front of everyone."
   d. "Someone posted a picture of me on Facebook—I look so fat in that picture!"

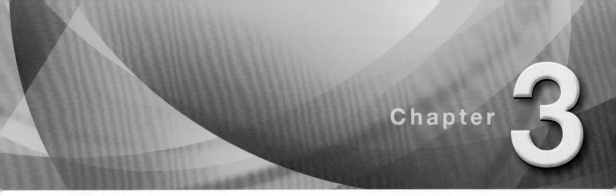

Chapter 3

Theories of Personality Development

⊙ Learning Objectives

After learning the content in this chapter, the student will be able to:

1. Define the concept of the personality.
2. Describe the factors that shape an individual's personality.
3. Define temperament.
4. Discuss the basic relationship between the behavior and the personality.
5. Identify the basic concepts of the common theories of personality development.
6. Explain the relationship between cognitive and moral developments.
7. Describe the nursing model of interpersonal development as described by Peplau.
8. Discuss the Family System theory and how it applies to mental health.

⊙ Key Terms

accommodation
anal stage
assimilation
behaviorism
central traits
concrete mental operations
conscious
conventional
countertransference
defense mechanism
ego
Electra conflict
equilibration
formal operations
genital stage
hierarchy
humanistic
id
interpersonal
latency stage

level of differentiation
Oedipal conflict
oral stage
personality
personality traits
phallic stage
postconventional
preconscious
preconventional
preoperational
pseudoself
psychosocial
secondary traits
sensorimotor
solid self
superego
temperament
transference
unconscious

Personality

Personality is defined as an enduring pattern of perceiving, relating to, and thinking about oneself and the environment that is demonstrated in our social and interpersonal interrelationships. Integrated into this personal portfolio are established characteristics and consistent behavioral responses or **personality traits** that are unique to each person. This explains why everyone does not act the same in similar situations. **Central traits** are those general prominent features that are most often descriptive of the person, some of which are seen in all the behavior patterns. **Secondary traits** are those that may surface in some circumstances, or situations. For example, one could be referred to as someone who has a quick temper or one who gets excited easily.

From the moment of conception, human development is influenced by forces that ultimately shape the way in which we respond to the world around us. A person's natural tendencies are the result of a combined genetic transmission of personality traits from both parents. A unique blend of multigenerational family patterns is inherited through this genetic factor. There are also many societal and environmental forces that influence personality. Patterns of behavior are formed as one responds to the awareness and perception of the self as autonomous and capable of individual control.

Although there are many theories about what shapes a person's personality, **humanistic** theories view the person as a whole, a totality of the physical, emotional, spiritual, intellectual, and social aspects of life that influence us toward reaching our potential. This holistic view of human beings not only applies to understanding personality and its development but also is the foundation of the nursing model of comprehensive care.

Individual Needs and Behavior

Abraham Maslow, a humanistic psychologist, theorized that one acts in response to a perceived internal or external force determined by certain needs that are unchanging and innate in origin. He defined these needs as a **hierarchy** in which some needs are more basic or more powerful than others. As the more basic needs are satisfied, we can move upward to meet other higher needs. Physiological needs form the first level, or those considered essential for basic functioning (Fig. 3.1).

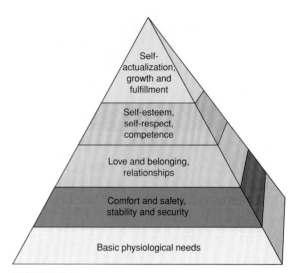

FIGURE 3.1

Abraham Maslow—hierarchy of needs.

These include oxygen, food, sleep, elimination, and sex. Comfort, safety, stability, and security are sought once the physiological needs are met. The need for a sense of being loved and belonging is achieved through relationships with others. Feeling loved and accepted promotes a feeling of self-respect and esteem that leads to confidence in oneself. Self-actualization, growth, and fulfillment emerge as one achieves this level of the hierarchy. It was Maslow's opinion that we cannot move to a higher level need unless the previous level of needs is satisfied. He believed that a personal identity is formed as we make conscious choices to seek certain things that provide value or meaning in our life. These experiences and choices may cause us to vacillate between levels and disrupt personal growth toward self-fulfillment.

William Glasser, the founder of Reality Therapy and Control Theory, described four basic psychological needs that determine our behavioral response in any given situation (Box 3.1).

He theorized that we will seek to satisfy their void in our lives on a continual basis. He identified these as the need for love and belonging, power

---

BOX 3.1

Glasser's Control Theory: Four Basic Psychological Needs

- Love and belonging
- Power and control
- Freedom and choice
- Fun and relaxation

and control, freedom and choice, and fun. The need to love and belong is internal, a hunger or void that may be filled by other people, pets, or even inanimate objects. Our drive for power often conflicts with our need for love as we seek to exert control over our world. Glasser asserts that we desire the freedom to exercise this control over our existence and that when this drive is hindered, we will respond or behave to regain the power that provides a psychological homeostasis. He also theorizes that a measure of fun and playtime evens out the personality. In an effort to meet these needs, Dr. Glasser advocates that we have a choice regarding how to behave. From the moment of birth, we accumulate mental pictures from our experiences with the environment. This photo album provides the basis for our choices to behave in response to a given situation. Our behavior is a constant attempt to decrease the incongruence between what we want (pictures in our head) and what we have (our perception of the situation). Glasser asserted that we tend to deny the reality of a situation instead of meeting our needs in a way that is responsible and within the boundaries of social norms and morality. He found that mental health is improved when we learn to meet our needs with responsible choices.

Just the Facts

Perseverance and determination are two personality traits that can help us to achieve success in life situations.

Temperament

We might ask why one person would respond to a situation with anger but diffuse it quickly, while another may show a milder emotional reaction and others no reaction at all. Variances in character, including how one thinks, behaves or reacts, and the intensity and extent of feelings are defined as the **temperament**. Temperament or disposition is the innate aspect of the developing personality and influences our interpersonal relationships. Studies describe three types of temperament in babies. *Easy* babies, who comprise the largest group, are seen as playful and adaptable. By contrast, a smaller number of babies are seen as *difficult* or irritable and unable to adapt well. A third group of *slow-to-warm-up* babies shows lower activity levels and slower adaptation to any new situation. As children develop, their

environment grows increasingly more complex it expands beyond the basic family unit to include the influence of society and culture of their world. The change and growth in personality have been the focus of much research from which theories have been developed to provide a basis for understanding of this process.

Mind Jogger

What adult behaviors might reflect a slow-to-warm-up or a difficult temperament?

Theories of Personality Development

Have you ever wondered why you think and behave in the way you do? This very issue leads to an integral concept in the study of psychology. Sigmund Freud was the first of many who studied and developed theories about the human mind and behavioral response to environmental forces. These theories are the foundation of therapeutic approaches to the treatment of mental illness.

Sigmund Freud (Psychoanalytic Theory)

Sigmund Freud is considered the founder of psychoanalytic theory. Although some of the theories he developed in the late 19th and early 20th centuries have been criticized by other theorists and health professionals, his work laid an important foundation for the development of other theories.

The Role of the Unconscious

Freud proposed that the psyche is made up of three components: the **conscious** or present awareness, the **preconscious** (also referred to as subconscious) or that which is below current awareness but easily retrieved, and the **unconscious**, which he cites as the largest body of material. The unconscious includes past experiences and the related emotions that have been completely removed from the conscious level. This level is largely responsible for contributing to the emotional discomfort and disturbances that threaten us, even though we are unaware of unconscious thoughts and feelings.

Freud also identified the concept of **transference** or the unconscious transfer of feelings and attitudes from a person or situation in one's past to a person or situation in the present. It may be a current expression of a previous experience or need (e.g., client may transfer romantic feelings to the therapist or nurse that was once felt for a previous person in his or her life). Freud indicated that clients tended to unconsciously transfer distressing thoughts and personal feelings to the therapist as the content was being analyzed. **Countertransference** is the response that is elicited in the person receiving the transferred feelings or communications. It is important for the recipient to be aware of the exchange in order to maintain insight into the client's problem.

Personality Components

Freudian theory also divides personality formation into three parts. The **id**, which operates on the pleasure principle and demands instant gratification of drives, is present at birth and contains the instincts, impulses, and urges for survival. These drives include hunger, aggression, sex, protection, and warmth. The **ego** begins to develop during the first 6 to 8 months and is fairly well developed by 2 years of age. The ego is the conscious self, which develops in response to the wishes and demands of the id that require appropriate exchanges with the environment. It is here that sensations, feelings, adjustments, solutions, and defenses are formed. The **superego**, often referred to as the conscience,

starts developing at about 3 to 4 years of age and is fairly well developed by the age of 10 to 11 years. It controls, inhibits, and regulates those impulses and instinctive urges whose unrestricted expression would be socially unacceptable. The values and moral standards of parents are incorporated into this control along with the norms and moral codes of the society in which one lives and grows. The superego operates at both the conscious and unconscious levels, decides right from wrong, and offers both critical self-evaluation and self-praise.

When environmental stressors create conflicts between the id and the superego, the ego is the peacemaker and balance between the instinctual drives and the societal demands influencing the superego (Fig. 3.2). For example:

Id—I want a piece of chocolate cake.
Superego—There are too many calories in that cake.
Ego—Be satisfied with a small piece.

Ego-Defense Mechanisms

The constant need for the ego to reconcile the conflicts between the id and superego leads to increased anxiety. This anxiety creates a dilemma in which stability is needed to preserve our sense of self. Freud theorized that for the ego to remain in control, automatic psychological processes called **defense mechanisms** are mobilized to protect us from anxiety and the awareness of

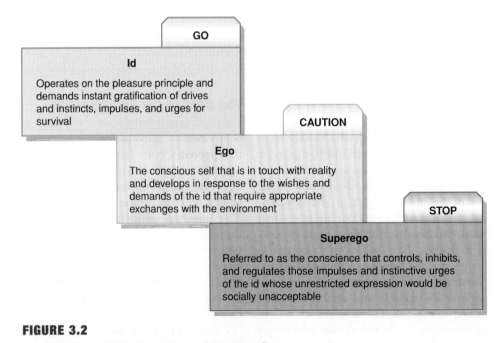

FIGURE 3.2
Freud's psychoanalytic theory: divisions of the personality.

TABLE 3.1   Ego Defense Mechanisms—Freud

MECHANISM	DESCRIPTION AND EXAMPLE
Sublimation	A socially acceptable behavior replaces one that is not acceptable or attainable. Primitive impulses are not acceptable to the ego and are rechanneled into a constructive outlet. (Aggressive desire to attack another person is rechanneled into a sport activity such as football.)
Intellectualization (isolation of feelings)	Person using reasoning and facts or logic to block unconscious conflict that creates stress and uncomfortable emotions. (Woman explains the signs of abuse to another woman while ignoring her own painful abusive situation.)
Suppression	Voluntary exclusion from conscious awareness anxiety-producing feelings, thoughts, or situations. (Nurse who argues with a family member during breakfast sets the incident aside while caring for patients at the hospital.)
Humor	Temporary reprieve of laughter to ease an anxiety-producing situation or stressor. (Individual who is told he is fired from his job laughs and says, "You are kidding of course.")
Denial	Conscious act of rejecting reality or refusal to recognize facts of a situation. Ego refuses to see the truth because it causes severe mental pain. (Wife whose husband dies continues to set the table for two as if he will be present for dinner.)
Displacement	Transfer of hostility or other strong feelings from the original cause of the feelings to another person or object. (Person who has a confrontation at his place of employment goes home and argues with his family.)
Fantasy	Conscious distortion of unconscious wishes or needs by using imagination to solve problems. (Young child who sees father physically abuse mother may imagine he is attacking a wild animal and saves his mother from harm.)
Repression	Involuntary distancing of events or thoughts that are too painful or unacceptable to one's ego into the unconscious level. These feelings can continue to influence behavior into adult years if unresolved. (Person who was sexually abused as a child is unable to achieve a meaningful intimate relationship as an adult.)
Regression	Personality returns to an earlier more comfortable and less stressful stage of behavior. (Child who is weaned returns to drinking from a bottle during hospitalization.)
Projection	Emotionally unacceptable traits, feelings, or attitudes are attributed or blamed on something or someone else. The person refuses to admit own weakness or accept responsibility for own actions. (Person who drinks alcohol blames his wife for doing something to make him get drunk.)
Compensation	Emphasizing capabilities or strengths to make up for a lack or loss in personal characteristics. (Person who is not talented in athletics excels in scholastic achievement.)
Introjection	Unconsciously integrating ideas, values, and attitudes of another into own mannerisms and actions. (Without awareness, a daughter begins to talk and act like her mother who is a pro-life advocate.)
Reaction formation	A conscious attempt to make up for feelings or attitudes that are unacceptable to the ego by replacing them with the opposite feelings or beliefs. (Mother who secretly dislikes her child becomes overprotective and outwardly affectionate toward the child.)
Conversion	Transfer of emotional conflicts into physical symptoms. (Person who dislikes her boss at work develops migraine headaches to avoid going to work.)
Undoing	A positive action is initiated to conceal a negative action or to neutralize a previously unacceptable action or wish. (Employer offers to take his secretary to lunch after verbally attacking her earlier in the day.)
Rationalization	Substituting false reasoning or justification for behavior that is unacceptable or threatening to the ego. This ignores the real reason for the behavior with falsehoods and avoids responsibility for the behavior. (Employee who is not given a promotion tells co-workers he really did not want the position.)

internal or external stressors (Table 3.1). Most of these mechanisms are mobilized at the unconscious level. High levels of anxiety can disturb perception and performance, which compromises the ability to problem solve and learn. These unconscious defense tools provide us with protection from unacceptable thoughts and impulses while continuing to meet personal and social needs in acceptable ways.

According to Freud, defenses are a major means of managing conflict and emotional response to environmental situations. These mechanisms differ from one another and may be adaptive as well as maladaptive. Used short-term, defense mechanisms can be mobilized in an adaptive way that allows us to work toward a realistic outcome or solution. Maladaptive defense mechanisms, on the other hand, may lead to distortion of reality and actual self-deception that can interfere with personal growth and interaction with society. For example, a person may continue to abuse alcohol using the mechanism of projection to blame his spouse and children for his behavior, while using denial to avoid self-blame and damage to his own ego. This maladaptive use of mechanisms interferes with an honest self-appraisal of reality and the detrimental effects of substance abuse. By contrast, a woman may temporarily deny her husband's extramarital affair by telling herself and others that he is just busy, yet project her feelings for her husband onto her children by punishing them for things they did not do. Unlike the person in the first example, when this woman realizes that she is projecting, she apologizes to her children and changes her behavior. The determinant for the effective and healthy use of defense mechanisms is based on the frequency, intensity, and length of time they are used.

Human beings sometimes behave in ways that provide a means of escape from the realities and responsibilities of life. These patterns of adjustment are common to everyone and are used to resolve conflicts and provide relief from the anxiety and stress of everyday existence. Most of the time, we are not aware that a defense mechanism is being used to adapt to a situation. However, when this escape becomes habitual, it becomes a dangerous inability to deal with reality and constitutes a psychiatric problem.

> ### Just the Facts
> Ego-defense mechanisms help us to justify our behavior in a seemingly logical way that allows us to retain self-respect. However, habitual use can cloud our view of reality.

Theory of Psychosexual Development

Freud believed that as the personality develops, there is an increasing self-identification and changing self-perception of sexuality and sexual identification. In his psychosexual theory, he proposed four major stages of development. The **oral stage** occurs during the first 2 years as the child seeks pleasure from sucking and oral gratification of hunger. The **anal stage** takes place from 2 to 4 years of age, during which pleasure is achieved as the child develops an awareness and control of urination and defecation. In the **phallic stage**, around the age of 4 years, the child discovers pleasure in genital stimulation and also struggles to accept a sexual identity. According to Freud, this gives rise to the **Oedipal conflict** (boys) and the **Electra conflict** (girls) in which the child begins to feel romantic feelings for the parent of the opposite sex but fears the wrath of the parent of the same sex. The child resolves the conflict by identifying with the parent of the same sex and redirects the feelings for the opposite sex parent into developing this gender role. Freud believed these feelings are put into the **latency stage** during middle childhood when the sexual desires remain subdued. The **genital stage** occurs as the child enters puberty and adolescence. It is at this stage that Freud believed sexual feelings reemerge and become directed toward establishing a relationship with a person of the opposite sex.

According to Freud, at any point during psychosexual development, the child can become fixated and frustrated, resulting in exaggerated adult character traits that reflect the arrested growth (Table 3.2). Although it has been the subject of much controversy regarding its sexual orientation, Freudian theory laid the groundwork for future developmental theories.

Erik Erikson (Psychosocial Developmental Theory)

Erikson viewed personality **psychosocial** (related to both psychological and social factors). His theory proposes that we develop in a pattern of eight psychosocial stages throughout our lifespan (Box 3.2). Each stage consists of a period of vulnerability when a person must face a developmental crisis. Resolution of this critical period will enhance a healthy continuation of the process. If unresolved, the progression to subsequent stages of development could be adversely affected. Erikson's view emphasizes, however, that failures at one stage can be corrected by successes at a later stage.

Stage I: Trust Versus Mistrust (Birth to 1 Year)

A sense of trust results in a feeling of comfort and reassurance that the world is a safe and pleasant

> **BOX 3.2**
>
> ### Erik Erikson: Eight Stages of Psychosocial Development
>
> - Trust versus mistrust
> - Autonomy versus shame and doubt
> - Initiative versus guilt
> - Industry versus inferiority
> - Identity versus role confusion
> - Intimacy versus isolation
> - Generativity versus stagnation
> - Integrity versus despair

TABLE 3.2   Adult Behaviors of Stage Theory Development

	SIGNS OF SUCCESSFUL RESOLUTION	INDICATORS OF DEVELOPMENTAL PROBLEM
Freud (Psychosexual)		
1. Oral stage	Satisfaction—gratification	Dependent on and easily influenced by others, manipulative cocky attitude, gullible
2. Anal stage	Giving, openness, self-control	Stinginess and orderliness Stubborn and rigid meticulousness
3. Phallic stage	Sexual identity accepted	Vanity and brashness, flirtatious
4. Latency	Sexual urges suppressed—expansion of social contacts beyond family	Unsuccessful attempts at expanding social relationships
5. Genital	Sexual energy channeled toward peers of opposite sex	Unconscious sexual conflict and inability to form intimate sexual relationship
Erikson (Psychosocial)		
1. Trust versus mistrust	Hope	Suspicion and fear of people and relationships Extreme self-doubt and fear of independence
2. Autonomy versus shame and doubt	Will	Sense of inadequacy and defeat
3. Initiative versus guilt	Purpose	Inadequate problem-solving skills
4. Industry versus inferiority	Competence	Manipulating others, no regard for the rights of others (such as in the workplace) Feeling unworthy, fear of failure
5. Identity versus role confusion	Fidelity	Uncertainty and loss of one who is in relationships with others
6. Intimacy versus isolation	Love and commitment	Emotional withdrawal into oneself
7. Generativity versus stagnation	Caring and giving	Inability to grow as an individual
8. Integrity versus despair	Wisdom	Disillusioned with life and inability to view death as reality
Piaget (Cognitive)		
1. Sensorimotor	Growth of abilities related to senses and motor skills Goal-directed behaviors Egocentric thinking	Focus only on what one wants without regard for possible consequences of those actions
2. Preoperational	Exploration motivated by magical and imaginative thinking	Decisions based on intuition, fantasy, or superstition with inability to make choices rooted in reality
3. Concrete	Base cognitive connections on actual events or objects Begin to think logically Think in terms of intentional moral response	Resistant to change with meager attempts at risk-taking strategies in which the outcome is unknown
4. Formal operations	Abstract thinking Problem-solving ability Symbolic reasoning with conceptual theoretical thinking	Unable to visualize possibility or solution to a problem Unwilling to formulate or accept reality-based decisions
Sullivan (Interpersonal)		
1. Infant	Satisfaction of needs	Anxiety develops as a result of unmet physiological needs Lack of bonding between infant and caregiver
2. Childhood	Self-control in gratification of needs	Increasing anxiety experienced with delay in gratification of own needs
3. Juvenile	Successful relationships with peer group	Difficulty in relating to others and developing interpersonal group relationships/workplace interaction
4. Preadolescent	Beginning appropriate interactions with persons of opposite sex	Inability to relate in a meaningful way to persons of the opposite sex
5. Early adolescent	Sense of personal identity in heterosexual relationships	Fear and withdrawal of relationships with persons of the opposite sex
6. Late adolescence	Satisfying intimate relationship with another	Inability to form a long-term intimate relationship with another person

place in which the child can live with minimum of fear and apprehension. The emphasis in this stage is on the oral-sensory gratification received during feeding through which the infant develops a trusting relationship with the parent or caregiver. Consistency and responsiveness by the parent in providing for the infant's needs of nourishment, comfort, and nurturing are essential to the development of trust. Babies who are not securely attached to their parent or caregiver are less responsive to him or her and show less effort in exploring the environment and world in which they exist.

Mind Jogger

How might failure to develop a sense of trust have implications in the establishment of adult relationships and one's interaction with society?

Stage II: Autonomy Versus Shame and Doubt (Ages 1 to 2 Years)

According to Erikson, children begin a period of increased self-confidence and independent striving to do more on their own. The most important event during this stage is toilet training. Children also try to do new things such as feeding or dressing themselves. It is essential that the parents positively reinforce these efforts while avoiding the urge to be overprotective and critical. Erikson believed that if parents do not show a consistent and reassuring attitude during this phase, children would experience too much self-doubt and shame about their abilities, resulting in a lack of confidence that would persist throughout life.

Stage III: Initiative Versus Guilt (2 to 6 Years)

During these years, children are challenged with an increasing responsibility to take care of their physical needs, their behavior, toys, pets, and so forth. This requires children to be assertive and creative in assuming the new tasks. The child is eager to do things, and it is essential that parents praise and recognize the child's efforts no matter how small they may be. On the other hand, children must also learn to accept that in their quest for independence, there are some things that are not allowed or safe for them to do. It is important they be reassured, however, that being imaginative

and pretending to take on adult roles are okay. If they are not given the chance to do things safely on their own and to be responsible, a sense of guilt may result. The child will learn to believe that what they want to do is not good enough or is always wrong.

Stage IV: Industry Versus Inferiority (6 to 12 Years)

In this stage of development, children are learning to be productive and to accomplish things on their own, both physically and mentally. This is a period when they master their ability to succeed in peer relationships, school, and activities. It is essential for children to receive encouragement and support in their drive for success from parents and others. Children learn by repeated efforts driven by self-confidence in their own ability. If children have difficulty relating to others outside of the home or in achievement of skills, a sense of inferiority and self-doubt may result.

Stage V: Identity Versus Role Confusion (12 to 18 Years)

During the years of adolescence there is a search for identity and answers to questions concerning a purpose in life. Erikson postulated that a basic sense of trust and self-confidence in oneself was necessary to provide the foundation for the adolescent to make conscious choices about a vocation, relationships, and life in general. Failure to resolve previous conflicts successfully would result in an inability to make these decisions and choices. As a result, adolescents might experience role confusion as to who they are and where they belong as they move into adulthood.

Stage VI: Intimacy Versus Isolation (Ages 19 to 40 Years)

In the years of young adulthood, the most important developmental goal is to form a committed relationship with another. A true intimate relationship requires sincerity and open sharing of feelings. Having a sexual relationship does not imply intimacy. A person can be sexually intimate without feeling for and commitment to the other person. Love relationships are strengthened by the ability of partners to relate on a deep personal level. The young adult who is unable to be open and committed to another may retreat into isolation and fear a giving and sharing relationship.

Stage VII: Generativity Versus Stagnation (Ages 40 to 65 Years)

As we enter middle adulthood, the task is related to parenting and supportive involvement in providing for the next generation. This role includes being an active participant in issues that will make this world a safer and better place for the future. The inability to nurture and to give whatever is ours to give in an attempt to ensure this progressive stability for our children may lead to stagnation and decreased meaning for one's life.

Stage VIII: Integrity Versus Despair (Over 65 Years)

The important event during these years is seen as a reflection on and acceptance of our life. According to Erikson, a positive outcome is demonstrated by a sense of fulfillment about a life lived and acceptance of death as an inevitable reality. This involves accepting responsibility for and being satisfied with choices that have been made over a lifetime. The older adult who has successfully reached this stage is able to put the past in perspective and achieve a sense of self-satisfaction with the present. Those who are unable to reach this sense of fulfillment and wholeness will despair about life accomplishments and fear death.

Erikson maintained that if each developmental crisis was not resolved in sequence, the personality would continue to manifest this conflict into the adult years (Table 3.2). Although critics of the stage theory say that psychological development may be influenced and altered by experiences throughout life, many have found Erikson's theory useful for continued study of personality development.

Just the Facts

The aim of progress in emotional development is not to get rid of the negative personality quality but to move toward the health quality as a dominant trait.

"Burdened and Alone"

Anthony is a 32-year-old male client who is being seen in an outpatient clinic for symptoms of depression and anorexia. He states he has had no success in finding a job and his girlfriend "ditched" him several months ago. Anthony states he has been living out of his car and on the street since his girlfriend left him. When asked about his family, he states, "I basically don't have one." His next comment of, "I can't seem to get along with anyone—they all act like they are out to get me one way or another," leaves you wondering where his feelings of self-guilt originated.

Based on Erikson's theory of psychosocial development, at what point might Anthony's personality development have been disrupted?

_____

_____

How is this preventing him from advancing according to Erikson's theory?

_____

_____

What other questions might you ask?

_____

_____

According to the hierarchy of needs, what would be a priority for this client?

_____

_____

Case Application 3.1

Jean Piaget (Cognitive Development Related to Personality)

Piaget theorized that personality is the result of increasing intellectual ability to organize and integrate experiences into behavior patterns. His observations led him to conclude that this organization tended to occur at certain age groups. Movement forward relies on four interdependent factors. Physical and psychological growth or maturation occurs in the child during a specific stage as the child thinks and experiences interaction with the environment. As the child begins to distinguish the self as a separate being, social experiences become a part of this learning. According to Piaget, **equilibration** occurs as the child brings all these factors together to build mental schema or connections that lead to a cognitive balance. Children are motivated to seek this balance by a perceived imbalance between what they already know (existing schema) and something new. Piaget refers to the ability to incorporate new ideas and experiences as **assimilation**, while **accommodation** is the ability to alter existing schema to incorporate the new information.

Piaget proposed that cognitive development occurs in four stages (Box 3.3).

In the first 2 years of life, the **sensorimotor** stage involves the growth of abilities related to the five senses and motor functions. Early responses are primarily reflexive in nature, with a gradual increase in skill as children adapt to their environment. These responses tend to reflect only a perception of that which is visible to the child. The perception that what is gone from view still exists (object permanence) begins to develop at about 9 months of age and is well developed by 1 year.

The **preoperational stage** of development occurs from 2 to 7 years. The mental schema developed during the earlier stage emerges into communication of thoughts that is largely egocentric without regard for another point of view. Language and actions reflect a focus on thinking that the world exists solely to meet the demands of the child's ego. As children grow, they explore and try out many new activities motivated by increasing magical and imaginative thinking.

Just the Facts

Most children in the preoperational stage are impulsive and cannot distinguish between actions and feelings. Unable to understand that others may see their actions differently than they do, they react to conflict with egocentric hitting, shoving, whining, and hiding behaviors.

From 7 to 12 years of age, Piaget saw children as able to perform **concrete mental operations** on their accumulated thoughts and memories. The phrase "seeing is believing" is descriptive of the child's need to base these cognitive connections on actual events or objects. Facts and routines with one way of doing things are a characteristic of this age group. The child begins to think logically, classify objects, and recognize that objects and people can have more than one label (e.g., daddy can also be a husband, a brother, and an uncle all at the same time). Although they are capable of thinking more logically, children of this age still depend on concrete cues to develop these thoughts.

According to Piaget, the person moves into the stage of **formal operations** during the years of 11 to 12 and older. This period of growth involves abstract thought processes, problem solving, and systematic purposeful mental relationships. Adolescents are capable of symbolic thinking and comprehension of theoretical concepts. They are able to visualize beyond what is known and formulate hypothetical reasoning.

Piaget maintains that once the child has entered a new stage, the process is irreversible, with each stage building on the previous level of development.

Lawrence Kohlberg (Theory of Moral Development)

In his research on cognitive development, Piaget concluded that changes in the child's level of thinking also affect the moral decisions the child makes. Motivated by Piaget's studies, Kohlberg developed his own theory based on six stages of moral reasoning included in three levels.

BOX 3.3

Jean Piaget: Theory of Cognitive Development

- Sensorimotor: Birth to 2 years
- Preoperational: 2 to 7 years
- Concrete: 7 to 11 years
- Formal operations: 11 years and older

BOX 3.4

Lawrence Kohlberg: Moral Development Theory

Preconventional Level: Values indicate environmental pressure
  Stage 1: Acts or behaves to avoid punishment
  Stage 2: Is motivated by personal reward (what is in it for me?)
Conventional Level: Influenced by societal pressure
  Stage 3: Values and acts to meet the expectations of others (peer group)
  Stage 4: Is motivated by the laws of society/legal system
Postconventional Level: Influenced by standards and shared principles
  Stage 5: Acts for the good of society or the most people (e.g., U.S. Constitution)
  Stage 6: Bases actions on moral principles and ethical values (the right thing to do)

Box 3.4 outlines these levels and stages. Basic to Kohlberg's theory is his belief that the choices one makes do not determine the stage of moral logic, but rather the reasons one gives to justify the behavior establish the level of ethical development. Like Piaget, Kohlberg believed that the intellect and the child's emotional development occur in a parallel pattern of stages during which the child changes his or her concept of self in relation to interaction with others. The level of cognitive development determines how the child perceives a situation and what is learned from that experience. Each of the three levels builds on the one prior with increasing complexity in the individual view of a moral issue.

Harry S. Sullivan (Theory of Interpersonal Development)

Nurses in the mental health setting develop therapeutic relationships with clients in an attempt to help them develop the skills to interact successfully with others. Sullivan believed that behavior and personality developments are the direct result of these **interpersonal** relationships. Unlike Freud, who believed that all behavior is the result of unconscious drives and unfinished agendas, Sullivan believed that human behavior could be seen in the social interaction between people. The major concepts of his theory include the following:

- Anxiety is a major force that develops as a result of unmet needs and interpersonal dissatisfaction.

- Fulfillment of needs occurs when all physiological, comfort, and security needs are met.
- The *concept of self* incorporates those experiences and behaviors developed to protect the child against anxiety and provide security for the self. As a result, three images of self develop:
  - *Good-me* develops in response to a positive feedback
  - *Bad-me* develops in response to criticism from caregivers
  - *Not-me* develops in response to intense anxiety and dread with resulting denial and repression of the situation to avoid the anxiety (this avoidance of emotions can result in mental disorders in the adult)

Sullivan divided development into six stages. During *infancy* (birth to 18 months), the child is concerned with oral satisfaction of needs. In *childhood* (18 months to 6 years), children learn to delay personal gratification with a minimum of anxiety. The *juvenile* (6 to 9 years) is learning to develop satisfaction in relationships with the peer group, while the *preadolescent* (9 to 12 years) is striving to develop successful interactions with persons of the same sex. During *early adolescence* (12 to 14 years) a sense of personal identity is formed as relationships with persons of the opposite sex are sought. In *late adolescence* (14 to 21 years) the person is working to develop satisfying and meaningful long-term relationships with others.

Sullivan believed that the attainment of successful interpersonal relationships was dependent on the formation of interaction skills at each level of development (Table 3.2).

Hildegard Peplau (Psychodynamic Nursing)

Peplau applied the interpersonal theory to nursing and the nurse–client relationship. She saw the stages of developmental growth as the basis for therapeutic interaction with clients, including many whose behaviors reflect a failure to understand their own feelings and actions, and the results of those actions.

Peplau's theory identified four stages of development. In *infancy*, the child is learning to count on others, while the *toddler* is learning to delay self-gratification. At the same time, the toddler derives much pleasure in a positive response from others to his or her actions. *Early childhood* is a time of developing the skill of behaving in a way that

Case Application 3.2

"Defeated"

You are interacting with Denise, a young female client who repeatedly apologizes for saying "the wrong thing." In response to your question about her family, she answers, "I really don't have a family. I'm sorry, that was a bad thing to say." She goes on to say that she has never done anything good enough for her parents. She feels that regardless of how hard she tries, she is always telling them she is sorry for disappointing them. Denise states that she is so afraid of failure that she is unable to follow through with a job application and cancels them before the scheduled appointment.

What other information about Denise's interpersonal relationships might be important?

_____

_____

How are past relationships with her parents affecting her present interpersonal relationships?

_____

_____

How is Sullivan's theory of interpersonal development reflected in this situation?

_____

_____

How would you follow up to continue the conversation?

_____

_____

---

is acceptable to others, preceding *late childhood* in which the child learns to compromise, compete, and cooperate in participation and interactions with others. Learning to practice self-control and compromise in our relationships with others is a precedent to living successfully and interacting as a member of society.

Mind Jogger

What do the stage theories have in common? How do they differ? What are the implications of interpersonal relationship development in the nurse's interactions with clients?

Murray Bowen (Family Systems Theory)

The Family Systems theory asserts that a person is able to change behaviors based on an awareness of the impact that present and past family patterns of behavior have on the choices one makes. This awareness can lead to an intentional desire to make changes and a refusal to function in the

way that has been perpetuated by members of the family.

Family is defined as the nuclear family of origin and extending to past relationships and family histories. Bowen saw this family as a single emotional unit composed of relationships that intermingle over several generations. He felt the dynamics of these family relationships held the key for understanding current behaviors. Integral in Bowen's theory is the biological, genetic, psychological, and sociological factors in the determination of behavior. Actions are seen as preceded by feelings that to some degree can be controlled by the ability to think. People are able to predict their own patterns of response based on an awareness of the dynamics that are evident in the family system.

Bowen identifies two major variables that affect our behavior in terms of relationships (Box 3.5). Anxiety is an individual reaction to stress that is seen as directly correlated to the person's **level of differentiation**, or the degree to which we define the self in terms of values and beliefs. The person whose behavior is based on internal

BOX 3.5

Murray Bowen: Family Systems Theory

- Level of differentiation: Degree to which one defines the self
- Solid self: Behavior based on internal convictions, values, and self-imposed beliefs
- Pseudoself: Behavior reflects external locus of control

convictions and principles is defined as a **solid self**, as opposed to the **pseudoself** whose behavior reflects an external locus of control. Individuals described as a solid self are more adaptable, more flexible, and more effective in coping with stressful situations, while those defined as a pseudoself are less adaptable, less flexible, and less able to rely on internal sources of strength to cope with anxiety.

People tend to seek partners of similar differentiation levels, breeding relationships that are either open or closed systems. An open family system is made up of persons who are predominantly a solid self. This promotes flexibility and exchange of ideas within an accepting environment. They are comfortable with being visible and are free to clearly define themselves and their belief system. By contrast, individuals who are willing to compromise their values when pressured by external sources make up the closed family system. The result of these relationships is one of dysfunction, fusion, and rigid standards in which one person gains control and the other loses self. An increase in fusion increases the anxiety within the system. As anxiety escalates, the emotional ties of family members become frayed and one or more persons feel overwhelmed. The family members who feel out of control tend to be the ones who give in to reduce tension in others. This absorption of the family anxiety issue leaves the individual most vulnerable to psychological problems and dysfunction. Some people deal with the anxiety through emotional distancing and cutting ties with parental conflict, which eventually results in continuation of the conflict. Those who attempt to reduce tension in their current family relationships by distancing from the nuclear family issues will eventually see the patterns they are trying to escape emerging in their present relationships. Triangles are created that draw a third party into the conflict, further dismantling the homeostasis of the family unit. The interactive patterns in a tri-

angle tend to shift with two members being close and "inside" and one being excluded and "outside." Involving others tends to make the situation more complicated and resolves nothing. Those within the triangle tend to become emotionally involved and take sides in the conflict.

The differentiation of people within the family system is projected onto other members of that family, creating a spiral effect as children marry and create another generation with similar characteristics and value systems. Marital conflict may result as a second generation of dysfunction is shaped. A union that pairs one spouse who repeatedly yields to a controlling or abusive partner in order to prevent family discord will result in the dysfunction of that individual. In addition, one or more children of the family will absorb the tensions and anxiety that perpetuate the dysfunction and demonstrates the continuation of the cycle.

Just the Facts
Within a family, a change in one person's functioning is typically followed by give-and-take changes in the behavior of others.

Mind Jogger
In what way do children become involved in a triangle formed by marital conflict between parents?

This theory provides a way for us to understand how families function and how people are affected by the dynamics in this multigenerational process. Once clients are aware of how they are influenced by dysfunctional patterns of behavior, they can be supported in an effort to effect change and break the cycle.

Other Theories

In addition to the theories discussed in this chapter, other approaches are very integral to the overall understanding of human development and behavior. Behaviorist theory, social learning theory, and cognitive-behavioral theory are among those that are embedded in the view that our actions are deeply rooted in our development. These theories are central to the current treatment approach to mental health treatment and are described in Table 3.3.

TABLE 3.3   Other Theoretical Approaches to Personality and Behavior

THEORY	THEORETICAL CONCEPTS
Behavioristic Theory **B. F. Skinner**	• **Behaviorism** is based on the concept that thinking, feeling, and interpersonal relationships are irrelevant and that all behavior is observable or learned behavior in response to a stimulus from the environment. • Behavior is the result of conditioning shaped by a system of reward, punishment, and reinforcement. • Human personality is formed in response to these stimulus-response situations. The personality includes both adaptive and maladaptive behavior as a result of reinforcement. • People show consistent patterns of behavior that will continue if action is rewarded by a response. If no reinforcement is given, the behavior will decline. • Conditioning strengthens and weakens behaviors automatically without regard to the conscious thought processes.
Social Learning Theory **Albert Bandura**	• Personality is largely shaped through learning by actively seeking out and processing information about the environment in response to a need for a positive outcome. • People can act to change their surroundings as a result of both internal and external forces that influence each other. • Social learning is based on observation and imitation of others. Both children and adults tend to imitate people they like or respect more than those whose persona is less appealing. • Models whose behavior leads to an approved outcome are also more likely to be copied. • Self-confidence develops as the belief that performance of behaviors should lead to the expected outcome becomes reality in the actions of that person.
Cognitive-Behavioral Theory **Aaron Beck**	• Focus is on the person's abilities to think, analyze, and decide on certain behavior rather than acting on feelings. • Actions are the result of distorted perceptions and thoughts that can be changed. This is unlike Freud who saw mental disturbances as being the result of childhood experiences. • Self-defeating behaviors are maintained because of irrational thoughts and erroneous beliefs. • Self-concept and evaluation of social image is affected by how people think others see them. Self-talk is used to praise or criticize and interpret situations. This is reflected in both normal behaviors and mental disorders as well. • Negative self-talk can be changed into more positive thoughts, leading to a more positive self-image and more productive outcomes.

Summary

• Personality is a combination of characteristic patterns of our perceptions, our relation to, and our thoughts about ourselves and the world in which we exist. Patterns are the result of genetics and the influence of social and environmental forces throughout the lifespan.

• The humanistic view sees the developing person as a whole inclusive of physical, emotional, spiritual, intellectual, and social components.

• Maslow theorized actions are in response to a perceived internal or external force determined by a hierarchy of needs that are innate and unchanging, ranging from basic survival requirements to a desire for self-fulfillment.

• Glasser identified the basic needs of power, freedom, love and belonging, and fun as the driving forces that drive us to interact with the environment in a constant attempt to decrease the incongruence between what we want (needs) and what we have (perception of a situation).

• Temperament defines those variances in character that influence the development of personality and our interpersonal relationships. These are identified as the easy or adaptable character, the slow-to-warm-up disposition, whose adaptation to new situations is at a slower pace, and the difficult or irritable and unadaptable disposition.

• Personality development is most often described by stage theories that divide the lifespan into age-related periods that correlate with physical growth and development.

• Freud proposed the psyche is made up of three parts: the conscious (current awareness), the preconscious (just below the awareness and easily retrievable), and the unconscious (buried and removed from conscious awareness and responsible for much of our emotional discomfort).

• Freudian theory divides the personality into three parts: The id, present at birth, operates on the pleasure principle, demanding instant gratification of drives, impulses, and urges for survival. The ego is the conscious self that develops in response to the wishes and demands of the id that require boundaries for appropriate exchange with the environment. The superego, or the conscience, develops between the ages of 3 and 11 years to control, inhibit, and regulate the impulses and urges of the id, which, if unleashed, may be socially unacceptable.

- For the ego to remain in control, automatic psychological processes called defense mechanisms are mobilized to protect from anxiety and awareness of internal or external stressors.
- Freud proposed five stages of psychosexual development.

- Erikson proposed a series of eight psychosocial stages of development. Each stage consists of a developmental crisis, indicating a period of vulnerability. Erikson proposed that if each development crisis is not resolved in sequence, the personality would continue to show this conflict into the adult years.
- Piaget theorized that personality development is the result of increasing intellectual ability to organize and integrate experiences into behavior patterns. Cognitive growth occurs as the child thinks and experiences interaction with the environment.
  - Piaget's cognitive theory proposes that mental connections or schema are formed by incorporating new ideas and experiences into existing mental information. Equilibration is the cognitive balance that results as learning takes place.
  - Piaget proposed four stages of cognitive development that align with chronological age periods; sensorimotor, preoperational, concrete mental operations, and formal operations.
- Kohlberg focused his theory on the moral development, dividing growth into three levels that center on the reasons one gives to justify choices and behaviors.

- In the preoperational level, values indicate environmental pressures to avoid punishment and receive personal reward. The conventional level demonstrates influence by societal pressures to meet the expectations of others or the legal system. The postconventional level reflects influence by ethical values and shared moral principles that show actions for the good of society or most people.
- Sullivan postulated that behavior and personality develop as a direct result of interpersonal relationships. Anxiety is the major force that results from unmet needs and dissatisfaction.
  - Sullivan's concept of self incorporates experiences and behaviors developed to protect against the anxiety and provide security. Positive response builds the "good-me," while negative criticism creates a sense of "bad-me" that over time can lead to repression and avoidance of emotions.
- Peplau applied the interpersonal theory to nursing and the nurse–client relationship with a focus on client behaviors that reflect a failure to understand their own feelings, actions, and the results of those actions.
- In Family Systems theory, Bowen asserts that a person is able to change behaviors based on an awareness of the impact that present and past family patterns of behavior have on the choices one makes. Level of differentiation refers to the degree to which we define the self in terms of values and beliefs. Behavior based on internal convictions and principles defines the solid self, while a pseudoself reflects an external locus of control.
- Behaviorist, social learning, and cognitive-behavioral theories contribute significantly to the overall current views underlying the current approach to treatment of mental health and illness.

Bibliography

American Psychiatric Association. (2013). *Diagnostic and statistical manual of mental disorders* (5th ed.). Washington, DC: Author.

Sternberg, R. J. (1995). *In search of the human mind.* Fort Worth, TX: Harcourt Brace & Co.

Varcolaris, E. M., & Halter, M. J. (2010). *Foundations of psychiatric mental health nursing* (6th ed.). St. Louis, MO: Saunders Elsevier Inc.

Weiten, W. (2011). *Psychology themes and variations* (9th ed.). Florence, KY: Wadsworth Publish.

Student Worksheet

Fill in the Blank

Fill in the blank with the correct answer.

1. Patterns of perceiving, relating to, and thinking about ourselves and the world around us define the concept of _____.

2. _____ describes the variances in character that influence the development of personality and interpersonal relationships.

3. The process by which we bring factors together to build mental schema or connections that lead to a cognitive balance is called _____.

4. According to Piaget, _____ is the ability to incorporate new ideas and experiences into our existing mental schema.

5. Once new experiences are encountered, the ability to alter the existing schema to incorporate the new information is referred to as _____.

6. The person whose behavior is based on internal convictions and principles is defined as a _____.

Matching

Match the defense mechanism with the appropriate behavior.

1. _____ Rationalization
2. _____ Denial
3. _____ Repression
4. _____ Regression
5. _____ Projection
6. _____ Displacement
7. _____ Reaction formation
8. _____ Sublimation

a. Unhappy with her boss for his criticism, Clara turns around and takes her anger out on her husband.

b. David is unable to remember a boating accident in which his friend was killed.

c. After going to the movie the night before an exam, Molly states that she failed the exam because she did not study the right chapter.

d. An adolescent wants his mother to stay with him during a hospital stay.

e. Confined to a wheelchair, Jack becomes a computer specialist.

f. A young man who secretly desires to harm his wife appears on a television show against spousal abuse.

g. When Martha is confronted about her alcohol problem, she states she can quit anytime she chooses.

h. After taking funds out of their savings account to buy golf clubs, Hank tells his wife that the bank must have made a mistake.

Multiple Choice

Select the best answer from the multiple-choice items.

1. A 70-year-old client states to the nurse, "My life is a pile of shambles with nothing to show for it." The client is demonstrating what Erikson would term:
   a. Doubt
   b. Inferiority
   c. Despair
   d. Stagnation

2. A 4-year-old boy tells the nurse, "When I grow up I am going to marry Mommy." Which stage of psychosexual development is portrayed by this statement?
   a. Phallic
   b. Anal
   c. Latency
   d. Genital

3. According to Piaget, children who seek to control their world from a centrated point of view would be in which stage of cognitive development?

a. Sensorimotor

b. Preoperational

c. Concrete

d. Formal operations

4. A person refrains from telling the truth to a friend whose partner is having an affair with a coworker to avoid hurting his friend. According to Kohlberg, this demonstrates which level of moral development?

a. Preconventional—stage 2

b. Conventional—stage 3

c. Postconventional—stage 5

d. Conventional—stage 4

5. Al has been arrested for physical assault of another individual. He has a history of an abusive childhood and previous aggressive offenses. Behavioral theory would explain this behavior as:

a. Feelings of repressed hostility

b. A diminished sense of self-esteem

c. An innate impulsive drive for survival

d. Reinforcement of early learning experiences

6. Surveys show that cigarette smoking and alcohol consumption are common among the adolescent population. These results reflect peer behavior and provide support for which of the following theories?

a. Social learning theory

b. Conditioning theory

c. Psychosexual theory

d. Behavioristic theory

7. A client tells the nurse that he realizes that most of the things that happen to him are the result of his choices. He indicates a desire to make changes that will lead to better outcomes. According to Bowen, this client tends to have:

a. A strong superego

b. An internal locus of control

c. A strong pseudoself

d. Strong unconscious drives

8. A young adolescent client is seen in the emergency room after she was raped by her brother. Calm and laughing she says, "I don't know why the big deal. Nothing happened." The nurse would assess this as probable use of which defense mechanism?

a. Projection

b. Conversion

c. Denial

d. Rationalization

9. A client is being seen who is unable to maintain employment. He states there is always an ulterior motive in company policies that affect him. Which of the following psychosocial stages is likely unresolved?

a. Trust versus mistrust

b. Autonomy versus doubt

c. Initiative versus guilt

d. Industry versus inferiority

10. A juvenile has been apprehended by law enforcement officials following a raid of a party involving underage drinking of alcohol. When questioned by his father, the juvenile states, "Everyone else was doing it too." According to Kohlberg, this response reflects which level of moral development?

a. Preconventional—stage 2

b. Conventional—stage 3

c. Postconventional—stage 5

d. Preconventional—stage 1

Chapter 4

The Delivery of Mental Health Care

⦿ Learning Objectives

After learning the content in this chapter, the student will be able to:

1. Identify individuals who have contributed to the advancement of mental health.
2. Describe legislative actions that have impacted care of those with mental illness.
3. Identify cultural and socioeconomic barriers to accessing mental health care.
4. Identify how client rights are preserved in mental health settings.
5. Differentiate between types of admission to psychiatric treatment.
6. Discuss ethics and legal issues involved with client confidentiality.
7. Identify areas of nursing accountability in the mental health setting.
8. Define criteria for the use of seclusion and restraints.
9. Describe practice settings for mental health care.
10. Apply concepts of mental health care to clients in nonpsychiatric settings.
11. Describe the role of the nurse in the deliverance of mental health care within a correctional facility.

⦿ Key Terms

Affordable Care Act
Americans with Disabilities Act (ADA)
chemical restraint
Client Bill of Rights
confidentiality
ethics
holistic
informed consent
involuntary commitment
manipulation

Mental Health Act of 1983
Mental Health Parity and Addiction Equity Act of 2008
Omnibus Budget Reform Act (OBRA)
physical restraint
powerlessness
seclusion
voluntary commitment

Historical Advancement of Mental Health Care

Mental health nursing can be viewed in the context of the nursing process as the assigning of nursing diagnoses and planned intervention in response to actual or potential mental health problems. It has evolved as a specialized area of nursing practice, applying scientific theories of human behavior and focused nursing skill. Mental health care providers have met with numerous challenges in their effort to provide a vision of wellness for those with mental illness and to increase public awareness of its existence. Historically, the journey to provide this humane and therapeutic approach to those with mental alterations has been a difficult one.

Early Civilizations

Before the advent of psychotherapeutic drugs now used extensively in the treatment of mental issues, the available options for control of symptoms were few. Those with bizarre behavior were considered outcasts of society and harbored in asylums for the remainder of their lives. Many of the more violent patients were referred to as "lunatics" often becoming a spectacle for public viewing. The first institution for the mentally ill was opened in London as the Bethlehem Royal Hospital in 1247. "The insane" as they were called, received cruel and inhumane treatment and were often required to wear metal arm and leg irons as they begged for food in the streets.

During the Renaissance in the early 1400s, there was a growing interest in what led to various abnormal behaviors. Early classifications of depression, neurosis, mania, and psychosis were developed by scholars and physicians according to what they saw in those displaying the behaviors. Despite the increased interest in what caused these illnesses, the care given to those with the disorders did not improve.

It was perhaps during the 17th century that conditions reached their lowest and most horrific point. Those with symptoms considered to be insanity were locked in cells, starved, brutally beaten, and helpless. In the late 1700s, psychiatry emerged as a separate division of medical science. Those connected with the specialty began to question the way those with mental problems were treated. Along with those in Europe, the US colonies began to open asylums to house individuals

with mental illness along with prisoners and orphans. It was considered a place for the rejected of society. Care was provided by the poor and included such practices as bloodletting, purging, and confinement chairs. Although the study of psychiatry continued, the actual treatment of those with behavior problems remained unjust and cruel.

The Beginning of Change

An early 19th century physician by the name of Benjamin Rush (1745 to 1813) became the first American to advocate change in the conditions for individuals with mental illness. A professor of chemistry and medicine, he theorized that there was a connection between blood circulation and diseases of the mind. He advocated that conditions for those with these diseases should include cleanliness, good air, lighting, and food. In addition, he felt that kindness and improved interaction between the patient and care provider would have curative effects.

Just the Facts

In 1812, Rush, referred to as the "Father of American Psychiatry," wrote the first American textbook of psychiatry.

About the middle of the 19th century, we began to see a change in perspective toward the care provided to those with mental illness. Dorothea Dix, a 19th century schoolteacher, began to question the treatment of both prisoners and individuals with mental illness. She began a tireless effort to expose these conditions and provoke legislation to help in the construction of mental hospitals with standards for care.

Just the Facts

Psychiatric-mental health nursing had its beginning in the late 19th century.

During the late 19th and early 20th centuries, training programs for nurses were created and provided an option for those interested in caring for the sick. There was also an increasing social awareness of the problems that related to mental illness. Although the need for trained nurses was recognized, caring for "the insane" was not seen as a fit occupation for women. Linda Richards (1841 to 1930) became a pioneer as the first trained nurse in America. Several years later, she traveled to England to receive more training at St. Thomas' Hospital in London, the hospital established by Florence Nightingale in 1860. Here she met and trained under Florence Nightingale. Nightingale encouraged Richards to continue her studies in Europe after which she returned to the United States and began to establish training curricula for schools of nursing. In 1882, Richards opened the Boston City Hospital Training School for Nurses to specialize in training nurses to care for those considered mentally ill. Although this was a beginning, it was not until 1913 that the first psychiatric content was included within the curriculum of a nursing school. Gradually, as the addition was phased into all schools of nursing, the specialized training hospitals were closed.

Just the Facts

Harriet Bailey wrote *Nursing Mental Diseases,* the first psychiatric nursing textbook, in 1920.

Mind Jogger

How does this early picture of nursing curricula reflect the holistic-centered approach to nursing today?

Twentieth Century Progress

Slowly, a component of psychiatric nursing was included in all nursing curricula. The well-known National Mental Health Act of 1946 was the first legislation to provide funds for research, advanced nursing degree programs, and improved community service for individuals with mental illness. In 1955, the Joint Commission on Mental Illness and Health was established to conduct a study on the guidelines used by mental institutions to provide care for their clients. Funding became available for research and improved treatment programs. Funds were appropriated by Congress for the National Institute of Mental Health (NIMH), established in 1949, for its support and continued research in the field of mental illness.

These political and social changes were beginning to influence the present and future roles of psychiatric nurses. Although most clients with mental illness were still institutionalized in state mental hospitals, there was a growing trend toward the provision of community-based treatment

at inpatient hospital units that specialized in the care of mental illness. This meant a growing need for trained nurses to fill both new and expanded roles. By the 1950s, many steps were taken toward improved conditions and treatment methods. In 1953, the National League for Nursing endorsed the inclusion of psychiatric nursing in all nursing programs.

It was during this period that the first psychotherapeutic drugs were introduced. These drugs provided relief of symptoms and put an end to the need for physical restraint in straightjackets and for lobotomies to remove portions of the brain to control behaviors. Sedatives were developed that quieted clients, and lithium carbonate was found to be effective in controlling mood swings. In 1956, the first antipsychotic drugs were introduced to control the bizarre behaviors seen in some disorders. Shortly thereafter, antidepressants and antianxiety drugs were developed.

Just the Facts

Thorazine was the first antipsychotic drug to be used in the treatment of these disorders.

As this new era of treatment emerged, the movement to deinstitutionalize clients with mental illness was in motion. Between 1950 and 1980, the number of institutionalized clients dropped from more than 500,000 to less than 100,000.

Community-Based Care

As the need for community-based mental health care gained recognition, federal legislation emerged to create funding for the establishment of centers that would offer these services. The Mental Retardation Facilities and Community Mental Health Centers Act of 1963 and the Community Health Centers Amendment of 1975 made it possible for clients to receive a variety of treatments designed to shorten hospital stays. Clients were returned to their homes with follow-up counseling and therapy on an outpatient basis. The trend toward improved and more compassionate care for those with mental illness was under way.

In 1982, the Omnibus Budget Reconciliation Act provided funds to support the treatment of those with drug additions and other mental disorders. This bill was further legislated in 1987 when the **Omnibus Budget Reform Act (OBRA)** prevented the inappropriate placement of mentally ill clients into nursing homes. The **Mental Health Act of 1983** addressed the rights of people admitted to psychiatric hospitals, including their right to refuse being admitted to a psychiatric facility against their will and their rights while in treatment, following discharge, and during community follow-up.

The 1990s were declared the "Decade of the Brain" by President George H.W. Bush. In this proclamation, he specified the need for specialized studies to find ways of reducing the impact and prevalence of diseases affecting the brain. At the same time, the **Americans with Disabilities Act (ADA)** was signed; it was the first federal civil rights law to prohibit discrimination against persons with mental and physical disabilities. This legislation protects those persons with disabilities in the employment setting, while using public transportation or facilities, and in areas of mass communication. The National Mental Health Parity Act was signed into law in 1996 by President Bill Clinton; this law made it mandatory for insurance companies to provide annual and lifetime benefit limits for mental illnesses comparable to those allotted for physical illnesses. An amendment to expand this act was proposed in March, 1998, to prohibit limitations on cost sharing applied to the cost of mental health care. Although this act did not eliminate all barriers to discriminatory treatment, it was an important initial step.

Throughout these legislative changes to prohibit limitations on cost sharing applied to the cost of mental health care, modifications have been made in the treatment of clients, both in hospital-based units provided care and those with outpatient services. The focus has been on providing treatment and support systems that provide normalization and allow the client to return to a home setting or structured living situation. Integral to this approach has been the need to define a logical and orderly way to fulfill the nurse's role in the treatment process. The expanded philosophy of mental health nursing was based on a scientific and systematic approach, later referred to as *the nursing process*. The work of Hildegard Peplau (1909 to 1999) laid the groundwork for the interpersonal and interactive processes so integral to the nurse–client relationship. When working with the psychiatric client, Peplau believed that the nurse acts as a resource person, counselor, role model, and support person for the client. In 1994, the American Nurses Association adopted standards of clinical practice for psychiatric-mental health nursing.

> **Mind Jogger**
>
> In what way does the nurse serve as a role model to those with mental illness?

Current Issues in Mental Health Care

The access to care and the way in which mental health care is delivered has undergone many changes and reforms. However, even today in the 21st century, there remains a stigma and lack of social awareness of the effects these disorders have on both those who have the illness and those who share the responsibility for their care. Two prominent issues in modern mental health care involve ensuring equality in access to mental health care and covering the costs of care.

Access to Care: Cultural Disparities

Although mental illness is present in all racial and ethical groups within our society and around the world, the disparities in providing treatment for all who are burdened by these illnesses are all too real. Inequalities exist both in the availability and in the utilization of mental health services. The disparities result both from barriers to seeking mental health care and from a lack of cultural preparedness in the health care system.

Barriers to Seeking Care

According to the latest report of the Surgeon General of the United States (1999), mental illnesses affect all populations, regardless of race or ethnicity. Although there may be an acute need for mental health care, findings show those in most minority groups are less likely to seek treatment, and those who do often receive a lower quality of care. People may not seek treatment because of cultural differences in how groups view symptoms of mental disorders. There is also much variance in willingness to seek treatment versus relying on family, spiritual, or folk remedies for the discomfort of these symptoms. If the family does seek treatment, it is often sought late in the course of the illness.

Although some people in minority groups may be successful in accessing services, they may not always receive the care needed. Lower socioeconomic status, lower educational levels, and limited income, together with the stressors created

"Cultural Dilemma"

While enrolled in a mental health nursing class, you are invited to study at the home of a classmate who is Hispanic. Being an Anglo-American, you are unfamiliar with many of the cultural traditions and customs you encounter. The family members are primarily Spanish speaking, although your classmate communicates to you in English. As you enter the home, your friend tells you that she has a brother who has a mental problem. Relating that he hears voices, she also mentions that he talks a lot to those who have passed on. She asks you not to say anything about this as the family is very protective of him. She admits that she is ashamed and feels that he is this way because of things their father has done. During your study time, you ask your classmate if they have taken her brother to get treatment for his mental illness. She replies, "Oh no, my mother would never allow that. She believes the *curandero* is the only one who can help. My grandmother also is a 'healer.' She uses her healing ability to cure him and he seems to get better for a while." While thinking about what you have heard, you debate in your mind what you should say or do next.

What additional information would you need to collect?

_____

_____

What cultural issues may be a deterrent to available treatment for this client?

_____

_____

What steps might you take to encourage treatment by health care professionals?

_____

_____

Case Application 4.1

by these factors, all serve as barriers to accessing the mental health treatment offered in our health care system. The existence of these barriers may be seen by some as discrimination.

In addition, whether perceived or inferred, racial and cultural bias and stereotyping during encounters with mental health workers often elicit hostility and breed feelings of prejudiced treatment. Immigrant and minority families alike often demonstrate a lack of trust in the system and fear the outcome. Many immigrants have endured trauma and were perhaps refugees before coming to the United States. According to NIMH, age at the time of immigration appears to affect the onset of mental disorders. Statistics demonstrate the younger the individual on arrival, the higher the incidence of psychiatric disorders. Studies show, for example, a greater incidence of childhood psychiatric disorders and substance abuse in Asian and Latino immigrants who arrived prior to age 12, while mood disorders increased in those arriving in the United States around age 40. The stigma attached to mental illness still exists and often continues to hinder the road to treatment and improved quality of life for these groups.

Mind Jogger

What factors may contribute to the public attitude toward those with mental illness?

Cultural Unpreparedness Within the System

Cultural incompetence among mental health providers and professionals is perhaps the single most pivotal barrier to equality in the delivery of mental health care. Problems arise when the context of mental illness is addressed without considering the cultural bridge to mutual understanding. American physicians are only beginning to understand the symptoms of mental illness found in other countries that might be viewed as a physical illness in the United States. For example, headaches or seizures might be seen by some cultures as the result of the mind being possessed by a demon. In other cultures, the psychiatric professionals must diagnose mental illnesses that clients first report as physical ailments.

Multicultural education is needed to prepare those who treat and care for those with mental illness. Studies continue to examine the diverse cultural traditions, beliefs, values, and adjustments to societal living. Clinicians must recognize the importance of communicating in the individual's first language and establishing a therapeutic relationship that includes modifications respectful of cultural traditions. The significance of cultural awareness and sensitivity in treatment is inherent in bridging the gap between the numbers of minority groups who need mental health care and those who receive treatment.

Cost of Care

The impact of managed-care delivery of health care has been dramatic on mental health units. Many psychiatric units are closing owing to a lack of operational funds. The paradox of this trend is the growing population of those who need these services but are unable to secure them. Those living in community settings need ongoing management and support. Without these services, clients often become unstable and treatment becomes ineffective. In addition, many who do receive services are inconsistent with compliance making it difficult to manage treatment effectiveness. The success rate in the treatment of depression and other mental illness is approximately 80% if supervised care is uninterrupted.

In February 2007, a bill was introduced and passed to provide parity between health insurance coverage of mental health benefits and those for medical and surgical services. Legislation and debate continued on this issue and in October 2008, the Paul Wellstone and Pete Domenici **Mental Health Parity and Addiction Equity Act of 2008** (H.R. 1424) was signed into law by President George H.W. Bush as part of the Emergency Economic Stabilization Act of 2008. The MHPAE was designed to create parity in group health insurance coverage by requiring coverage and benefits for mental health and substance abuse equal to those for other physical disorders and diseases. However, the federal law does not mandate equal parity to the same extent as state laws which allow many discrepancies in the level of benefits provided. In 2010, the **Affordable Care Act (PPACA)** was passed into law, which expands the federal mental health parity requirements and creates a mandated benefit for the insurance coverage of mental health and substance abuse disorders that includes Medicaid plans and those plans offered through the individual market. The controversy over this healthcare legislation is ongoing as of this writing.

Mind Jogger

How have the changes in the provision of mental health services affected your community?

More negotiation is needed to ensure that millions of people across the country will have the right to nondiscriminatory mental health coverage, including many under self-funded plans who are not protected by state parity laws. Lack of access to treatment has disastrous implications for the person with mental illness, their families, and to society as a whole. The cost of lost productivity and income is paid by everyone, including the public health care community. A guaranteed coverage at parity for both mental and substance use diagnoses and services will help to provide equal access to the mental health system.

Legal and Ethical Considerations in Mental Health Care

As the road is being paved toward equal access to care, laws and standards have been put in place to protect the rights of clients and set guidelines for mental health care providers.

Many decisions of health care professionals involve matters that include both legal and ethical issues. The term **ethics** refers to a set of principles or values that provides dignity and respect to clients. Like any other aspect of the system, the care of clients with mental disorders involves a certain standard of principles and values. This set of beliefs also provides a guiding philosophy for the nursing profession and protects clients from unreasonable treatment. In some instances, nurses and other mental health care professionals must make decisions that involve conflicting standards and values. There are guidelines that assist in resolving these issues, but the pathways are nonetheless complicated and difficult. In these situations, the individual client must remain the most important factor in the decision.

As members of the health care team, nurses must be familiar with current laws and ethical governance of mental health care delivery. This includes understanding the rights of clients. In addition, the nurse is responsible for maintaining standards within the nursing profession itself. Through attention to this set of values, the nurse facilitates the therapeutic relationship and improves the self-esteem of the client. Integrating positive values into client care improves the self-esteem of clients and facilitates the therapeutic relationship.

Client Rights

All clients entering a treatment facility have certain rights that have been documented in the **Patient Bill of Rights**. Those that apply to the client with mental illness were declared in the Mental Health Systems Act Bill of Rights passed by the U.S. Congress in 1980. Clients are given the opportunity to read these rights at the time of admission for treatment. This document is usually displayed in a prominent area of the client service units so that it is available to clients and families. It is a nurse's responsibility to be knowledgeable of these rights and to ensure that they are preserved and protected for the client.

> **Mind Jogger**
>
> In addition to being a responsibility, how does knowledge of client rights protect the nurse?

Appropriate Care

Although the nurse is not directly responsible for deciding where or what treatment is provided, an integral part of the nurse's responsibility is to ensure that the client receives appropriate care. All clients are entitled to receive care based on a current and individualized treatment plan that includes a description of the services that are available and those that are offered upon discharge. Included in the Patient Bill of Rights are the rights to:

- be treated with dignity, concern, and respect at all times.
- expect quality care provided by trained and competent professional providers.
- anticipate complete confidentiality within the limits of the law and to be informed of legal exceptions to this standard.
- know the qualifications of the professionals who will be involved in the treatment process.
- receive explanations of treatment and be involved in the planning of their care.

- refuse to be a part of experimental therapy or treatment methods.
- understand the effects of prescribed medications along with any potential adverse effects.
- be treated in the least restrictive setting—one that prevents excessive restraint within a confined atmosphere.
- be involved in the decision-making as to which treatment options are best for them.
- refuse treatment unless there is a court order that dictates reasons for admission.

> **Just the Facts**
>
> Least restrictive environments can include locked or unlocked hospital units, community living centers, or outpatient treatment centers, depending on the individual needs of the client.

Informed Consent

Prior to admission to any health care setting, the client receives an explanation of client rights and institutional policies from the agency. In the case of an incompetent or incoherent client, a family member or legal guardian should be given this information. (Box 4.1 provides information about legal determination of decision-making ability.) These full explanations give the client, or those who may have legal guardianship for the client, the ability to make an informed choice. **Informed consent** is the client's grant of permission to undergo a specific procedure or treatment after being informed about the procedure, risks, and benefits. The agency providing the services is protected by getting a signed statement of understanding from the client. At the same time, the client has the right to refuse any aspect of treatment and may elect not to sign the consent.

> **BOX 4.1**
>
> ### Legal Guide to Decision-Making Capability
>
> - Adults are seen as capable of making informed decisions unless determined "incompetent or incapacitated" by a court of law
> - If it is determined that a person lacks the ability to make informed decisions about health care, another person other than the client will make the decisions
> - A durable power of attorney for health care allows a person to designate whomever they choose to make health care decisions in the event the person is unable to do so

At the time of admission for mental health services, the client receives an explanation of policies regarding available services, visitation, phone usage, unit rules, and physician contact. The agency representative also explains insurance benefits or payment options, as well as the contracts between the treating professionals and third-party payment reimbursement. The client should be afforded the opportunity to discuss treatment options with a physician or other health care providers. Suggested topics for the client to discuss with their mental health professional are listed in Client Teaching Note 4.1.

Confidentiality

Confidentiality refers to the client's right to prevent written or verbal communications from being disclosed to outside parties without authorization. To facilitate a client's trust, nursing students and licensed nurses must assure them that all communication is confidential and will not be communicated to anyone not participating in their care. The Nurse Practice Act of each state's Board of Nursing requires nurses to protect the client's right to privacy by maintaining confidentiality. Every member of the treatment team has a duty to uphold this ethical standard. The privacy and confidentiality provisions of the Health Insurance Portability and Accountability Act (HIPAA) of 1996 went into effect in April 2003. This law ensures that security procedures protect the privacy and confidentiality of this information. Clients have the right to know the content of their medical records, what information is being disclosed for payment benefits or other treatment reasons, and to whom any disclosures are being given.

Protecting the client's record from unauthorized personnel is a nursing responsibility. Health care providers who are not consulted by the physician or providing direct client care do not have the privilege of viewing the medical record without permission. Student nurses who are involved in observation or interaction with clients should be cautious not to disclose any clinical information that is used for education purposes. Another way of providing privacy is to conduct the nursing report in a private area where other clients and uninvolved hospital staff cannot hear what is being said. Report sheets should be kept in a discreet place and shredded before leaving the nursing unit. At no time should the nurse discuss a client's problems or treatment with another client. Acknowledgment of a client admission should not occur via telephone to outside parties unless a policy and system exists that can be used to ensure confidentiality. Some psychiatric facilities have codes that are provided to individuals that the client approves. In some situations, it may be legally required that client information is disclosed. These may include the following:

- Intent to commit a crime
- Duty to warn endangered individuals
- Evidence of child abuse
- Initiation of involuntary hospitalization
- Infection by human immunodeficiency virus (HIV)

It is important to let clients know that information they disclose may be shared with other team members if it is relevant to their well-being and treatment progress.

Mind Jogger

In what way might confidentiality raise more of a concern to the client in a psychiatric unit than the client on a medical or surgical hospital unit?

Appeals and Complaints

Regardless of the setting in which clients receive mental health services, they have the right to receive information about how to channel complaints about their care or the professionals providing their treatment. This should be explained to the clients at the time services are anticipated, whether in a hospital unit or an outpatient setting. Should the person wish to file a complaint to a professional board, the person should be advised of the procedure to do so. Some clients may wish to appeal decisions on payor systems and should be given the name and address of the appropriate contact. (See Client Teaching Note 4.2 for locating mental health services.)

CLIENT TEACHING NOTE 4.2

Locating Mental Health Services

- Substance Abuse and Mental Health Services Administration (SAMHSA) http://mentalhealth. samhsa.gov/databases/ (Accessed 3-17-09)
- NIMH http://www.nimh.nih.gov/index.shtml (Accessed 3-17-09)
- Veterans Administration (VA) Medical Center
- Health Resources and Services Administration (HRSA) http://www.hrsa.gov/ (Accessed 3-17-09)

Use of Seclusion and Restraint

Seclusion and Restraint

Because some mental health disorders may cause a person to become extremely agitated or even act violently, seclusion or restraints may sometimes be necessary if other interventions or therapies are ineffective. The Joint Commission on Accreditation of Healthcare Organizations (JCAHO) and the federal government regulate the use of seclusion and restraints by health care workers. **Seclusion** refers to the placement of a client in a controlled environment in order to treat a clinical emergency in which the client poses an immediate threat to themselves or to others. Many times this refers to placing a client inside a room with a locked door away from stimuli of the nursing unit. **Physical restraint** refers to the use of mechanical devices to provide limited movement by the client. Physical restraints are used to prevent harm to self or others and require careful monitoring. These may consist of padded leather or cloth devices for the wrist, ankles, waist, or fingers. **Chemical restraint** refers to the use of medication to calm a client and prevent the need for physical restraints. Chemical restraint is less restrictive and is generally the initial choice unless the situation warrants otherwise.

Just the Facts

Seclusion should never be used when a person is suicidal.

Just the Facts

Restraints are applied only with a physician's order and under the supervision of a registered nurse.

These methods are only used when verbal interventions or less restrictive methods of treatment have failed or are not available. It is essential that nurses attempt to de-escalate aggressive behaviors before these measures are necessary. Many times the environmental situation or other clients have provoked the behavior. In this case, removing the client to another area of the unit may allow the client to regain control without further intervention. If seclusion or restraints are employed, the client is usually given sedating medication to provide a calming effect and assist in behavior control. Continuous monitoring of the client in restraints or seclusion is mandatory. These methods are discontinued at any time they are seen as ineffective or at the earliest possible indication that the client has regained control. Time limits are a part of many state and institutional statutes.

Nurses should be familiar with the legal implications involved in the use of seclusion and restraint. It is important to know the qualifications and training of any person that is delegated the task of assisting with restraint. The nurse should know the facility rules and state laws regarding this procedure to avoid any probable cause of wrongful liability. Clients who are confined without justification or who are subject to inappropriate use of seclusion or restraint can be viewed in a civil court as having been falsely imprisoned. The restraint of clients with inappropriate use of force can be viewed as assault and battery. Having an awareness of how, when, and why to use confining methods will help the nurse avoid litigation for these circumstances.

Nurse Accountability

Student and licensed nurses are accountable for the care they provide, which means they must take responsibility for what they do. Each level of nursing is responsible for adhering to the standard of care that is acceptable for that particular level. The Nurse Practice Act of each state identifies the scope and minimum standards of practice for both the (LPN/LVN) and (RN). If a question arises with regard to a statute contained in the practice act, the nurse should contact the board of nursing for the state in which he or she is practicing.

Nurses have an obligation to maintain current licensure and educational requirements required by their board of nursing. In the area of psychiatric-mental health care, the nurse is also responsible for knowing institutional and governmental policies regarding client admission and rights. If uncertainty exists, the nurse is responsible for securing the correct information from other sources such as procedure manuals, textbooks, other health care professionals, or network resources.

Nurses may be held accountable and liable to any client for an act of incompetence or negligence in the deliverance of care. All actions on the part of the nurse to facilitate appropriate treatment of the client should be documented to provide a written record of events. The nurse also has a legal and ethical responsibility to act as a client advocate to protect the clients and those rights that are legally afforded to them.

> ### Mind Jogger
> How would the nurse's role as client advocate pertain to the client who is mentally incompetent?

Practice Settings for Mental Health Care

Mental health care is a multifaceted integration of varied approaches that have developed in an attempt to meet the needs of people with mental disorders and their families. Although many clients with mental disorders are seen in mental health treatment centers, these same individuals or others with psychological or emotional symptoms may be seen in additional health care settings (i.e., outpatient clinics, hospital outpatient/inpatient units, correctional institutions, long-term care facilities, and home-health care). The ability to recognize the symptoms and initiate appropriate interventions is important in any situation encountered in any practice setting.

A client has the right to receive treatment in the least restrictive environment that would promote safety and therapeutic care. The type of facility and level of care provided depend on several factors. The client's history has a strong influence on the treatment methods that will be used. The circumstances that led to the current admission also contribute to the treatment and nursing care that will be needed. The family physician or psychiatrist makes the determination whether the client will need to receive inpatient or outpatient treatment and the appropriate setting in which that care can be provided.

Inpatient Psychiatric Settings

Depending on the urgency, a need for immediate intervention may be referred to a hospital emergency room or inpatient facility. A client experiencing acute symptoms of a mental disorder may be brought for evaluation by law enforcement officers after an arrest or other altercation with the law. Others may be brought by family members out of fear or concern for the welfare of the individual or themselves. In addition, sometimes the client makes an individual decision to seek treatment as an inpatient. Clients may recognize that they are out of control or fear that they will harm themselves or others. In these instances, an admission to inpatient services is usually indicated.

Many clients with mental health problems request admission to a psychiatric center for treatment. A **voluntary commitment** occurs when the client is admitted based on his or her chosen willingness to comply with the treatment program. In this situation, the physician writes the order for admission and the client signs and agrees to the terms of treatment. The person is then allowed to sign the appropriate documents and leave when treatment is complete. Policies vary among facilities, but most states have an initial period (e.g., 72 hours) that allows the physician and other members of the treatment team the opportunity to assess the situation before the person can leave voluntarily. If the client leaves prior to this time or without a discharge order from the physician, he or she may be asked to sign an Against Medical Advice (AMA) form that releases the facility from any liability related to the person leaving treatment.

An **involuntary commitment** occurs when a person is admitted to a psychiatric unit against his or her will. The amount of time a person can be detained is determined by law, which varies from state to state. For an involuntary admission to occur, an evaluation statement that clearly indicates the person's mental state is a danger to self or others is necessary. This is a time-consuming and sometimes difficult process. The order for protective custody (OPC) is given by a court official. The client can be detained on an emergency status against his or her will for an interval of 48 to 72 hours. At the end of that period, the client must be discharged, given voluntary admission status, or receive a court hearing to determine if there is a need for continued involuntary treatment. Laws may vary from state to state on these options. Involuntary commitment is most commonly used in an inpatient setting but can be ordered on an outpatient basis, such as in substance-abuse programs.

Outpatient Mental Health Settings

In some situations, a referral may be made by a medical physician to a community mental health center, social service agency, or private clinic or facility where various treatment options are available without having to admit the client for services. Residential facilities are also available for clients who need to reside in a therapeutic environment for extended periods of time. In other circumstances an individual may seek treatment from a private psychiatrist, psychologist, or personal counselor.

The purpose of outpatient mental health care is to provide services to individuals, families, and the community that will promote mental health and quality of life in their day-to-day functioning. These services may include psychiatric consultation along with psychotropic medication evaluation and management. Consultation by a trained professional is focused on helping individuals to better understand themselves and their behaviors, and to facilitate changes that help the individual to achieve greater satisfaction and happiness. Outpatient therapy may include the following:

- Individual therapy
- Marriage and family therapy
- Child and adolescent therapy
- Divorce therapy
- Group therapy
- Psychological evaluation
- Stress reduction and relaxation
- Assessment for various mental disorders
- Grief and loss support
- Addictive behaviors and codependency therapy
- Parenting therapy

Nonpsychiatric Health Care Facilities

The **holistic** concept of nursing care incorporates the entire scope of human needs, addressing the physical, psychosocial, cultural, and spiritual issues of the individual client. Nurses practice in a variety of nonpsychiatric settings that provide an array of situations in which the emotional and psychosocial needs of clients may emerge. Settings may include hospitals, physician's offices, long-term care facilities, home health care, and hospice care among others. In some instances, mentally healthy individuals may experience temporary mental instability as a result of a situational cri-

---

BOX 4.2

Factors Affecting One's Ability to Cope

- **Individual factors**, such as age, personality, intelligence, values, cultural beliefs, and emotional state
- **Environmental factors**, such as support system and financial stability
- **Illness-related factors**, such as type of illness, rate of progression, functional impairment, and prognosis

---

sis, such as rape, trauma, abuse, or environmental disaster. Crisis intervention and supportive nursing strategies can make a major difference in the ability of the client to access and mobilize coping resources at a time when life seems to be unraveling. In many situations, the nurse is the health care worker who observes and assesses these feelings or behaviors that may demonstrate symptoms of mental health dysfunction. Box 4.2 identifies some factors that may affect one's ability to cope.

Among the most common emotional and psychological responses to trauma, physical illness, or loss are depression, fear, anxiety, denial, withdrawal, anger, apathy, regression, and dependency. Levels of these emotions may accelerate as a person feels a loss of control over what is happening when pain, disability, hospitalization, or death may loom in the unknown. The stage of illness and the possible treatment options will be a factor in this reaction. The economic impact of health care in any setting can also produce an overwhelming flood of emotions and fears. Fear of the "unknown" is especially threatening to the client who is experiencing an emotional or psychological crisis. In addition, a projection of these fears is often demonstrated by the client in self-centered, demanding behaviors such as unreasonable requests of health care providers. Regardless of the setting, the nurse should be prepared to initiate interventions to address the psychosocial needs, as well as the physical needs, of each client.

Mind Jogger

Can you think of some ways that "fear of the unknown" could escalate anxiety to severe levels?

Outpatient Health Care Settings

Clients who experience the psychological effects related to a physical illness are seen in many

TABLE 4.1	Psychological Factors that Affect Medical Conditions
PSYCHOLOGICAL FACTOR	**EFFECTS ON MEDICAL CONDITIONS**
Mental disorders	Disorder such as bipolar, schizophrenia, or major depression may affect the client who has a myocardial infarction, renal disease, asthma, or surgery
Psychological symptoms	Symptoms such as apathy or a depressed state can significantly affect the course or treatment of the medical condition or recovery from surgery
Personality traits or coping styles	Personality traits that are controlling or hostile may interfere with post myocardial infarction treatment progress. Maladaptive coping strategies that deny the need for a diagnostic procedure or surgery
Maladaptive health behaviors	Behavior practices such as unsafe sexual practices, lack of exercise, or excessive use of food, drugs, or alcohol
Stress-related physiological response	Might initiate increased incidence of hypertension, cardiac arrhythmias, angina, migraine headache, or respiratory crisis

outpatient practice settings. The *DSM-V* addresses psychological factors that may affect or alter the course of an existing medical condition, resulting in an exacerbation of the illness or a delayed recovery. Sometimes the factors may interfere with treatment of the medical condition such as continued noncompliance with diet or medication therapy in the client with diabetes, or continued smoking by the client with chronic pulmonary disease. Each problem is addressed based on the individual issue that is present (see Table 4.1).

A physical illness that imposes a severe threat to a person's health status and lifetime of chronic disease may elicit a grief response to this real or perceived loss. The disease process may restrict the person's lifestyle and socioeconomic status, which may threaten both the self-esteem and

sense of security previously enjoyed. Future goals and family roles may be shattered by the imposition of the physical and psychological effects of the symptoms. Box 4.3 lists some physical illnesses or surgeries that have the potential to elicit major psychological effects on the client and the client's family. Various means by which people cope with the impact of physical illness are listed in Box 4.4.

The lack of control over the devastating effects imposed by many of these conditions may be described as a state of helplessness or **powerlessness**. This may be true of both the person who has the illness and the family involved. The nurse should assume an empathetic and supportive role as the emotional and psychological defenses of those persons are attacked by the decision making and coping necessary to deal with the illness or surgery. The nurse should plan to include time for active listening, allowing and encouraging the release and expression of feelings and concerns. Explanations concerning diagnostic tests, procedures, permits, and consent forms are vital to allow the person to make informed decisions regarding their situation. A sense of empowerment is returned to the client when he or she is included in planning to meet care needs and

---

BOX 4.3

Physical Illnesses and Surgeries with Major Psychological Effects

- Alzheimer's disease
- AIDS/HIV disease
- Diabetes mellitus
- Parkinson's disease
- Multiple sclerosis
- Lou Gehrig's disease
- Hemophilia
- Stroke (CVA)
- COPD, asthma
- Cancer/chemotherapy
- Myocardial infarction
- Hemodialysis
- Mastectomy
- Prostatectomy
- Colostomy, ileostomy, nephrostomy
- Amputation
- Quadriplegia or hemiplegia
- Radical facial/neck surgery

BOX 4.4

Common Coping Strategies in Clients Experiencing Psychological Effects from Physical Illness

- Asking questions to obtain information and guidance for treatment
- Sharing concerns and finding support from others
- Change in emotional climate with light-hearted humor
- Suppression of fears and "what ifs."

has the opportunity to make choices about those needs. The nurse's sensitivity to the anxiety the client is experiencing will also be a major factor in the client's ability to adapt to the situation.

Just the Facts

Nurses can strengthen a client's coping strategies with positive reinforcement.

Mind Jogger

How does informed decision making help to defuse the anxiety of the client?

An assessment of the client's emotional reaction to the diagnosis, past and current coping abilities, and available support resources provides the nurse with a baseline for intervention to facilitate adaptation as the outcome. A basic guide to the client's emotional response is provided in Box 4.5. Consistency of caregivers in providing the needed help also provides a sense of security during a time when ego defenses are weakened and the client needs a sense of stability to allow and encourage trust in the environment. It is most important to teach the client problem-solving skills and provide support for self-care efforts. The increase in self-care responsibilities as appropriate helps to preserve self-esteem and provides a sense of control over a situation that may seem overwhelming.

Mind Jogger

How can the nurse assist in strengthening the client's support system? What referrals could be utilized?

BOX 4.5

Guide to Emotional Responses in a Psychological Crisis

- *Adaptive coping behaviors* are seen when the client demonstrates the ability to mobilize internal and external resources to adapt to a situation.
- *Maladaptive coping behaviors* are demonstrated when the client is unable to mobilize internal and external resources resulting in disorganized and destructive behaviors.
- *Crisis level* describes a situation in which the client's available coping mechanisms are inadequate.

Acute Care Settings for the Client with Dual Diagnosis

The client with a diagnosed mental illness who is hospitalized can present a nursing challenge. Whereas the nurse may prioritize the medical–surgical needs of the client, the secondary mental illness diagnosis must be considered in all aspects of care planning. Critical thinking leads the nurse to ask questions such as the following: How will the client mentally view this procedure? What environmental stimuli could be misinterpreted? What explanations will be needed to reinforce reality to the client with a psychotic disorder? How might this client misperceive pain? What approach could be used if the client exhibits delusional thinking or hallucinations? What psychological signs and symptoms might be anticipated in a client with schizophrenia or major affective disorder who is diagnosed with a serious medical or surgical condition?

Nurses facing the challenge of a dual-diagnosis situation such as this can use the nursing process to identify the problems related to both physiologic and psychological issues. Communication techniques and nursing interventions for altered thought processes are critical to the outcome in the client's situation. An altered psychological state complicates compliance with treatment and overall recovery from the surgery itself. Both the physiological and psychological needs of the individual client must be assessed and met. Acute assessment skills and creative interventions are needed to avoid complications and promote the client's return to a state of wellness and discharge from the hospital. Nursing diagnoses that may apply to the medical–surgical client with a diagnosed mental illness are listed in Box 4.6.

Correctional Facilities

There are many theories and assumptions as to why individuals commit acts against society that secure them time living behind walls and locks of a prison. What happens? Is it related to environmental factors, or is it fostered by a predisposition to engage in behaviors that defy the legal boundaries that define right from wrong? In his book, *Inside the Criminal Mind*, Stanton Samenow describes the criminal's irresponsible pattern of behavior as predominant "throughout his life." All associations including school, work, family, and friends all fall victims to the **manipulation** or behavioral tactics of deceit, devious thinking, and actions used to meet the criminal's self-serving

"More Than One Problem"

John, a 48-year-old unemployed mechanic is admitted to the emergency room with the following symptoms: acute upper left abdominal pain, abdominal distention, febrile, elevated WBC, nausea, and vomiting. Initial medical assessment leads to a diagnosis of a perforated diverticulitis of the splenic flexure with peritonitis. The patient also has a diagnosis of chronic schizophrenia, undifferentiated type and has lived in a group home milieu for the past 6 months. John is given sedation prior to the emergency abdominal surgery performed. When John returns to the medical–surgical unit, he has a nasogastric tube connected to intermittent suction, a left triple-lumen subclavian IV line, a right jugular IV line with TPN infusion, and an open abdominal incision with wet-to-dry packing secured with ABD pads and Montgomery straps.

Because John also has a diagnosis of schizophrenia, his behavior may be altered by the events of anesthesia and surgery. What response might the nurse expect as John emerges from sedation and anesthesia?

_____

_____

How might he misinterpret the array of "tubes" connected to his body?

_____

_____

Do you think John will understand that the pain is related to his surgery? What approach might the nurse use to help John understand the reality of the pain?

_____

_____

The second postoperative day, John begins to question the invasive equipment lines entering his body. The nurse enters his room to find him drinking water with his nasogastric tube lying on the floor beside the bed. He tells the nurse he was thirsty, and "that hose was siphoning all the water out of my body to water the plants neglected by my inability to turn the shower on, and I got some water so I can water the shower."

What type of psychotic behavior is seen in John's actions?

_____

_____

coercive views of the world. Feeling no obligation to anyone, criminals believe that people, their property, and society in general exist for their own benefit. Criminals will do virtually anything to acquire whatever they want. They have a voracious and ruthless need for power, caring very little about whom they injure or things they destroy as they manipulate others. Samenow states, "They have an inflated self-image in which they regard themselves as special and superior and assume that people will do their bidding."

Characteristic Behavior Patterns

Although there are some types of crimes that are viewed by psychiatric professionals as the result of mental instability, it must be considered that all criminals think differently. In a distorted form of logic, they think their behavior is acceptable as long as it benefits them. Correctional facilities have continuously sought ways to reform and rehabilitate those whose thinking is dominated by devising ways to be a better criminal. Prison is an environment where antisocial thoughts and behaviors are the norms, and the exchange of crime-related ideas is fostered by the commonality of narcissistic and self-serving personalities. The same behaviors demonstrated on the street are continued in prison. The incarcerated person usually uses the system to his or her favor, continuing manipulative and power-seeking behaviors. Fear, remorse, or regret may be temporarily displayed by the inmate new to the system. However, the

What physical assessments related to his surgical care would be import to report?

_____

_____

How should the nurse respond to John's altered thinking?

_____

_____

The nurse assesses that bowel sounds are present and that no nausea or vomiting has occurred with the oral intake. The physician orders a liquid diet for John. While passing his room several hours later, the nurse hears John talking. When entering the room, no one is present except John. The water faucet in the sink and the shower are both turned on with hot water running. John tells the nurse, "It can't flow through me if it is not running. Don't turn it off or I will shrivel up!"

How could the nurse use the IV and TPN fluid to divert John's delusional thinking back to reality?

_____

_____

The nurse proceeds to change the packing and dressing on John's abdominal incision. John tells the nurse, "If you take that off, the water will become contaminated and kill the plants."

What misperception does John have concerning the open abdominal incision?

_____

_____

How could the nurse use the wet-to-dry packs to reinforce reality?

_____

_____

hard-core truth of survival leads many to play the game of toughness in an atmosphere where stabbing, rape, gang warfare, and rioting are common. There is a constant struggle within the confines of the prison walls to maintain some sense of self. Inmate complaints are common, along with selfish requests and expectations, and charges that their rights are being violated when their wishes are denied, all the time ignoring the fact that their present situation is the result of their own choices.

For those who know aggression and crime as a way of life, it is understandable that incarceration with a living environment where privacy, dignity, and individuality are absent further contributes to the underlying hostility. The obvious sense of powerlessness stimulates the inmates to search for power and control within the system. This search for a sense of importance or personal significance is often the motive for the inmate seeking medical attention. Continued evaluation and treatment of medical or mental illnesses the inmate had prior to incarceration are often the reason the client is seen. While these and any new medical problems are legitimate health care needs, there is often an additional manipulative effort by the inmate to acquire personal gain from the medical personnel, such as special privileges, medications, or personal articles.

Mental Healthcare Issues

A psychiatric evaluation process is required by the American Correctional Association, the national accrediting body for prisons and jails. This is done

BOX 4.6

Nursing Diagnosis for Clients with Psychological Needs Related to Medical Illness

- Adjustment impaired, related to chronic illness
- Anxiety, related to situational crisis
- Alteration in self-image, related to functional changes imposed by illness
- Coping ineffective, family; related to inability to care for client
- Coping ineffective, individual; related to situational crisis
- Denial, ineffective; related to fear or anxiety
- Grieving, anticipatory; related to potential for loss
- Hopelessness, related to chronic illness
- Powerlessness, related to situational crisis
- Role performance alteration, related to change in health status
- Self-care deficit, related to effects of medical or surgical condition
- Self-esteem, situational low, related to increased dependence on caregivers
- Social isolation, related to factors imposed by illness

at the time the inmate first arrives at the correctional facility. Data collected in this process may include the following:

- Previous counseling or psychiatric treatment
- Current or previous use of psychotropic medications
- Any history of inpatient psychiatric treatment, either court mandated or voluntary
- Family history of psychiatric problems
- History of seizures or head trauma
- History of suicide attempts
- Any hallucinations or delusional thinking
- Any objective psychotic symptoms
- History or current use of illicit drugs
- Any criminal history as a juvenile
- Convictions for sex offenses
- History of violence, assault, or destructive behaviors
- History of being the target of violence while incarcerated

Further diagnostic evaluation is recommended and referral is warranted if the inmate demonstrates symptoms or behaviors of psychiatric illness, has a history of previous mental health treatment, voices current suicidal ideation or prior suicidal gestures, indicates affective distress, is at high risk for problems with adjustment to confinement, or the offense committed is of an unusual nature.

Any psychological symptoms voiced by an inmate or observed by prison personnel are referred to the psychiatric counselor for evaluation and/or treatment. Nursing staff members are often the recipient of the complaint while doing an assessment or when aberrant behavior is reported to them. An inmate may complain of hearing voices or seeing things that are not real in order to gain special attention or access to psychotropic medications. Medications are coveted and requested for both actual and nonsensical reasons. The medical division of a correctional facility also is one of the bargaining bases for the inmates. Real or perceived ailments become a means to seek special privileges and excuses from assigned labor and regimental routines. The need for treatment must be separated from the exploitative methods devised by the criminal to assure that any legitimate condition receives the appropriate medical attention.

Many of the prison population are presently dealing with or have a history of some type of substance abuse. Risk behaviors related to drug use give rise to the growing numbers of those who test positive for HIV. Hepatitis B and C are rampant within the system. A portion of the population has developed AIDS. Regardless of whether a person is a prison inmate, the psychological impact and verdict imposed by hearing that one has tested positive for these diseases is the same. The result is devastating. Nurses within the prison system do the same counseling for these victims as for those in the outside world. For this victim, the nurse may be the sole support system. There are no families or friends from whom consolation and sympathy can be sought. Silence is absolute to avoid the harassment of fellow inmates. Although treatment is available, the cold reality of another sentence engulfs their being.

Nurses who work in a correctional facility must learn to separate what is real from what is a manipulative endeavor by the inmate. A calm, but firm and matter-of-fact approach is essential to command compliance with rules and policies of the institution. Security is always present in the medical department and the same standards of behavior are expected from the inmates regardless of where they are in the prison. The empathy and compassion that is so integral to other areas of nursing may quickly be seen by criminals as an opportunity for their con games. While it is important to accept the inmate as a person with human feelings and needs, the nurse must be vigilant to avoid being victimized by these actions.

Summary

- Early treatment of the mentally ill was inhumane and unjust.
- Dorothea Dix was a 19th century pioneer in advocating improved standards for mental hospitals and those with mental illness.
- In 1882, Linda Richards opened the Boston City Hospital Training School for training nurses to care for individuals with mental illness.
- National Mental Health Act of 1946 was the first legislation to provide funds for research, nursing degree programs, and improved community service for those with mental illness.
- OBRA prevented the inappropriate placement of mentally ill clients into nursing homes.
- The Mental Health Systems Act Bill of Rights of 1980 afforded the client seeking mental health care certain rights to appropriate treatment.
- The Mental Health Parity and Addiction Equity Act of 2008 was designed to create parity in insurance coverage by requiring benefits for mental disorders and substance abuse equal to those for other physical disorders and diseases.
- Clients receiving mental health care should be given an explanation of client rights and institutional policies to give them the ability to make informed consent.
- The Nurse Practice Act of each state and the HIPAA of 1996 hold mental health care professionals to a legal and ethical responsibility of confidentiality.
- Situations that may legally require disclosure of information include intent to commit a crime, duty to warn endangered persons, evidence of child abuse, initiation of involuntary hospitalization, and infection by HIV.
- The client receiving mental health care has the right to report a complaint against any professional involved in providing treatment. It is the responsibility of the health care team to provide the contact information to the client.
- Nurses are accountable for adhering to the standard of care outlined in the Nurse Practice Act for the level in which they are practicing.
- The nurse has a legal and ethical responsibility to act as a client advocate to protect clients and the rights legally afforded to them.
- A voluntary commitment to inpatient mental health care indicates the client's willingness to comply with the treatment program.
- Involuntary commitment occurs when the client is admitted to a psychiatric unit against his or her will. This requires an OPC issued by a court official.
- Under federal guidelines, the client receiving mental health care must be cared for in the least restrictive environment possible.
- Seclusion refers to placement of a client in a controlled environment to treat a clinical emergency in which the individual may pose a threat to themselves or to others. Continuous monitoring and time limits are required with discontinuance if ineffective or at the earliest indication the client has regained control.
- Restraining a client can include physical restraints such as the use of mechanical devices, or chemical restraints, which refers to the use of medications to calm the client and prevent the need for physical restraint.
- Nurses should be familiar with the legal implications, facility rules, and state laws of seclusion and restraint to avoid any probable cause of wrongful liability.
- The purpose of outpatient mental health care is to provide services to individuals, families, and the community that will promote mental health and quality of life.
- Nurses encounter those who need emotional and psychosocial care in a variety of health care settings other than psychiatric units.
- Physical illness can create a psychological response that may interfere with treatment, result in an exacerbation of the illness, or delay a recovery.
- Clients with a dual diagnosis of a medical condition and a mental illness require that needs related to both situations are assessed and met in systematic care of the client.
- Nurses who work in a correctional facility must learn to separate manipulative behavior from that which is a legitimate health care need in the client who is confined within the criminal justice system.

Bibliography

AGS Foundation for Health in Aging. (2012). Making your wishes known. Accessed October 30, 2014, from http://www.healthinaging.org/making-your-wishes-known/

American Mental Health Counselors Association. (2010). *AMHCA Code of Ethics* (Revised 2010). Retrieved December 14, 2013, from www.amhca.org/code/

American Psychiatric Association. (2013). *Diagnostic and statistical manual of mental disorders* (5th ed.). Washington, DC: American Psychiatric Publishing.

Barry, C. L., Huskamp, H. A., & Goldman, H. H. (2010). A political history of federal mental health and addiction insurance parity. *The Milbank Quarterly, 88*(3), 404–433. Retrieved December 15, 2013, from http://www.ncbi.nlm.nih.gov/pmc/articles/PMC2950754/

National Institute of Mental Health (NIMH). *Getting help: Locate services.* Retrieved December 14, 2013, from www.nimh.nih.gov/health/topics

Samenow, S. E. (1984). *Inside the criminal mind.* New York, NY: Random House, Inc.

Simon, R. I. (2001). *Concise guide to psychiatry and the law for clinicians.* Washington, DC: American Psychiatric Publishing, Inc.

Stefan, S. (2001). *Unequal rights: Discrimination against people with mental disabilities and the American Disabilities Act.* Washington, DC: American Psychological Association.

Texas Department of State Health Services. Patient's bill of rights. (*Updated December 20, 2011*). Retrieved December 15, 2013, from http://www.dshs.state.tx.us/mhsa-rights/

Student Worksheet

Fill in the Blank

Fill in the blank with the correct answer.

1. The development of _____ medications allowed behaviors and symptoms to be controlled without restraints and surgery.

2. _____ was the first trained psychiatric nurse in the United States.

3. _____ refers to a set of principles or values that provide dignity and respect to clients.

4. _____ _____ is a signed statement of understanding that provides protection for both the client and the agency providing the services.

5. _____ refers to the client's right to prevent written or verbal communications from being disclosed to outside parties without authorization.

6. Although some types of crimes are viewed by psychiatric professionals as related to mental instability, the common link between criminals is the difference in their _____.

Matching

Match the following terms to the most appropriate phrase.

1. _____ Omnibus Budget Reform Act
2. _____ Thorazine (chlorpromazine)
3. _____ Accountability
4. _____ Nurse Practice Act
5. _____ Seclusion
6. _____ Chemical restraint
7. _____ Manipulation

a. Purposeful self-serving behavior directed at getting needs met
b. Placement in controlled environment
c. First antipsychotic drug developed
d. Taking responsibility for own actions
e. Prevented inappropriate placement of mentally ill in nursing homes
f. Use of medication to control behavior
g. Defines the scope of nursing practice

Multiple Choice

Select the best answer from the multiple-choice items.

1. Which of the following pioneers worked diligently to secure legislation to help in the construction of mental hospitals with standards for care?
   a. Dorothea Dix
   b. Linda Richards
   c. Florence Nightingale
   d. Harriett Bailey

2. In which of the following situations would obtaining an OPC be appropriate?
   a. Client is hallucinating
   b. Client is exhibiting sexually inappropriate behavior
   c. Client's mental state is a danger to self or others
   d. Client is angry and verbally hostile

3. The nurse is caring for a client who has recently been diagnosed with leukemia. Which of the following should the nurse include in a psychological assessment of this client?
   a. Available coping behaviors
   b. Relaxation techniques
   c. Consistency of caregivers
   d. Explanation of diagnostic tests

4. The nurse is doing a psychiatric evaluation for an inmate of a correctional facility. Which of the following factors would indicate a need for referral and further evaluation?
a. Has difficulty sleeping well
b. Anger toward the justice system
c. Previous treatment for depression
d. Ambivalent feelings about other inmates

5. A client who is seen in the emergency room for acute symptoms of anxiety and situational crisis. The examining physician asks that arrangements be made to refer this client to a mental health clinic for counseling. This action by the physician recognizes which of the client rights to appropriate treatment?
a. To accept or refuse treatment
b. Know qualifications of professionals involved in care
c. To receive explanations of treatment
d. To be treated in least restrictive setting

6. In which of the following situations would it be considered legally appropriate to disclose client information?
a. Wife of client calls and asks for medications her husband is receiving
b. Court hearing for client with a history of mental illness who is charged with rape
c. Nurse who works part-time on your unit asks about a client's progress
d. Media inquires if person involved in accident has been admitted for treatment

7. A nurse working on an inpatient unit hears a client shouting at other clients in the hallway. Knowing the client has a history of aggressive behavior, which of the following actions should the nurse initiate initially?
a. Check the physician's orders for sedative medication directive
b. Warn the client seclusion will be necessary if action continues
c. Attempt to de-escalate the situation and redirect other clients
d. Allow the clients to work through the conflict on their own

8. After repeated attempts to secure cooperative behavior from a client who is aggressively acting out, the nurse notifies the physician for restraint orders. Which of the following restraint orders would be the least restrictive?
a. Antipsychotic and sedating medication
b. Seclusion until behavior is controlled
c. Sedation followed by seclusion
d. Five-point physical restraints

9. For which of the following behaviors would the nurse recognize seclusion as an inappropriate intervention for behavior management?
a. Continued verbal aggression toward staff and other clients
b. Physical aggression toward nurse and other personnel
c. Client who continues to threaten suicidal intent
d. Disruptive behavior during sessions of group therapy

10. The nurse is admitting a client with bipolar disorder to the psychiatric unit. The nurse assesses a lack of orientation and delusional thought processes during the admission process. When explaining client rights and unit policies, it would be important for the nurse to do which of the following?
a. Go over the information more than once to reinforce content
b. Wait until a later time when client is more rational
c. Include a family member or guardian in the explanation
d. Ask a co-worker to witness the conveyance of information

Chapter 5

Treatment of Mental Illness

⊙ Learning Objectives

After learning the content in this chapter, the student will be able to:

1. Describe the goals of treatment in the mental health setting.
2. Identify socioeconomic and cultural barriers to seeking treatment for mental disorders.
3. Define what is meant by a therapeutic milieu.
4. Differentiate between roles and responsibilities of the mental health team members.
5. Discuss the role of the nurse in the psychotherapeutic process.
6. Identify the basic principles of common psychotherapeutic treatment methods.
7. Identify the function of psychopharmacology in the psychotherapeutic treatment regimen.
8. Name five classes of psychotropic drug agents.
9. Describe relationship between psychotropic drugs and neurotransmitters.
10. Discuss effects of psychotropic agents in older clients.

⊙ Key Terms

behavioral therapy
biofeedback
biomedical therapy
clinical psychologist
cognitive therapy
contracting
electroconvulsive therapy (ECT)
group therapy
humanistic therapy
neurotransmitter

postsynaptic receptors
presynaptic compartment
psychiatrist
psychodynamic therapy
psychotherapy
psychotropic
reuptake
synaptic cleft
telemental health
therapeutic milieu

Treatment of mental health issues aims to reduce the symptoms of mental disorders and to allow the person with mental illness to live and function in society with improved personal and interpersonal skills. Trained professionals help clients to identify and change current behavior or thought patterns that adversely affect their lives. This treatment gives the client the opportunity to set realistic goals for living. Specific treatment goals are set collaboratively by the health care team and the client.

Various approaches to treatment have evolved to meet the individual needs of clients and their families. Treatment methods may include medications, counseling, various types of psychotherapy, or other means that are available. This chapter will discuss the components of mental health treatment. Integral to the development of a treatment plan in mental health care are the therapeutic milieu, the professionals who serve as members of the treatment team, and the more common modalities or types of therapy that are used in the psychotherapeutic process.

Establishing a Therapeutic Milieu

In mental health care, a **therapeutic milieu** is a safe and secure structured environment that facilitates the therapeutic interaction between clients and members of the professional team. This combination of a social and encouraging environment provides a supportive network in which there is a sense of common goals. In one situation, this setting might be the client's individual room, or in another, it could be a dayroom designed to encourage interaction between clients and the support team. Dayrooms often include overstuffed comfortable furniture; tables and chairs for games, puzzles, reading; and arcade games such as air hockey or pool tables. These types of activities lend themselves to fulfill goals of participation in acceptable social behaviors and communication skills. Group activities are scheduled that maximize the functional ability of each client, and clients are encouraged to be as independent as possible during treatment. The nurse is often in a position to maintain the milieu as a place where dignity and acceptance allow the client to practice skills without reprisal.

Because of time spent with the client, the nurse is also a role model for social behaviors and communication skills, which reinforces the trusting relationship needed for successful treatment. The nurse is seen as someone who will listen and assist the client with difficult situations that arise in his or her day-to-day efforts toward improved mental functioning. The support provides an encouraging climate for growth and change.

To establish a safe and structured therapeutic milieu, rules are often needed. In the inpatient setting, explaining unit rules or policies to the client and significant others during the admission process helps to establish a sense of client trust. These rules may vary from facility to facility but usually include topics such as the following:

- Hours of visitation and client approval for certain persons to visit
- Types and times for therapy sessions
- Personal free time
- Mealtimes and bedtime
- Caffeine restrictions, available food or snack items
- Shaving or cosmetic items
- Sharp items, cords, and belts
- Violent or threatening behaviors
- Medication schedule
- Activities
- Telephone privileges

Close supervision is necessary to maintain compliance with all unit rules. It is important for each member of the mental health team to maintain consistency in enforcing these rules to establish limits and boundaries for behavior. Clients are encouraged to comply with all the rules and to attend all activity and therapy sessions.

In outpatient settings such as therapeutic community groups, nurse leaders give clients the opportunity to voice complaints, concerns, or feedback regarding the staff, other clients, or the environment in general. The security of a safe environment to express these feelings is essential. The group leader establishes and maintains guidelines for behavior in a consistent manner. This structured milieu helps the client toward improved social skills and functioning as a member of society. The client learns how to express concerns in a rational and acceptable manner as well as tolerance and acceptance of the views of others.

Client behaviors such as aggression and physical violence, foul language, or inappropriate confrontation are not tolerated in a therapeutic milieu. Clients are encouraged to express thoughts and feelings they experience during times when these actions occur. Interventions are used to help the client identify the unacceptable behavior and develop constructive approaches to deal with similar situations in the future. This provides the client with a way to effectively manage self-control toward behavior modification.

Just the Facts

Nurses assess both adaptive and maladaptive behaviors and collaborate with clients to identify behaviors that need to change.

Mind Jogger

What benefit could there be to moving a client who has been discharged from an inpatient setting to a group home milieu instead of returning to the general social climate?

Treatment Team

Within the various mental health care settings, health and social service professionals work together to provide a diversified treatment plan of care with a common goal. Each team member has a specific role in the treatment process. Because each of the members may have contact with the client in a different circumstance, it is important to have collaborative meetings in which each member can provide insight and any new information about the client (Fig. 5.1). Such meetings enhance the holistic approach to optimize the

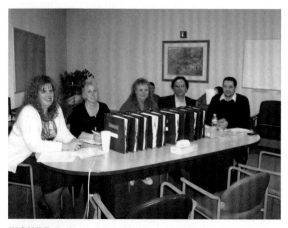

FIGURE 5.1

This treatment team, which includes a social worker, recreation therapist, nurse, psychiatrist, and clinical psychologist, meets regularly to coordinate client care. (Photo used with permission from Allegiance Behavioral Health, Plainview, Texas.)

BOX 5.1

The Mental Health Treatment Team

- Psychiatrist
- Clinical psychologist
- Registered nurse
- Licensed practical/vocational nurse
- Mental health technician
- Social worker
- Licensed professional counselor
- Case managers and outreach workers
- Therapeutic recreation specialist
- Occupational therapist
- Religious advisor

---

treatment pathway. The frequency of the meetings will depend on the individual needs or problems the client is experiencing, but they are often daily or weekly meetings. The exchange of ideas focuses on what will be the best approach to facilitate a positive outcome for each person. Discharge planning is also a topic during the meeting. From time of admission, all strategies are aimed toward discharge as an outcome.

Interdisciplinary Team Members

While the physician or psychiatrist is considered the foundation of the treatment team approach, there are many other professionals who contribute to working toward the best possible outcome for any particular client. Box 5.1 lists members of the treatment team.

Psychiatrist

A **psychiatrist** is a licensed physician who specializes in psychiatric or mental disorders. A board-certified physician has passed the examination of the American Board of Psychiatry and Neurology. A psychiatrist can evaluate, diagnose, and treat all types of mental illness, including pharmacological, biomedical, and psychotherapeutic interventions. Some psychiatrists subspecialize in the pediatric, adolescent, or geriatric populations. Others may specialize in the area of substance abuse and addiction disorders. As physicians, psychiatrists are licensed to prescribe medications in addition to providing individual psychotherapy. The settings in which they offer services may include hospitals, outpatient clinics, geriatric-psychiatric units, private practice offices, or schools and other institutions, in which they work on a consultation basis.

Clinical Psychologist

Clinical psychologists administer and interpret psychological testing that can be used in the diagnostic process. Most licensed clinical psychologists have received a master's or doctoral level degree specializing in psychology with advanced training and field requirements. A clinical psychologist also provides individual, family, marital, and group therapies to assist in the resolution of mental health issues. Licensed psychologist can work independently or as a member of the mental health team. They work in private practice settings, hospitals, outpatient clinics, schools, research institutions, and other settings that provide mental health services.

Just the Facts

Clinical psychologists often refer clients to psychiatrists for medication to accompany the counseling or treatment being provided.

Psychiatric Nurse

Psychiatric nursing is a specialized area of nursing practice that focuses on the prevention and treatment of mental health–related problems. Most psychiatric nurses are registered nurses (RNs), with some advanced-practice nurses (APRNs) working in specialized areas such as geriatric psychology, consultation, and administration.

- The RN may have an associate degree, diploma, or bachelor's degree in nursing. APRNs have at least a master's or doctoral degree in nursing. In the psychiatric setting, the RN is accountable for both the physical and mental health care of the client. The RN is responsible for developing the individualized care plan and ensuring that it is implemented within a safe and therapeutic environment. APRNs may diagnose and treat mental illnesses in some settings.
- The licensed practical/vocational nurse (LPN/LVN) has received a certificate in practical/vocational nursing from an approved college-based, technical, or hospital-based program. The LPN/LVN assists in all aspects of the nursing process, and may be responsible for basic nursing care such as observing behaviors and collecting data, administering medications, monitoring for medication side effects, participating in therapeutic communication

with clients, and documenting in the client record. The nurse is often able to establish and maintain a therapeutic relationship with the client while performing basic nursing interventions such as vital signs, dressing changes, or assisting with hygiene needs. The nurse works closely with other members of the mental health care team to facilitate the best possible rehabilitative efforts for the clients. (See the section titled Role of the Nurse later in the chapter for a more detailed discussion of specific nursing responsibilities.)

Mental Health Technician

A mental health technician assists clients with physical and hygiene needs as needed, monitors unit activities, and assists with group or recreational activities. Technicians usually receive on-the-job training and typically have at least a high school education. Some may have additional studies at the vocational, technical, or college level. Some people with baccalaureate degrees in psychology or related fields may also be employed in this capacity.

Social Worker

Licensed clinical social workers (LCSWs) are trained as client advocates and usually have a master's or doctoral level degree in their discipline. They are responsible for providing referrals, acting as a client liaison with government and civil agencies, and helping individuals with daily living problems and readjustments to living in society. The LCSW often works with placement agencies, such as community group homes and nursing homes, to secure a continued support and care system for the client who is unable to live in an independent or home setting. Some LCSWs specialize in specific areas such as domestic violence, rape and abuse, or substance abuse.

Licensed Professional Counselor

Licensed professional counselors (LPCs) have a master's level degree in psychology with specialized training and licensure in professional counseling. Counseling incorporates approaches that best meet the needs of the client to resolve problem areas toward a more satisfying and rewarding lifestyle. Counselors may specialize in areas such as marital and family counseling or substance abuse, and they may work in various community settings and schools or in private practice.

Case Manager and Outreach Worker

Agencies such as mental health centers, psychosocial rehabilitation programs, and government agencies employ case management and outreach workers to monitor and ensure that a client's needs are met. Most individuals with severe mental illness need medical care, social services, housing, and financial assistance. Case managers and outreach workers provide assistance in securing these services. They also provide follow-up support to ensure the client's ability to live in the community setting.

Religious Counselor

Pastoral or religious counselors provide spiritual support and counseling for clients and their families. They participate in treatment team meetings, therapy sessions, and discharge planning.

Therapeutic Recreation Specialist

Therapeutic recreation specialists use various approaches such as art, music, leisure education, and recreation participation to help clients make the most of their lives physically, mentally, and socially. These specialists have either a bachelor's or a master's degree, receive national certification, and are licensed or certified by the state in which they work. Recreation therapy provides ways for people to help themselves and to feel good about their improvements in the areas of concentration, decision-making, and completion of task-oriented projects. These accomplishments help to enhance the client's self-confidence and improve their ability to work in a team environment with improved social and communication skills.

Occupational Therapist

Occupational therapists have a bachelor's or master's level degree in occupational therapy and work with clients to improve their level of functioning for everyday living. Occupational therapists use activities such as cooking, money management, grocery shopping, and transportation to improve the client's self-esteem and promote a realistic level of independent living. Occupational therapists work with other members of the treatment team toward rehabilitation and discharge planning.

Dietician

Dieticians usually have a master's level degree in nutrition and serve as a resource person by providing nutrition information and counseling to clients with specific nutritional problems and needs.

Mind Jogger

What is the therapeutic benefit of a collaborative team approach to mental health care?

Role of the Nurse

At the hub of the mental health team, the nurse functions in a variety of different roles. The nurse assesses, evaluates, and interacts with clients on a day-to-day basis and also serves as a liaison between the client and therapist or physician. The nurse–client relationship provides multiple opportunities for the nurse to obtain information that is often a vital resource to other team members. The nurse is a vital component of maintaining a therapeutic milieu that supports and encourages clients in appropriate behavioral responses. In addition, the nurse models and assists the client with communication skills and social interactions with others in the milieu Fig. 5.2.

The nurse is an important source of unbiased and nonjudgmental support for the client. How the nurse perceives the client and the client's behavior can be influenced by the nurse's psychological state at the time of the assessment. The nurse is able to maintain an objective view of the client's situation by understanding his or her own feelings and emotional responses toward the client. Ongoing self-assessment, allows the nurse to separate reaction from therapeutic action and remain focused on ways to promote a positive outcome for the client and their family.

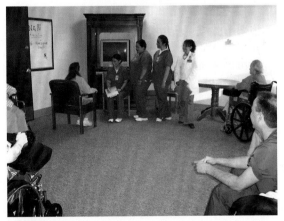

FIGURE 5.2

Student vocational nurses practice communicating with a client during clinical training. (Photo used with permission from Allegiance Behavioral Health, Plainview, Texas.)

> ### Just the Facts
> The nurse's psychological state can influence the nurse's perception of the client and the intended behavioral message.

The Nurse as Caregiver

The nursing process provides the foundation for the implementation of all nursing interventions. Basic to the nursing assessment is the observation of appropriate and inappropriate behaviors, noting both precipitating factors and situational reinforcers. The nurse documents this information in the client record and provides feedback for other members of the mental health care team for evaluating effectiveness and progress of the treatment plan. The nurse often observes a response to therapy while performing other nursing interventions such as medication administration, physical assessment, or personal care assistance. It is important for the nurse to positively reinforce appropriate behavior and encourage clients to participate in all aspects of the psychotherapeutic process.

The Nurse as Counselor

Nurses are often the person who is available and willing to provide an attitude of genuine concern for the client through active listening and therapeutic communication. The nurse should encourage the client to openly express feelings and thoughts without reprisal. Although not all behavior is acceptable, the nurse must separate inappropriate behavior from the client. Unconditional acceptance of the client as a person is imperative to a therapeutic outcome.

The Nurse as Educator

Nurses are often the link between clients and information about their illnesses and treatment. Compliance with treatment is more probable when clients are informed about the problem and how the treatment works. The nurse needs to provide education at the client's level of understanding through verbal explanation, demonstration, and printed materials about the illness and treatment regime. It is important for the nurse to evaluate the client's understanding of the instructions by verbal response or return demonstration.

The Nurse as Advocate

As a client advocate, the nurse functions to protect the rights of the client through acceptance and support for decisions that are made. Compliance with treatment usually improves as the nurse demonstrates an empathetic positive regard for client needs. Empathy involves the nurse's willingness to understand the situation from the client's perspective. By being willing to listen, the nurse is able to view a problem through the client's eyes and assist in providing the resources necessary for the client to make a decision.

> ### Mind Jogger
> How would the nurse support a client's decision if that choice is contradictory to the suggested treatment?

Types of Therapy

Specific types of therapies are selected based on the treatment plan and goals determined by the mental health treatment team and the client. Common types of treatment for psychiatric disorders include pharmacological treatment, psychotherapy, biomedical therapy, electroconvulsive therapy (ECT), and others. The most common treatment approach for individuals with mental illness is the use of psychotherapeutic drugs in conjunction with psychotherapy.

Psychotherapy

Psychotherapy is a dialog between a mental health practitioner and the client with a goal of reducing the symptoms of the emotional disturbance or disorder and improving that individual's personal and social well-being. The aim of this dialog is not to give advice, but to allow clients to learn about themselves, their life, and their feelings, and to make choices toward change. The intent is for clients to rediscover their own person, their priorities, and inner courage to act on these priorities. Credible psychotherapy fosters insight into feelings, behavior, and interpersonal skills with success resting in the quality, not the type, of therapy method used. Most clinical licensed mental health practitioners embrace an eclectic theoretical orientation, meaning their belief is in using components of many types of therapies, which they in turn, use in their practice. People are complex beings with diverse and unique individual problems that are more successfully addressed by a flexible approach.

Today, there is a current trend toward the use of psychological **telemental health** or telehealth interventions that use a focus on web camera–based intervention. Telemental health is the use of electronic and telecommunication technology to manage long-distance health care to many rural and underserved areas. In mental health, there is growing research that suggests this type of therapy may be more successful, especially with children and adolescents, than traditional face-to-face intervention.

When telemental health is initiated, a face-to-face intake history, identification, and head-to-toe assessment are usually done by a psychologist or physician. Once the client is established, video and audio technology can be used to monitor progress toward goals and review medication effectiveness. The client, family, and/or other significant individuals are in a room with a video–audio camera. The screen is visible to the physician or therapist who can also interact with the client and/or family via the camera. This allows the physician to view behavior and/or symptoms that relate to that client's situation. In the case of children, there may be specific toys or tables that allow the clinician to observe development and other behaviors. For those who are reluctant to seek traditional psychotherapy, telemental health may offer a more cost-effective alternative by which the client can answer questions more honestly on a camera or computer than face-to-face. On the other hand, some clinicians are concerned that camera-based intervention lacks the ability to establish an effective rapport with the client that in turn promotes a successful clinical relationship and compliance with treatment.

Regardless of the method used, psychotherapy is successful when issues in the person's life are uncovered and energy and power are released to allow constructive change. An important variable in this success is the relationship between the client and therapist, as well as how the client views this relationship. Various types of approaches have proven to be comparably effective, although each may have its advantages and disadvantages in different client situations.

Just the Facts

Therapeutic intervention begins with the assumption that everyone can experience functional growth in interpersonal relationships and the demands of daily living.

Individual Psychotherapy

There are five main approaches to individual therapy: psychodynamic, humanistic, behavioral, cognitive, and contracting. **Psychodynamic therapy** is primarily based on psychoanalytic theory, or the assumption that when a client has insight into early relationships and experiences as the source of his or her problems they can be resolved. It is further assumed that these experiences can be analyzed to resolve current emotional problems. This Freudian-based therapy characteristically lasts several years with biweekly sessions.

Humanistic therapy centers on the client's view of the world and his or her problems. The goal is to help clients realize their full potential through the therapist's genuineness, unconditional positive regard, and empathetic understanding of the client's point of view, which foster the client's sense of self-worth. This therapy is nondirective but focuses on helping the client to explore and clarify his or her own feelings and choices, while emphasizing potential and individual strengths.

Behavioral therapy does not foster awareness but emphasizes the principles of learning with positive or negative reinforcement and observational modeling. The goal is to bring about behavioral change within a relatively short time. In this therapy, the behavior or symptom is the problem. The underlying belief is that the original causes of maladaptive behavior may have little to do with present factors invoking the behavior. It is primarily used to treat mood and anxiety disorders, but can also be used successfully in other disorders such as attention deficit hyperactive disorder (ADHD) and some addictive conditions.

The therapist formulates and executes a plan of treatment, often with a variety of exercises for the client to perform between sessions. Gradual exposure or systematic desensitization to an anxiety-producing situation (such as in phobias) may be used along with relaxation exercises (e.g., breathing, visualization, or meditation). The therapist teaches and models skills for real-life situations with emphasis on what works best in specific symptom situations. Other techniques that may be used include contracting based on positive reinforcement or reward for desired behaviors, and role-playing behaviors. It is important that reinforcement schedules, limits, and consequences be consistently followed.

Cognitive behavioral therapy (CBT), is based on the cognitive model that focuses on identifying and correcting distorted thinking patterns that can lead to emotional distress and problem behaviors. Cognitive therapists believe that clients respond in stressful situations based on their subjective perception of an event. Once the misperception is identified, clients can change their behaviors by changing their maladaptive thinking about themselves and their experiences.

Albert Ellis was the first to consider the client's irrational thoughts as the cause of existing psychological problems. He developed the pioneering form of CBT called rational emotive behavior therapy (REBT). REBT is based on the idea that it is primarily our thinking about the world around us that leads to our emotional and behavioral distress. These irrational thoughts tend to be in the form of "musts," "oughts," or "shoulds" that create anger, depression, low self-esteem, and other psychological problems. Hence, we often choose to respond to these unreasonable thoughts with behaviors in which we actually create our own consequences and disappointments. REBT therapists attempt to help clients to identify and change these unrealistic thoughts and beliefs and replace them with positive rational thinking that can lead to a more reasonable and satisfying way of living.

Aaron Beck also based his cognitive therapy on this premise that how we think influences our feelings and actions. CBT is a combination of using this approach to help the client modify his or her dysfunctional thinking which will subsequently change the client's feelings and behavior. CBT therapists teach clients problem-solving skills and stress-reducing methods. Techniques may include self-monitoring logs and homework that work toward mutually set goals. Clients learn that their psychological difficulties or problems can be solved through cognitive processing.

Contracting is a behavioral technique in which the client and therapist draw up a contract to which both parties are obligated. The contract requires the client to demonstrate specific behaviors that are included in the therapy. In exchange, the therapist will give certain rewards the client has requested. The criteria for success are clearly outlined in the contract.

Mind Jogger

In what situations might contracting be beneficial for managing problem behavior?

Group Therapy

In **group therapy**, a trained and competent therapist leads a small group of people with similar problems who discuss individual and common issues. Group sizes range from 3 to 4 up to 20. Remedial groups are concerned with individuals who are not coping effectively with the stresses and strains of living. These groups can assist individuals in learning age-appropriate ways to manage behavior or regain self-control, skills for conflict resolution, problem solving, and interpersonal socialization and communication. Groups often must work through negative content before positive results can surface. The success of the group interaction depends on the degree of trust, openness, and interpersonal risk taking among the members. Interaction between members allows each to hear from others about their perceptions and behavior, either confirming or contradicting these self-views. Arguments and debates often indicate the attempt of each member to validate his or her own sense of reality.

Couples therapy is a highly effective group model used in helping couples resolve interpersonal conflict and initiate enhanced communication skills. In cases of marital conflict, the therapy tends to be most effective if the differences are of short-term duration. The therapist facilitates by listening to points of view and reality expressed by both partners.

Family therapy involves discussions and sessions designed to assist members with problem-solving skills within the family system. The problem may lie with all family members (e.g., troubled communication among family members) or center on the behavior of one particular person. The underlying belief is that individual problems originate from the family system. To treat the basic issue, the whole family must undergo therapy. The goal is to facilitate and encourage the family to work together, listen to, and respect each other as they gain an understanding of how their behaviors affect the entire family.

Biomedical Therapy

Biomedical therapy is the use and application of biological and natural sciences to treat psychological disorders. A form of biomedical therapy using psychopharmacotherapy has benefited many clients with mental disturbances and disorders. The use of drugs is often combined with psychotherapy for a more successful outcome. The medication prescribed depends on the disorder being treated and the client's overall medical condition.

Electroconvulsive Therapy

Electroconvulsive therapy (ECT) is a biomedical treatment using low-voltage electric shock waves passed through the brain to induce short periods of seizure activity. The seizures appear to aid in restoring a chemical balance within the brain, which helps to relieve the serious symptoms of mental illness. Some conditions where this type of therapy may be used include major depression, psychosis, bipolar disorder, catatonia, and severe suicidal ideation. ECT is generally reserved for clients with severe mental illness that is unresponsive to medications and other forms of therapeutic intervention. Treatment is voluntary, and the client must give informed consent.

During ECT, the electric shock is given for several seconds to cause the seizure activity. It is administered along with general anesthesia and muscle relaxants to minimize the risk and negative impact on the client. The adjunctive use of medication helps to prevent the seizure from impacting the entire body, and to prevent severe muscle contractions that can inadvertently result in fractures or dislocated bones. ECT is usually given two to three times a week, typically lasting no longer than 6 to 12 treatments. Use of therapy may vary in the electrode placement and the type and exposure time of the electrical stimulus. Adverse effects include temporary memory loss, headache, hypotension, tachycardia, and confusion. Most confusion clears within hours after the treatment, while memory loss may be more persistent. Studies continue regarding the long-term effects of ECT.

Other Types of Therapy

Biofeedback is a training program used for specific types of anxiety that is designed to develop the client's ability to control heart rate, muscle tension, and other autonomic or involuntary functions of the nervous system by using monitoring devices during situations that trigger this reaction. This is followed by an attempt or feedback that allows the person to reproduce the desired change and control these body functions under the anxiety-producing emotional circumstances. Biofeedback works best if used consistently. Neurobiofeedback is currently being used in the treatment of attention deficit disorder.

Agitation therapy may be used in problematic and aggressive people who do not respond positively to other therapies. The person is exposed to external agitation from other clients in a controlled atmosphere. This is designed to increase that person's self-awareness of maladaptive behavior and limitations. The goals of this therapy are to teach sublimation of aggression and anger impulses with insight and a willingness to change. The desired outcome is for the client to achieve control over his or her behavior and assume responsibility for emotional and social growth. It is often used in combination with other types of therapy.

Play therapy is often used with children and allows the therapist to treat the child during the dynamic process of play. The therapist assesses the child's internal affective state and psychological response during the various stages of the treatment process. With the activity techniques used, the child can more easily express emotions and feelings if they are unable to do in words.

The attachment that is formed between humans and animals has led to the use of *pet therapy*. Old and young alike are drawn to the unconditional response and affection of animals. An animal can stimulate a client to interact with another person by creating a subject for conversation. Petting the animal also brings the comfort of touch and the acceptance the client feels from the animal. Pet therapy may be used in treating children and adolescents, and has widespread use in nursing homes and geriatric psychiatric facilities.

Other adjunctive therapies may include occupational, recreational, and creative art therapies. These provide a relaxed atmosphere in which the client is often able to express emotions and feelings that may be subdued during other forms of therapy. Recreational therapy provides an outlet for sublimating frustration and internal drives of emotion, along with encouraging social interactive skills. In the clinical setting, participation in all forms of therapy sessions is encouraged to provide the client with every opportunity for maximum benefit of treatment.

Pharmacological Agents and Mental Illness

Throughout history, there have been efforts that aim to treat psychiatric disorders using both drugs and various approaches in psychotherapy. Early pharmacotherapy used plants (e.g., the purple fox-glove, *Digitalis purpurea;* the opium poppy; and the antimalarial compound quinine from the bark of the cinchona tree), mineral salts, and herbs. Over time, a more scientific approach evolved in under-standing the molecular components of drugs taken from natural sources. These advances in chemistry and human physiology led to the modern branch of pharmacology and laboratory origin of most drugs.

Today, the major approach to the treatment of psychiatric disorders is the use of psychothera-peutic drugs used in conjunction with psycho-therapy. Developing drugs to treat the cause of a particular psychiatric disorder is difficult because the actual causes of most disorders have not been identified; in most cases, a pattern of both genetic and environmental factors predisposes a person to the development of a particular illness. Regardless of the etiology, the psychiatric disorders are con-sidered to be medical illnesses with typical signs and symptoms. Therefore, drug developers have focused on treating the symptoms of these disor-ders, rather than the cause.

Symptom Categories of Psychiatric Disorders

Medically, the disorders tend to present an aggre-gate of symptoms often referred to as a *syndrome.* Much as a group of symptoms characterize the ill-nesses such as diabetes or gastroesophageal reflux, the symptoms of the psychiatric disorders are rec-ognizable and linked to the particular disorders as described by the *DSM-5.* The most common symptoms fall into the following categories:
- Mood alterations
- Irritability and anxiety
- Altered thought processes
- Misperceptions of the environment
- Impaired and illogical communication or interaction patterns
- Disorientation and confusion

Since the 1950s, the development of drug agents for psychiatric disorders has provided symptomatic relief for many people. **Psycho-tropic** agents, also called **psychoactive** drugs, have their impact on target sites or receptors of the nervous system to induce changes that affect psychiatric function, behavior, or experience. **Psychopharmacology** refers to the study of the changes that occur as the drugs interact with the chemicals in the brain. These drug agents have provided a sense of normalcy for many clients

with altered feelings, perceptions, and thinking. The use of psychotropic agents has also expanded our understanding of how the brain and mind are affected by psychiatric disorders. These drugs do not cure or resolve the underlying problem. Rather, they are used in combination with coun-seling and other therapeutic modalities to reduce the disabling symptoms and promote restoration of a manageable and functional level of existence. Most clients with psychiatric disorders require a combination of two drugs to maintain stability.

> **Mind Jogger**
> How does the nurse play a key role in enhanc-ing the benefits of psychotropic drug agents for the clients who take them?

Classification of Psychotropic Drug Agents

Drugs used to treat mental disorders fall into five major categories.
- Antianxiety agents
- Antidepressants
- Antimanic agents
- Antipsychotic agents
- Antiparkinson (anticholinergic) agents

Although each drug has an individual chemical composition, each group of psychotropic agents includes drugs that are similar in their desired effect, side effects, adverse effects, and related properties. The categories and their characteris-tics, along with normal dosage ranges and related nursing responsibilities or interventions, will be discussed in Chapters 9, 10, and 11.

Action of Psychotropic Drugs on Neurotransmitters

Psychotropic drug agents have their primary effect on neurotransmitter systems of the body. **Neurotransmitters** are the chemical messen-ger proteins stored in the **presynaptic compart-ment** located before the nerve synapse. There are many types of neurotransmitters that combine with individual receptors of the body. Once the neurotransmitter is mobilized into the **synaptic cleft** (the space between two neurons) it will con-tinue to activate a response in the **postsynaptic receptor** (a cell component located in the neuron distal to the synapse) until the neurotransmitter

TABLE 5.1	Basic Relationship of Neurotransmitters to Mental Disorders

NEUROTRANSMITTER	RELATIONSHIP TO MENTAL DISORDER
Acetylcholine	Decreased in Alzheimer disease
Dopamine	Decreased in Parkinson disease Increased in schizophrenia
Gamma-aminobutyric acid (GABA)	Decreased in anxiety disorders
Norepinephrine	Decreased in depression Increased in mania
Serotonin	Decreased in depression Increased in mania

is inactivated. Neurotransmitters can be inactivated either by enzymatic action or by **reuptake**. In the case of reuptake, the neurotransmitters are absorbed back into the presynaptic compartment of the previous neuron.

Psychotropic drugs are effective because they either enhance or decrease the brain's ability to use a specific neurotransmitter. Some drugs, such as the antiparkinson agents, cause the release of the neurotransmitter **acetylcholine**, which is thought to contribute to the transmission of nerve impulses at the synapse and myoneural junctions. Others, such as the antipsychotic agent clozapine, interfere with the binding of chemical messengers to the intended receptors in the brain. Lithium carbonate, a drug used in the treatment of bipolar disorders, accelerates the destruction of monoamine neurotransmitters (dopamine, norepinephrine, and serotonin), inhibits their release, and decreases the sensitivity of postsynaptic receptors. Table 5.1 identifies the link between the specific neurotransmitters and the deficiency or excess seen in common mental disorders.

infusion into the brain tissue. The selectivity of the barrier between the blood and the brain further protects the brain by regulating the extent to which the drug penetration can occur. Drugs such as alcohol, heroin, and diazepam have high lipid solubility and are readily absorbed into the cerebral cells through the blood–brain barrier, increasing their potential for abuse. By the same token, the rate at which a medicinal agent is absorbed affects its efficacy. Scientists continue to study the specific effects of individual psychotropic drugs on psychological processes and the use of these drugs in treating psychiatric disorders.

Psychotropic Drug Agents and the Older Client

For older clients who have dementia-related aggression, distressing repetitive behaviors, catastrophic reactions, delusions, hallucinations, or agitation, the use of antipsychotic drugs has become a common approach to reducing and managing the incidence of these symptoms. The Omnibus Budget Reconciliation Act (OBRA) of 1987 limited the use of psychotropic medications for residents in long-term care facilities. These guidelines have been modified but with specific diagnostic and monitoring specifications. Antipsychotic medications can cause serious side effects such extrapyramidal symptoms and tardive dyskinesia. The newer generation of psychotropic drugs is associated with fewer side effects, and they have thus become drugs of choice for older clients. Guidelines set by OBRA specify that these drugs can only be used for specific diagnoses and when behavioral and environmental measures are unsuccessful in managing symptoms. Research data on the safety and response of the older client to psychotropic medications is limited further suggesting a cautious approach to the use of these drugs.

Just the Facts

Monoamine neurotransmitters stored in presynaptic compartments of neurons in the central nervous system (CNS) include the chemical messengers norepinephrine, dopamine, and serotonin.

Senior Focus

In the elderly or older adult, the half-life of a drug tends to increase by as much as five to six times increasing the risk of toxicity. The effects accumulate slowly and may not be apparent for days or weeks following the initiation of the drug.

All drugs do not penetrate the brain cells equally. The chemical property known as *lipid solubility* is a major determinant of a drug's molecular

The impact of age-related physiological changes on antipsychotic drug therapy accounts for many of the serious side effects that occur in older adults. Many antipsychotic drugs, either by themselves or in interaction with other drugs, can cause the very symptoms they are prescribed to treat, such as agitation or delusions. Because many older clients commonly take medications for several illnesses, this situation is all too familiar. In addition, the adverse effects of one drug can be mistaken as a symptom of another condition and needlessly treated. Because older adults have a higher body fat-to-lean ratio, less serum albumin, less total-body water, fewer brain cells, and slower liver metabolism and renal clearance than young adults, they need far less of these drugs to produce a therapeutic effect. The higher fat composition of tissue increases retention of the drug resulting in effects and side effects that persist longer, sometimes even after the drug is discontinued. Because older clients have less protein to bind with the drug, more of the drug is free to circulate. A slowed metabolic rate and renal excretion time allow the drug to remain in the body longer. Table 5.2 shows these physiological changes and their imposed risk when administering a psychotropic agent.

All of these factors highlight the importance of monitoring the response to and recognizing the adverse effects of psychotropic agents in the older

TABLE 5.2   Age-Related Physiological Changes and Drugs in Older Clients

PHYSIOLOGICAL CHANGE	DRUG RISK
Higher-body fat-to-lean ratio	Increased risk of cumulative effects
Less serum albumin and protein-bound drug	More free drug in bloodstream
Less total-body water	Dehydration increases concentration of drug in body
Decreased liver metabolism	Clearance of drug is delayed or slowed
Decreased renal elimination	Slowed elimination of drug from system

client. It is extremely important that all alternative approaches be considered before the use of drugs, and that, if used, treatment is discontinued if the person is adversely affected by the drug.

Senior Focus

In the older client, always consider a new symptom or behavior may be related to drug therapy.

Summary

- Mental health care includes an umbrella of therapeutic treatment methods directed toward relieving the symptoms of mental illness and empowering the individuals to live and function within society.
- A therapeutic milieu describes an environment that provides a setting conducive to providing therapeutic interaction between clients and members of the professional team. Within this atmosphere, there is a supportive network to help the client establish common goals within safe and secure surroundings.
- The treatment team consists of professionals who work together to provide a diversified approach toward a common outcome of improved access and outcome to mental health care.
- The physician or psychiatrist is considered the foundation of the team approach, with each team member having a specific role in the holistic approach to treatment. With diversified client contact in various

circumstances, the members come together to have a collaborative meeting in which each can provide insight from their perspective.
- Collaborative team meetings are held daily or weekly to discuss new and continuing needs or problems of individual clients. The exchange focuses on the best approach to facilitate a positive outcome for each person.
- The nurse often serves as a liaison between the client and therapist or physician.
- The psychological state of the nurse can influence how the client or client behavior is perceived. Understanding these feelings and emotional responses will assist the nurse in maintaining an objective view of the client situation.
- Nursing functions in the treatment milieu include caregiver, counselor, educator, and client advocate.
- Various types of psychotherapy are used to allow clients to interact with practitioners toward a goal

of reducing the symptoms of the emotional disturbance or disorder and improving the individual's personal and social well-being.

- Therapeutic intervention begins with the assumption that everyone can experience functional growth in interpersonal relationship and the demands of societal living.
- Regardless of the method, psychotherapy is successful when issues in the person's life are uncovered and energy is released to allow constructive change.
- Biomedical therapy uses psychotherapy and pharmacological means to provide treatment. ECT may be used to treat clients with severe mental illness unresponsive to other methods of treatment.
- Other types of therapy may include biofeedback, agitation, play, pet, occupational, recreational, or creative art therapy, all of which are designed

to support varied opportunities for the client to improve his or her functioning.

- Psychotropic drug agents affect psychiatric function, behavior, or experience. They are not curative, but are used in combination with counseling and other therapeutic modalities to reduce the disabling symptoms to a manageable and functional level, allowing them to function in an adaptive role within society.
- Psychotropic drugs have a primary effect on neurotransmitter systems, either enhancing or decreasing the brain's ability to use a specific neurotransmitter.
- All psychotropic agents are used with caution in the older client because of age-related physiological changes. The drug effects persist longer and remain in the body longer. Careful monitoring is mandated to avoid the adverse consequences of their use.

Bibliography

Agens, J. E. Jr. (2010). Chemical and physical restraint use in the older person. *British Journal of Medical Practitioners, 3*(1), 34–39. Retrieved December 29, 2013.

Carbon, M. (2013). Rational use of generic psychotropic drugs. *CNS Drugs, 27*(5), 353–365. Retrieved December 28, 2013.

Davis, D., Corrin-pendry, S., & Savillo, M. (2008). A follow-up study of the long-term effects of counseling in a primary care counseling psychology service. *Counseling & Psychotherapy Research, 8*(2), 80–84. Retrieved December 28, 2013.

Levy, S., & Stachan, N. (2013). Child and adolescent mental health service providers' perceptions of using telehealth. *Mental Health Practice, 17*(1), 28–32. Retrieved January 12, 2014.

Mancama, D., & Kerwin, R. W. (2003). Pharmacogenomics; mental illness – treatment. *CNS Drugs, 3*(17), 143. Retrieved December 28, 2013.

Martens, W. H. (2001). Agitation therapy. *American Journal of Psychotherapy, 55*(2), 234–250. Retrieved December 28, 2013.

Merck Manual On-Line for Health Care Professionals (Last Revision October 2013): Pharmacokinetics in the elderly. Retrieved December 28, 2013, from http://www.merckmanuals.com/professional/index.html.

Moretti, F., Biondini, A., Bernabei, V., Dalmonte, E., Caretto, V., DeRonchi, D., & Atti, A. R. (2012). Use of psychotropic drugs in the elderly, data from an Italian population based study. *European Psychiatry, 27*(1 Suppl), 1–1. Retrieved December 28, 2013.

Perle, J. G., Langsam, L. C., Randel, A., Lutchman, S., Levine, A. B., Odland, A. P., Nierenberg, B., & Marker, C. D. (2013). Attitudes toward psychological telehealth: Current and future clinical psychologists' opinions of internet-based interventions. *Journal of Clinical Psychology, 69*(1), 100–113. Retrieved January 12, 2014.

Pinelli, E. (2003). Client-therapist relationship. *American Journal of Psychotherapy, 56*(3), 357–363. Retrieved December 28, 2013.

Sienaert, P. (2011). What we have learned about electroconvulsive therapy and its relevance for the practicing psychiatrist. *Canadian Journal of Psychiatry, 56*(1), 5–12. Retrieved December 28, 2013.

Stahl, S. M. (2012). Psychotherapy as an epigenetic 'drug': Psychiatric therapeutics target symptoms linked to malfunctioning brain circuits with psychotherapy as well as with drugs. *Journal of Clinical Pharmacy & Therapeutics, 37*(3), 249–253. Retrieved December 28, 2013.

Sternberg, R. J. (2001). *In Search of the Human Mind* (3rd ed.), Orlando, FL: Harcourt, Brace.

Wilson, B. A., Shannon, M. T., & Shields, K. (2014). *Prentice hall nurse's drug guide.* Upper Saddle River, NJ: Pearson Education, Inc.

Zervas, I. M., Theleritis, C., & Soldatos, C. R. (2012). Using ECT in schizophrenia: A review from a clinical perspective. *World Journal of Biological Psychiatry, 13*(2), 96–105. Retrieved December 28, 2013.

Student Worksheet

Fill in the Blank

Fill in the blank with the correct answer.

1. A therapeutic milieu combines a _____ and _____ environment.

2. _____ is described as a dialog between a mental health practitioner and the client with a goal of reducing the emotional symptoms and improving the client's personal and social well-being.

3. The role most closely associated with nurses is that of _____.

4. The process of working toward a common care goal that is mutually shared by the client is referred to as the _____.

5. _____ agents are drugs that affect psychic function, behavior, or experience.

6. The chemical property known as _____ is a major determinant of a drug's molecular infusion into the brain tissue.

7. Because of a higher body fat-to-lean ratio, the older client has an increased risk of _____.

Matching

Match the following terms to the most appropriate phrase.

1. _____ Neurotransmitter
2. _____ Synaptic cleft
3. _____ Therapeutic milieu
4. _____ Contracting
5. _____ Cognitive therapy
6. _____ ECT
7. _____ Behavioral therapy

a. Focuses on identifying and correcting distorted thinking patterns
b. Psychopharmacological and electroconvulsive methods of treating mental disorders
c. Behavioral method with a mutually obligated agreement between therapist and client
d. Supportive network providing a sense of common goals within safe and secure surroundings
e. Space between two neurons where neurotransmitter activity occurs
f. Chemical messenger proteins stored in presynaptic compartments
g. Fosters reinforcement and observational modeling to resolve problems

Multiple Choice

Select the best answer from the available choices.

1. The role of the nurse working with the client who has a mental disorder includes:
   a. Conducting psychological testing
   b. Daily individual psychotherapy sessions
   c. Monitoring behavioral responses to therapy
   d. Acting as a liaison with government and civil agencies

2. When caring for the client with outbursts of uncontrolled anger, which of the following nursing actions would most reinforce the desired outcome?
   a. Model an appropriate response to the situation
   b. Provide insight into the cause of the observed response
   c. Reprimand the client for the inappropriate actions
   d. Observe and document a detailed description of the incident

3. The nurse is working with a client who is to be discharged in the next few days. Which of the following mental health team members will be most involved in securing placement for the client?
   a. Mental health technician
   b. Licensed professional counselor
   c. Licensed practical/vocational nurse
   d. Clinical social worker

4. The nurse who demonstrates an empathetic positive regard for the client's needs is functioning in which of the following roles of the nurse–client relationship?
   a. Educator
   b. Advocate
   c. Counselor
   d. Caregiver

5. The nurse observes a client having thrusting tongue movements that were not present on admission and reports this to the charge nurse and the physician. In which of the following roles is the nurse functioning?
   a. Caregiver
   b. Counselor
   c. Educator
   d. Advocate

6. A client has contracted with a therapist to demonstrate decreased inappropriate language outbursts on the nursing unit. Which of the following nursing actions would best support the client toward a positive outcome?
   a. Ignore negative behaviors and report to the therapist
   b. Separating the client from other clients if outbursts occur
   c. Modeling appropriate ways to communicate feelings
   d. Reprimanding the client for language outbursts

7. A newly diagnosed client with bipolar disorder is prescribed several psychotropic drugs. Which of the following would best guide the nurse to teach the client about the actions of the medications?
   a. Psychotropic agents will resolve the underlying problems of the disorder
   b. They will reduce symptoms and assist to restore functional levels of living
   c. These drugs will restore the client to a symptom-free level of existence
   d. The medications can help to cure this illness if they are taken correctly

8. The nurse is caring for an older adult client who is taking a psychotropic agent. Which of the following is a contributing factor to the increased risk of adverse effects in this client?
   a. Slowed metabolic rate and renal excretion time
   b. Decrease in the fat composition of body tissue
   c. Increase in protein-bound drug in the bloodstream
   d. Increase in total serum albumin available for binding

9. A nurse working in an outpatient clinic is preparing an elderly client to be seen by the physician. Which of the following statements by the client would alert the nurse to a need for further questioning?
   a. "I just don't understand why I have to take all this medication."
   b. "I take so much medication every day but I just seem to feel worse later."
   c. "I just had my medication refilled so I hope the doctor doesn't change anything."
   d. "It takes me a long time to take all this medication since I take one or two at a time."

10. A nurse working in a long-term care facility is preparing to administer an antidepressant medication to an elderly client. Which of the following assessments would alert the nurse to an increased potential for accumulated effects of this drug?
    a. Client requires a walker for ambulation to the bathroom
    b. Client takes more naps than usual during the day
    c. Lack of interest in participating in group activities
    d. Dry skin with decreased intake of fluids

Chapter

6

The Nursing Process in Mental Health Nursing

⊙ Learning Objectives

After learning the content of this chapter, the student will be able to:

1. Identify the five steps of delivering nursing care using the nursing process.
2. Describe types of information obtained in a psychosocial assessment.
3. Determine applicable nursing diagnoses for identified client problems.
4. Evaluate client outcome of anticipated improvement in functioning and well-being.
5. Apply the nursing process to the care of the client in the psychiatric setting.

⊙ Key Terms

assessment
expected outcomes
evaluation
nursing diagnosis
nursing interventions

nursing process
objective data
prioritize
subjective data

Understanding the Nursing Process for Mental Health Nursing

The **nursing process** is a scientific and systematic method for providing effective individualized nursing care and serves as an aid in resolving client problems. The nursing process consists of five steps: assessment, diagnosis, planning, implementation, and evaluation (Fig. 6.1). This problem-solving approach allows the nurse to help the client achieve a maximal level of functioning and well-being. It is accepted by the nursing profession as a standard for providing ongoing nursing care that is adapted to individual client needs. Integral to this approach is an organized method of problem solving called the *care plan* or *clinical pathway*. Accountability to the client and communication between members of the mental health care team are enhanced as the care plan is developed. Use of the nursing process also allows nurses to share information that is important to the continuity of client care and treatment. The nurse can reevaluate each step of the nursing process to adjust, revise, or terminate the plan of care based on new or added information. It is important to remember that each client's response to therapy and treatment may be different. Adjustments can and will be made as the level of illness and dysfunction affects his or her independence and well-being.

Vital to the nursing process is the therapeutic climate of interaction between the client and members of the mental health team. The nurse is often the first member of the team that is in contact with the client. It is at this point that a therapeutic milieu is established. The environment is modified to create a setting in which the client feels safe, secure, and free to express feelings and thoughts without fear of rejection, retaliation, or punishment. The nurse can best build a relationship and establish a sense of trust by approaching the client in an accepting and nonjudgmental manner. A trusting link is vital to the successful outcome of the client's improved functioning and well-being.

As in other areas of nursing, the nursing process in mental health nursing is the foundation of providing care to the client through a systematic, organized approach. Since the mental health nurse is in frequent contact with the client, he or she is in an optimum position to provide new data, implement the care plan, and observe the response to treatment. In addition, the nurse is in a position to model the most effective and adaptive coping strategy available for clients through the problem-solving method used in the nursing process.

Psychosocial Assessment

Assessment, or the collection of data, begins when the client is admitted to a health care facility or contact is made for the first time, and it continues as the cycle of the nursing process progresses and new information is gained. A psychosocial assessment is usually conducted within the psychiatric setting. However, symptoms of psychosocial needs can be seen in any health care setting and, therefore are part of any nursing assessment.

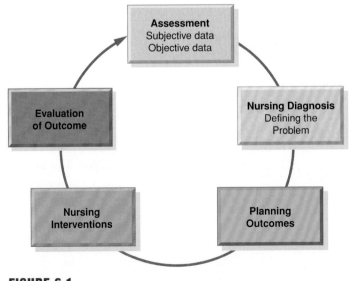

FIGURE 6.1

Steps of the nursing process.

Although the assessment is usually the responsibility of the registered nurse, assisting with the collection of data and observation is integral in the role of the licensed practical/vocational nurse.

A standard assessment tool is used to gather cognitive, emotional, and behavioral information and helps to categorize the information received he or she collects. Table 6.1 provides a summary of the components of a psychosocial assessment. (The Mini-Mental Status Exam is found

in Appendix B). A basic psychosocial assessment usually includes the client's history and mental or emotional status, and encompasses both **subjective** and **objective data**.

Subjective Data

Subjective data are provided by the client and typically include the client's history and perception of the present situation or problem, in addition to feelings, thoughts, symptoms, or emotions that he or she may be experiencing (Box 6.1). Sometimes the client's information is questioned or contradicted by information received from other sources and may need to be validated by family, friends, law enforcement officers, or others who are involved with the client.

Just the Facts

Input from the client's family can provide information about family dynamics, any present turmoil or disruption within the family, and how the client's problem may be affecting other members of the family.

When collecting subjective data, it is important for the nurse to be as accurate and descriptive as possible. Citing direct quotes from the client is a way of including what the client is saying without attempting to interpret the intended meaning. Using the client's own words to describe feelings or thoughts often provides insight into perceptual distortions or illogical thought processes.

The subjective information gathered during the initial assessment will allow the nurse to establish a baseline used to formulate the care plan. By asking direct, focused, and leading questions, the nurse gets a clear picture of certain problems or issues concerning the client. Providing a climate that ensures privacy and confidentiality affords the

TABLE 6.1	Components of Psychosocial Assessment
ASSESSMENT	**OBSERVATIONS TO INCLUDE IN DATA**
Appearance	Grooming, dress, hygiene, eye contact, skin markings, posture, facial expression
Motor activity	Pacing, slow, rigid, relaxed, restless, combative, bizarre, gait, hyperactive, retarded, aggressive
Attitude	Cooperative or uncooperative, friendly, hostile, apathetic, suspicious
Speech pattern	Speed, volume, articulation, congruence, confabulation, slurring, dysphasia
Mood	Intensity, depth, duration, anxious, sad, euphoric, labile, fearful, irritable, depressed
Affect	Flat or absence of emotional expression, blunted, congruent with mood, appropriate or inappropriate
Level of awareness	Level of consciousness, attention span, comprehension, processing
Orientation	Time, place, person
Memory	Recent or short term and remote or long term
Understanding of illness	Insight or ability to perceive and understand their illness and symptoms as related to the illness
Description of stressors	Ability to describe any internal or psychological/physical stress factors they are experiencing or an actual loss occurring in their life
Thought processes	Speed, content, organization, logical or illogical, delusions, abstract or concrete
Perception	Hallucinations, illusions, depersonalization, or distortions
Judgment	Problem-solving and decision-making ability
Adaptation	Available coping mechanisms, adaptive or maladaptive coping
Relationships	Attainment and maintenance of satisfying interpersonal relationships

client the freedom to communicate personal feelings openly. The nurse's willingness and ability to listen actively to the client are vital to the outcome of this step. Examples of leading questions that can be used to obtain data from the client during the assessment interview include the following:

- What brought you to the hospital today?
- Was there any situation that caused you to feel this way?
- How did you react to the situation?
- How you are feeling about being here?
- Where do you live?
- Who lives with you?
- What type of work do you do?
- Have you been able to work prior to admission?
- What causes the most stress in your life?
- What do you do to alleviate the stress?
- Do you blame yourself for bad things that happen to you?
- Are there things that overwhelm you each day?
- Are you currently taking medication to help you through the stressful times?

Objective Data

Objective data are observed and gathered by the nurse or provided by others who are familiar with the client including additional members of the health care team (Box 6.2). In most situations, a standardized assessment tool is used to compile this information. Assessments should include not only the factors that put the client at risk emotionally and psychologically (i.e., recent changes or stressors, history of mental disorder, drug use or abuse), but also those positive factors that suggest the likelihood that the client can recover from the current situation, such as positive coping

---

BOX 6.2

Examples of Objective Data

- Physical exam
- Behavior
- Mood and affect
- Awareness
- Thought processes
- Appearance
- Activity
- Judgment
- Response to environment
- Perceptual ability

---

strategies, a strong support system, and willingness to receive treatment.

Because the nurse is often the first person to do an admission physical assessment of the client, he or she has an opportunity to begin gathering information informally by observing nonverbal behaviors and using direct questioning. Objective data resulting from the physical assessment would include the client's medical history, past illnesses or surgeries, medication history, allergies, vital signs, height and weight, diet, and head-to-toe systems evaluation.

A psychosocial assessment is an important part of any nursing assessment, but for the mental health nurse, the purpose is to assist in specifically delineating any problems in the individual's life that could have a psychological impact on his or her immediate well-being. Social issues may include relationships, personal and or family history of mental illness, religious and cultural beliefs, and specific health practices. Often, the past medical and psychiatric histories help to identify potential problems related to the present situation.

Mind Jogger

How might a past medical and psychiatric history help to identify potential problems?

It is very important to note both verbal communication and nonverbal mannerisms, expressions, and emotions. The nurse should look for congruence between what the client is saying and what is displayed in the accompanying behavior. It is also important to recognize if the client poses any immediate threat or danger to self or others, in which case safety becomes a priority and must be secured.

Nursing Diagnosis

Establishing a nursing diagnosis from collected data is the second step in the nursing process. The nurse analyzes all data gathered and compares it to normal functioning or values to find out if a problem or a potential problem exists. A **nursing diagnosis** is not a medical diagnosis but an identification of a client problem based on conclusions about the collected data. A nursing diagnosis may be an actual or potential health problem, depending on the situation. The most commonly used standard is that of the North American

Nursing Diagnosis Association (NANDA). This is an approved list of problems that the nurse can legally address toward a measurable outcome. A list of nursing diagnoses approved by NANDA is found in Appendix C.

Formulating a nursing diagnosis consists of three parts: (1) the actual or potential problem related to the client's condition, (2) the causative or contributing factors, and (3) a behavior or symptom that supports the problem. A nursing diagnosis is correctly written as follows: (problem) risk for injury, related to (contributing factor) marital break-up, evidenced by (behavior) suicidal ideation and gestures. Although a medical diagnosis is not used as the etiology of a nursing problem, signs and symptoms of the condition may be reflected in the cause. This is illustrated by a client who has sensory perceptual alteration, related to auditory hallucinations, evidenced by talking to people who are not physically present. Determining the problem provides the groundwork for planning nursing interventions to meet the needs of the client for which the nurse is responsible.

Once applicable nursing diagnoses have been determined, they are **prioritized** according to the intensity and immediate urgency of the problem. Any health condition that endangers life will receive a high priority. Situations that are recurrent or chronic may be given a lower priority and will be addressed at a later time. A client with suicidal ideation or intent, for example, would have an immediate risk for self-injury. This problem would require the nurse's attention first. Based on Maslow's hierarchy of needs, basic physiologic needs such as oxygen, food, water, warmth, elimination, and sleep must be met before other higher level needs can be achieved. This model can be seen as a staircase in which a client may vacillate between steps. Given that the client can move up and then back down, the nurse should understand that the priority given to a problem can change at any time during the treatment process. To illustrate this concept, a client who has begun to identify strengths and display positive self-talk (self-esteem level need) is told by another client that she is stupid and ugly. The client has not refused to eat for two meals. At this point the nutritional needs of the client become the priority.

It is also important to give priority to the problem that the client is currently experiencing (actual) over a problem that may happen (potential). An actual problem has priority over one that could possible occur during the course of the illness.

Acute withdrawal symptoms in the client with multiple substance abuse would have priority over the potential for social isolation in that individual.

> **Just the Facts**
>
> Nursing diagnoses and care should be planned to include religious and cultural practices of the client.

Planning Expected Outcomes

The next phase of the nursing process involves planning measurable and realistic **expected outcomes** that anticipate the improvement or stabilization of the problem identified in the nursing diagnosis. These outcomes are defined in terms of short-term goals that address the immediate client's immediate unmet needs and long-term goals that achieve the maximal level of health that is realistic for the individual client at the time of discharge and as a member of society. These goals should be determined in collaboration with the client, so as to increase cooperation and compliance with therapeutic interventions.

Listed below are examples of both short-term and long-term outcome criteria for a common mental health nursing diagnosis: sensory/perceptual alteration, related to auditory hallucinations.

Short-Term Outcomes

- Client symptoms of auditory hallucinations will decrease within 48 hours.
- Client does not harm self or others in next 48 hours
- Client identifies feelings associated with hallucinations with each episode.
- Client reports a decrease in anxiety level within 24 hours.

Long-Term Outcomes

- Client demonstrates understanding of need for continued compliance with medication therapy by discharge.
- Client demonstrates awareness that hallucinations are the result of internal conflict within 1 week.
- Client identifies and demonstrates ways to maintain contact with reality at onset of symptoms by discharge.
- Client identifies environmental factors that precipitate the hallucinations by discharge.
- Client participates in activities that reinforce reality during hospitalization within 1 week.

Case ❻ Application 6.1

Scenario "Alone and Lost"

Matthew is a 26-year-old carpenter who up until 5 days ago was employed by a building contractor. At the time of his termination, Matthew was told by his supervisor that his work had not been consistently satisfactory and to avoid legal problems, he was being fired. Matthew has been living with his girlfriend and her two children for the past 3 years. Two days after he lost his job, his girlfriend told him she was seeing someone else and wanted him to move out. Matthew is brought to the emergency room by the police who state he was wandering around a parking lot at 2:00 AM, is disoriented and unable to tell them who he is or what he was doing in the parking lot. He told the police he is lost and doesn't know where he should go.

What subjective data should the nurse obtain from Matthew at the time of admission?

_____

_____

What objective data is available from those who know about his situation?

_____

_____

Using the nursing process, how would you develop the following nursing diagnoses?

_____

_____

Anxiety (severe), related to _____ **, evidenced by** _____.

Coping, ineffective individual, related to _____ **, evidenced by** _____.

Personal identity disturbance, related to _____ **, evidenced by** _____.

Implementation of Nursing Interventions

Nursing interventions are actions taken by the nurse to assist the client in achieving the anticipated outcome. It is important to plan actions that are appropriate for the individual client and take into consideration the level of functioning that is realistic for that person. What may be realistic for one person may be unattainable for another. The written plan is a collaborative effort between all members of the health care team and is communicated to each health care worker. This helps to ensure the continuity of care and consistency in the implementation of interventions by all personnel. Consistency is a vital component of the therapeutic milieu.

There are many clinical units that use standardized or computer-generated care plans or clinical pathways. In the current managed care concept, these are designed to be cost-effective and improve the efficiency with which treatment is carried out. Regardless of the method used, the care plan identifies the outcomes and interventions that are to be addressed by each discipline of the care team. Specifically, the nursing care plan identifies those interventions for which the nurse has responsibility. It is imperative that the unique needs and problems of each client are retained as central to that person's plan of care.

Nursing interventions that focus on mental health care do not involve intensive physical care nursing skills. Rather, the nurse focuses on observing behaviors and symptoms, improving communication strategies, and assisting the client in problem solving with improved overall functioning. Nursing interventions are implemented according to the nurse's level of practice. Achievement of the anticipated outcomes is difficult for psychiatric clients. Many require extensive reinforcement and reassurance to change behaviors and understand the underlying emotional issues. Box 6.3 provides a list of nursing intervention strategies for working with psychiatric clients.

BOX 6.3

Nursing Strategies for Mental Health Nurses

- Respect and accept each client as he is when he/she comes to you.
- Allow the client opportunity to set own pace in working with problems.
- Nursing interventions should center on the client as a person, not on control of the symptoms. Symptoms are important, but not as important as the person having them.
- Remember, *all behavior has meaning*—an attempt to prevent the occurrence or decrease the intensity of anxiety.
- Recognize your own feelings toward clients and deal with them.
- Go to the client who needs help the most.
- Do not allow a situation to develop or continue in which a client becomes the focus of attention in a negative manner.
- If client behavior is bizarre, base your decision to intervene on whether the client is endangering self or others.
- Ask for help—don't try to be a hero when dealing with a client who is out of control!
- Avoid highly competitive activities.
- Make frequent contact with clients—let them know they are worth your time and effort.
- Remember to assess the physical needs of your client.
- Have patience! Move at client's pace and ability.
- Suggesting, requesting, or asking work better than commands.
- Therapeutic thinking is not to think about, think for, but with the client.
- Be honest and truthful so the client can rely on you.
- Make reality interesting enough so the client prefers it to his/her fantasy.
- Compliment, reassure, and model appropriate behaviors.

Just the Facts

Nursing interventions are intended to encourage, maintain, and reestablish a level of mental and physical functioning that promotes the well-being of the client.

Mind Jogger

How might a client's desire and motivation to participate in goal achievement influence the manner in which the care plan is implemented?

---

criteria. Additional data also aid in the planning of ongoing nursing care.

Evaluation

During the **evaluation** phase of the nursing process, the nurse evaluates the success of the nursing interventions in meeting the criteria outlined in the expected outcomes: the goal has been achieved, some progress has been made toward the intended outcome, or no steps forward have been observed or documented. Specific client behaviors may be reviewed by the entire mental health care team to determine the overall success of the treatment plan. If a goal has been partially met, there may be supporting data to indicate continuance of the current plan of care. This approach recognizes that the client may need more time to make changes and adjust to them. A distinction must be made between a lack of client motivation and the need for continuance of the current plan to help the client achieve the outcomes. Some interventions may have been ineffective, and thus new strategies may be needed to help meet the client's needs. It is also important to reevaluate the outcome criteria; the expected outcome may not actually be achievable for this client.

The evaluation phase is a form of validation for the entire nursing process in the delivery of care to the client. Continued data collection may indicate new problems or alterations in the original nursing diagnoses. Criteria are reevaluated to clarify realistic and measurable terms for the individual client. Nursing strategies are reevaluated for effectiveness. This persistence in maintaining a therapeutic approach toward resolution of client problems provides the continuity needed to expedite the treatment process.

The implementation step of the nursing process should focus on helping clients rechannel their energies in a constructive manner. The nursing interventions should be based on scientific principles for resolution of the identified problem and should be safe for the client and others involved. Other chapters in this text will include appropriate nursing actions for clients with the various categories of mental disorders. As strategies are implemented and documented, a picture of client progress evolves. Data collection is continuous during this phase. Client response to interventions provides valuable information that assists the nurse in determining whether the client is making progress toward the defined outcome

Just the Facts

The nurse is the only member of the mental health team who can continuously evaluate client response to planned care.

Mind Jogger

How is documentation vital to the process step of evaluation?

Sample Application of the Nursing Process

As you study the various mental disorders and situations in this textbook, you will find a section in most chapters that reinforces the application of the nursing process. However, to facilitate your understanding of this process as it relates to the mental health setting, we need to apply this concept to an actual client situation.

Client Situation

Freda is a 47-year-old public school teacher who received word several days ago that her only child, 23-year-old Benjamin, was arrested for armed robbery. Benjamin is married and the father of two small children. Two months ago, Freda discovered that her husband of 26 years is having an affair. Freda blames herself for his indiscretion, stating that she is overweight and unattractive. She says that he would be better off without her anyway. She feels that she is a failure as both a mother and a wife. She is unable to concentrate in the classroom and has considered a leave of absence from her job. Last night Freda's husband told her he was leaving her and wanted a divorce. Freda was brought to the

emergency room this morning after being found unresponsive by her daughter-in-law, Andrea. Andrea gives the nurse an empty bottle of Xanax (alprazolam). She also tells the nurse that Freda has been drinking a lot of wine in the past few months. After initial treatment, Freda is admitted to the psychiatric unit with a diagnosis of depressive episode: situational crisis with suicide attempt.

Nursing Assessment

The mental health nurse obtains the following data:

Objective Data

- Suicide attempt with Xanax and alcohol
- Was found unresponsive by daughter-in-law
- Is overweight and has unkempt appearance
- Son has been arrested for armed robbery
- Has two small grandchildren she loves
- Husband has asked for divorce after several months of infidelity
- Has been drinking more in past few months

Subjective Data

- "I don't blame him for finding someone else. I am so fat and ugly."
- "He would be better off without me anyway. I'm such a mess."
- "I must have done something wrong for my son to be in so much trouble. I can't do anything right."
- "I can't even think clearly enough to teach my kids what I'm supposed to. I might as well quit."
- "The only good thing in my life is my little grandkids. They deserve better than me."

Table 6.2 demonstrates the application of the nursing process to Freda's situation for three applicable nursing diagnoses.

TABLE 6.2 Sample Care Plan			
NURSING DIAGNOSES	**EXPECTED OUTCOME**	**NURSING INTERVENTIONS**	**EVALUATION**
Risk for self-injury, related to suicide attempt, evidenced by suicide overdose with use of alcohol	Does not engage in self-destructive behavior while hospitalized Begins to explore reasons for substance abuse in 48 h Signs contract that she will not harm herself in 24 h	Monitor frequently for signs of oversedation Monitor vital signs every half-hour Assess for social withdrawal or isolation Assess for self-destructive thoughts Remove potentially dangerous items from room	Recovers from overdose without complications Expresses feelings about substance abuse Discusses harmful effects of substance use Participates in goal-planning sessions Identifies self-talk that is destructive

TABLE 6.2   Sample Care Plan (Continued)

NURSING DIAGNOSES	EXPECTED OUTCOME	NURSING INTERVENTIONS	EVALUATION
		Provide quiet, soothing environment Monitor mood, affect, and behavior	Has not harmed self during hospitalization Develops supportive network of family, friends, and support group
Coping, ineffective individual, related to life events, as evidenced by drinking more and inability to meet role expectations	Performs activities of daily living in next 2 d Communicates feelings about current situation in next 2 d Participates in determining goals for improvement in 2 d Implements one adaptive coping strategy by the end of 1 wk Identifies support systems available to him/her by the end of 1 wk	Help to perform activities of daily living Encourage to make decisions about self-care Encourage expression of feelings Help to identify internal factors of self-blame Teach and model adaptive coping strategies Encourage to use adaptive coping skills Praise efforts and successes in coping	Independently performs activities of daily living Makes independent decisions about self-care Openly discusses feelings and emotional response to live situations Identifies self-defeating thoughts and behaviors Demonstrates use of adaptive coping strategies
Self-esteem, situational low, related to inability to handle life events, evidenced by feelings of self-blame and inadequacy	Refrains from self-blame and negative self-talk by the end of 1 wk Participates in self-care with interest in self-improvement in 2 d Identifies positive life accomplishments and personal strengths in 3 d Identifies internal factors that harm self-esteem in 1 wk Participates in unit activities in 2 d Discusses realistic goals for self-improvement by discharge	Establish trusting relationship Provide safe and supportive environment Encourage to discuss life events Assist to distinguish between life situations over which he/she does and does not have control Help to recognize negative self-talk and self-defeating statements Encourage to keep journal of negative and defeating thoughts Encourage social interaction with others Assist to identify personal strengths and accomplishments Provide positive reinforcement for expression of positive feelings and thoughts	Demonstrates trust in mental health team Identifies realistic views of life events Demonstrates ability to recognize negative thought patterns Reframes negative self-talk with more realistic perspective Uses positive statements to describe self Identifies strengths and acknowledges accomplishments Interacts with others using positive approach

Summary

- The nursing process is a scientific, organized, problem-solving method of addressing those situations for which nursing can legally intervene.
- As a member of the mental health team, the nurse is responsible for assessing and communicating information concerning the current status of the client to the physician and other team members.
- A basic psychosocial nursing assessment usually includes the client's history and mental or emotional status including both subjective and objective data.

- Subjective information is provided by the client. This information includes a history and perception of the present situation or problem along with feelings, thoughts, and symptoms client may be presently experiencing.
- Objective information is observed by the nurse, acquired from past medical records, or provided by others familiar with the client. This includes the physical assessment, medical history, medication history, allergies, and psychosocial assessment.

- Nursing diagnoses are formulated by relating them to the cause or contributing reason for the symptoms.
- Planning measurable and realistic outcomes that anticipate the improvement or stabilization of the identified problem provides a strategy for nursing interventions to be developed.
- Nursing interventions are intended to encourage, maintain, and reestablish a level of mental and physical functioning that promotes the client's well-being.

- The evaluation phase is a form of validation for the entire nursing process in the delivery of care to the client. Continued data collection and revisiting the plan of care allows the nurse a system of addressing client problems in the most effective manner toward resolution.
- The nursing process is an ongoing continuum from admission to discharge and outpatient status.

Bibliography

Doenges, M. E., Moorhouse, M. F., & Murr, A. C. (2013). *Nursing diagnosis manual* (4th ed.). Philadelphia, PA: F. A. Davis.

Schultz, J. M., & Videbeck, S. L. (2009). *Lippincott's manual of psychiatric nursing care plans* (8th ed.). Philadelphia, PA: Lippincott, Williams, & Wilkins.

Student Worksheet

Fill in the Blank

Fill in the blank with the correct answer.

1. The nursing process is a _____ approach that assists the client in achieving a maximal level of functioning and well-being.
2. Information that is provided by the client is _____ data.
3. Information that is observed by the nurse or provided by others who are familiar with the client situation is referred to as _____ data.
4. A nursing diagnosis consists of a problem that is related to a _____ , and behavior or symptoms that support the problem.
5. Goals and outcomes should be planned _____ with the client.

Matching

Match the following terms to the most appropriate phrase.

1. _____ Assessment
2. _____ Prioritize
3. _____ Nursing diagnosis
4. _____ Nursing interventions
5. _____ Evaluation
6. _____ Expected outcome

a. Actual or potential problem the nurse can legally address
b. Measurable and realistic goal that anticipates the improvement or stabilization of the client
c. Collection of subjective and objective data concerning the psychosocial needs of a client
d. Defining immediacy or intensity of problems to determine the order in which they will be addressed
e. Actions taken to assist client to achieve anticipated outcomes
f. Determines success of strategies used in meeting anticipated criteria

Multiple Choice

Select the best answer from the multiple choice items.

1. The nurse is assessing a client with chronic schizophrenia who has stopped taking medication and is being admitted with acute psychotic symptoms. The client's perception of the present problem would best be documented by the nurse:
   a. Using exact words in client statements
   b. With information obtained from the family
   c. By observing behavior for several hours
   d. As interpreted from the client thoughts

2. Which of the following is most important in establishing a trusting environment for the organized delivery of nursing care to a client?
   a. Cooperation of the client
   b. A completed psychosocial assessment
   c. The client's perception of the current situation
   d. Accepting and nonjudgmental attitude of the nurse

3. Which of the following is a component of the client's mental status nursing assessment?
   a. Past medical history
   b. Mood and affect
   c. Medical diagnosis
   d. Nursing diagnosis

4. Which of the following terms would be descriptive of a client's attitude?
   a. Blunted
   b. Remote
   c. Retarded
   d. Apathetic

5. When gathering data concerning the present mental status of a client, the nurse would recognize which of the following as a perceptual disturbance?
   a. Persistent use of rationalization to explain present situation
   b. Describes reoccurring voices that are talking to him
   c. Inability to stay focused on question asked
   d. Retention of immediate happenings is decreased

6. The nurse is working with a client who is having difficulty understanding and associating present symptoms with the illness. In which of the following components of the mental status assessment would this information be documented?
   a. Insight
   b. Level of awareness
   c. Orientation
   d. Judgment

7. After teaching a client about a newly prescribed drug, the nurse asks the client to explain how he/she will take the drug and what side effects to watch for. The nurse is executing which step of the nursing process?
   a. Assessment
   b. Planning of nursing diagnoses
   c. Intervention implementation
   d. Evaluation

8. Validation of the nursing process in the delivery of care is most evident in which phase of the care plan?
   a. Assessment
   b. Nursing diagnosis and planning
   c. Interventions
   d. Evaluation

Chapter 7

Communication in Mental Health Nursing

◉ Learning Objectives

After learning the content of this chapter, the student will be able to:

1. Discuss how communication is used as a therapeutic tool to interact with clients.
2. Discuss techniques that facilitate communication between the client and the health care worker.
3. Describe what is meant by nonverbal communication as a therapeutic exchange.
4. Identify issues that affect the exchange of messages between the nurse and the client.
5. Explain how personal space is related to the effectiveness of communication.
6. Identify various ways in which communication can be nontherapeutic or blocked.

◉ Key Terms

active listening
blocking
circumstantiality
echolalia
flight of ideas
focusing
kinesics

loose association
neologism
objectivity
reflection
restating
validation
verbigeration

Communication in Mental Health Nursing

Communication is a process of exchanging information involving the person sending a message, the person receiving the message, and the message itself (Fig. 7.1). Thinking is the means by which a thought is developed, but thinking in itself does not communicate that thought. The thought content must be communicated by one of various methods which may be verbal or nonverbal. Verbal communication is the exchange of information using words, such as through speaking, listening, writing, or reading. Nonverbal communication is the exchange of information without using words, for example, through body language, space, or touch. These processes of communication occur as we respond to an instinctive drive for connection to other human beings.

In nursing, communication is purposeful and is centered on the needs and problems of the client. It is through communication that the nurse builds the therapeutic relationship and establishes trust. To do this effectively, the nurse must develop effective therapeutic communication skills, which are described in this chapter.

Speech Patterns Common to Clients with Mental Illness

Before discussing specific communication techniques, it is important to have an understanding of speech patterns that are common to the clients who have mental illness. These speech patterns often reflect distorted thoughts and processing flaws that occur as the person is attempting to transmit a message. Common speech patterns include the following:

- **Blocking**—The client unconsciously blocks out information, which results in loss of thought process and causes the client to stop speaking (e.g., "Then my father...What was I saying?").
- **Circumstantiality**—The client cannot be selective and describes in lengthy, great detail (e.g., when asked, "Do you have any physical illness?" client replies, "My head hurts, but my nose has been leaking, my hair just won't stay in place, I have this cramping in my joints...").
- **Echolalia**—The client vocally repeats last word heard (e.g., "Please wait here" is responded to with, "here, here, here, here...").

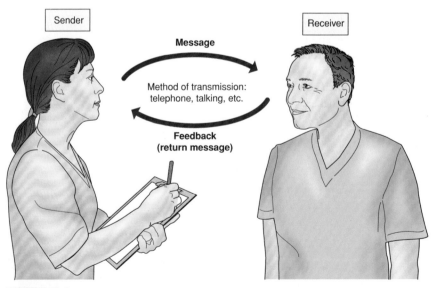

FIGURE 7.1

Communication is a process of exchanging information involving the person sending a message, the person receiving the message, and the message itself. Communication between a sender and receiver is part of the holistic human component. This interaction occurs both verbally and nonverbally as we respond to an instinctive drive for connection to other human beings.

- **Loose association**—The client exhibits continuous speech, shifting between loosely related topics (e.g., "Martha married Jim. You know Jim is a good cook. I can cook. Chickens are something we can cook. The cook comes here before daylight. I get up in the daylight. Do you know Jim?").
- **Flight of ideas**—The client rapidly shifts between topics that are unrelated to each other (e.g., "My cat is gray. Gray is day and day is gray. The food here is good. My hair needs a perm. Do you think my pants are too tight? What color should I dye my hair?").
- **Neologism**—The client coins new words and definitions (e.g., "Hiptomites are real powerful people" in reference to a husky mental health technician on the unit.).
- **Verbigeration**—The client repeats words, phrases, or sentences several times (e.g., when the nurse says, "It is time to take your medication," the client responds with, "Take your medicine, take your medicine, take your medicine, take your medicine...").

Not all of these speech patterns are exhibited by each client. As you learn about individual disorders, you will become familiar with those patterns that are more common to each.

Therapeutic Communication

Therapeutic communication is an interaction between the nurse or other team personnel and the client that is conducted with the specific goal of learning about the client and his or her problem. This type of skilled communication is learned and requires practice. Although the focus is on the client, the exchange is planned and directed by the nurse. The goal is to use both verbal and nonverbal techniques to facilitate active involvement by the client and to encourage the client to express feelings and thoughts that are contributing to his or her problem. In order to do this, it is important to view the relationship between the nurse and the client as part of a complex environment influenced by individual experiences, culture, values, and beliefs. There are many cultural and ethnic factors relating to both the client and the nurse that can compromise the quality of this exchange. In addition, educational background, gender, and personal emotions all impact the dynamics of this interaction. Each message within the communication exchange is filtered through the mental processes of both the sender and the receiver. Differences in communication style or expression of one's feelings can be easily misinterpreted and must be considered integral to establishing trust within the nurse–client relationship.

> ### Just the Facts
> **Objectivity**, or the ability to view facts and events without distortion by personal feelings, prejudices, or judgments, allows the nurse to remain unbiased and open to what clients say about their problems and about themselves.

The nurse must be vigilant, demonstrating awareness and sensitivity to the needs of the client. The perceived power of the nurse may at times relay a condescending attitude to the client. It is essential for the nurse to be constantly aware that manner of speech and actions are being observed and interpreted by the client. Many clients do not trust anyone and are especially suspicious of those in authority. Nurses are seen as authority figures. Keeping this in mind, the nurse must continuously monitor his or her own actions as well as the client's response to maintain a therapeutic climate within the relationship. It is important to be flexible and make the client physically and emotionally comfortable during the therapeutic interaction. Learn to anticipate the client's needs and meet them as completely and consistently as possible within therapeutic guidelines.

Verbal Communication

Verbal communication is enhanced by speaking clearly, using vocabulary the listener can understand, and avoiding ambiguous statements. Both the sound of our voice and the tone in which we convey the message have an impact on the way in which the message is received. Based on the variances of the participants, the meaning intended by the sender is never exactly the same as the meaning understood by the receiver. Meanings are interpreted based on individual experiences and knowledge. Verbal communication can be either enhanced or undermined by the nonverbal dynamics that accompany the verbalization.

When engaged in verbal communication with a client, *silence*, in which the nurse remains quiet with an attentive manner, conveys a willingness to continue listening. It allows both the nurse and the client time to collect thoughts. A client may also find that emotions override the ability to

TABLE 7.1 Effective Verbal Communication Techniques

EFFECTIVE TECHNIQUE	EXAMPLE	THERAPEUTIC EFFECT
Clarification	Nurse: "Did I understand you correctly…" "Let me see if I have this correct…" "I seem to have missed something. Could you repeat that…"	Clears up any possible misunderstanding and assures message intended is message received
Validation	Nurse: "You seem anxious about something…" "I get the feeling that something is bothering you…" "You look down this morning. Would you like to talk about it?"	Attempts to verify the nurse's perception of feeling conveyed by either verbal or nonverbal message of the client
Reflection (also called parroting)	Client: "I don't think my daughter will need me after she gets married." Nurse: "You are afraid you won't be needed after your daughter's marriage?" Client: "I am sick of all this mess." Nurse: "Sick of this mess?"	Shows nurse's perception of the client's message in both content and feeling areas—paraphrases the message that the client has conveyed to nurse
Restating	Nurse: "You have told me something about the problems between you and your wife…"	Repeats to the client the content of interaction and serves as lead to encourage further discussion
Focusing	Nurse: "Let's get back to the problem with your son…"	Helps the client concentrate on a specific issue
Using a general lead	Nurse: "Go on…" "And then…" "Continue…"	Shows the nurse is listening and interested—encourages the client to continue talking
Giving information	Nurse: "The doctor has ordered a new medication for you. Let me go over this information with you."	Increases client involvement in plan of care—helps to demonstrate team effort to improve the client's well-being
Using silence	Nurse remains silent with attentive manner.	Conveys willingness to continue listening—allows both the nurse and client time to collect thoughts
Explore alternatives	Nurse: "Have you considered taking a weekend for some time alone with your wife?"	Guides the client to possible options for problem solving
Offering of oneself	Nurse: "I will be here awhile if you wish to talk…"	Reassurance of interest and presence in the client's problem
Reinforcing Reality	Nurse: "I know you hear the voices, but I do not hear them. You and I are the only ones in this room."	Provides reassurance that voices are symptoms of illness—helps the client to trust the nurse as real

convey feelings verbally. Silence shows respect for the emotions and offers the client time to regain control and continue the conversation.

Table 7.1 describes some effective verbal communication techniques. These techniques are used with the specific intent of facilitating interaction with the client. The method used will depend on the situation and the client's ability to communicate verbally. For example, if the purpose is to encourage the client to discuss feelings about a current problem, the nurse would use methods of reflection or validation. On the other hand, if the nurse is unsure of the message being conveyed by the client, the nurse might choose clarification, restating, or focusing. Whatever the situation, it is important to consider what technique will best encourage a therapeutic outcome for the client.

Nonverbal Communication Techniques

Nonverbal communication is an exchange of information without the use of words, and can confirm, strengthen, or emphasize what is being said orally. It can add emotional color to words as well as contradict the message that is being sent. The behavior that accompanies a verbal message is often more important and more powerful than what is being said. The nonverbal message will go beyond verbal content and convey unconscious emotions or thoughts than can clearly negate the verbal message.

BOX 7.1

Nonverbal Communication in Action

- **Appearance**—remember, you are modeling socially appropriate behaviors.
- Watch **kinesics**—body movements can indicate emotions and moods.
- **Facial expression**—is it congruent with verbal message?
- **Gestures**—fingers and hands can sometimes say more than words.
- **Eye contact**—in Western culture, little or no eye contact indicates low self-esteem, while too much can be intimidating. (In some cultures [e.g., Hispanic, Asian, Middle Eastern, and Native American] a lack of eye contact does not mean the person is not paying attention; it may mean that prolonged eye contact is seen as a sign of disrespect.)
- **Position**—vertical conversations can be intimidating and block further communication, whereas lateral conversations at eye level are more inviting.
- **Personal space**—in most people, this is an arm's length which is about 2 to 4 ft; in others this may extend up to 12 to 25 ft.

Nonverbal aspects of a therapeutic exchange must convey a sense of genuine caring and interest in what the client has to say. Body movements or **kinesics** such as hand gestures, facial expressions, movement, arm placement, and other mannerisms can invite the trust of the client or block further interaction. Box 7.1 provides reminders of how kinesics can speak louder than words. Effective use of nonverbal techniques must be a conscious choice for the nurse to maintain a therapeutic relationship with the client.

Mind Jogger

What body posture would reflect an attitude of acceptance and genuineness?

Specific nonverbal techniques the nurse can employ to improve communication in a therapeutic exchange with the client include the following:

- Intermittent eye contact—helps provide reassurance that you are interested and concentrating on what the client is saying.
- A facial expression that is congruent with other gestures—assures the client of your interest and attention. Inconsistency between verbal and nonverbal messages leads to misinterpretation of the intended meaning.

- Arms or legs that are not crossed—conveys a sense of openness to the client. A seated position with legs together and both feet on the floor with arms uncrossed reflects an attitude of acceptance and genuineness.
- Respecting the physical or personal space between the client and yourself—helps the client feel safe. The anxiety level, suspiciousness, distorted thinking, and personal comfort zone of the client will all influence the proximity of this distance. Box 7.1 provides a good guideline for nurses to maintain unless otherwise indicated by the client's behavior.
- Use of touch—helps convey caring and understanding. However, when working with the client who has a mental illness, you must use caution and forethought about how the client might interpret your actions. A client who is suspicious, for example, might react with aggressive actions toward a simple pat on the shoulder. A client who is sexually preoccupied might misinterpret any form of touch as having seductive connotations. Some cultures (e.g., Islamic and Japanese cultures) may also view personal touch as inappropriate except in certain circumstances.

Active Listening

Active listening is a learned skill that includes observing nonverbal behaviors, giving critical attention to verbal comments, listening for inconsistencies that may need clarification, and attempting to understand the client's perception of the situation. Active listening by the nurse demonstrates care and a desire to help the client. It allows the client to express feelings and thoughts without fear of being judged or criticized. The nurse must constantly listen and cognitively review the comments and behaviors of the client before responding. Because clients tend to view the nurse as someone with power who cares and is available, the opportunities for interaction are more likely. Some responses by the nurse may not be effective or correct. The intended message can be misread by either the client or the nurse. It is important that both participants remain open to the possibility of error. Sometimes this actually allows the nurse to apologize and model appropriate behavior. Willingness to try another approach can also reinforce the genuineness of the nurse's efforts to help the client.

Case Application 7.1

"No Other Way Out"

Olivia is a 26-year-old married mother of three children who is brought to the emergency room of a local hospital following a suicide attempt using an excessive ingestion of a prescribed antidepressant. The nurse notes that Olivia is avoiding eye contact during the time the staff are implementing procedures to reduce the physical consequences of the ingested drugs. She turns her head to the side but it is observed that tears are consistently running down her cheeks. She tells the nurse in a quiet voice, "I never seem to do anything right. My family would be so much better off without me. Why don't you just let me die?"

What would be an appropriate reflection response by the nurse to Olivia at this time?

_____

_____

How can the nurse validate Olivia's feelings at this time?

_____

_____

What techniques would encourage Olivia to tell the nurse more about her feelings and thoughts leading up to her suicide attempt?

_____

_____

Just the Facts

Accept that as a nurse, you may have feelings of irritation and impatience toward a client. Looking at your own feelings and response to the client situation can help you to grow and be more effective.

Just the Facts

If a communicative response is intimidating, judgmental, or demeaning, it is NOT therapeutic.

Nontherapeutic Communication

It is important to recognize that there are also ways that communication can be sidetracked so that it does not accomplish the intended goal of helping the client. In contrast to effective therapeutic communication, nontherapeutic communication involves messages and behaviors that actually hinder the therapeutic process. For example, closed body language with arms folded and appearing busy or uncomfortable with the conversation would send a message to the client that the relationship is superficial. If the nurse interjects opinions or personal values, or minimizes the client's feelings, a condescending attitude is presented that puts the client on the defensive. This type of approach will deny the client the chance to trust the nurse as a resource of help and hope. Table 7.2 demonstrates how ineffective responses can block therapeutic communication along with suggested therapeutic alternatives.

In addition, there are a number of factors that can prevent an intended message from being understood. Variances in age, language, or ethnic and cultural differences can produce barriers to the correct interpretation of a message. Physical handicaps such as hearing or visual impairment can also interfere with the transfer of information. Background noise or confusion can produce a distraction when attentive listening is needed. Communication is only therapeutic when the client is actively involved in the process. The nurse must be alert to any indication that communication is being misunderstood and make provisions or adjustments to improve the outcome.

A supportive approach is needed to aid the client with mental illness in working toward resolution of his or her own problems. The nurse should refrain from offering advice or responding to the client with criticism. While the ability to be empathetic is necessary, the need to give appropriate feedback is just as important. Clients need to feel

TABLE 7.2   Blocks to Therapeutic Communication

INEFFECTIVE RESPONSE	EXAMPLE	BLOCKING EFFECT
Arguing/disapproving	Client: "I want to try to get my girlfriend back." Nurse: "Why would you want to do that after what she did to you?" Therapeutic Response: "Tell me more about that…"	Expresses opinions or interjects the nurse's values of right and wrong on the client's actions—may prevent the client from working through options in solving the problem
Giving advice	Nurse: "You should not be so hard on your kids." "If I were you, I would do what the doctor says." Therapeutic Response: "It seems your kids are a problem for you…" "Can you tell me what is bothering you about what the doctor has told you?"	Seemingly says that the nurse's values are correct and devalues the client's actions
False reassurance	Nurse: "You are going to be out of here before you know it." Therapeutic Response: "We are here to help you get stronger and feel better."	Minimizes the client's feelings and concerns—conveys superficial attitude
Use the word "why"	Nurse: "Why did you act that way?" "Why are you getting so upset?" Therapeutic Response: "Can you tell me what you are feeling right now?" "You seem to be upset about something. Can you tell me about it?"	Puts the client on the defensive—demands an answer Invasive and direct probing of issue
Closed-ended questions	Nurse: "Do you want to talk about it?" "Are you feeling better this morning?" "I don't think that's a good idea, do you?" Therapeutic Response: "Tell me about that…" "Tell me how you are feeling this morning…" "Let's talk about that…"	Allows a "yes" or "no" response without encouraging further information from the client (If the client replies with a "yes" or "no," nurse can use a more effective response to elicit more conversation)
Changing the subject	Client: "I really don't think I can handle going back home." Nurse: "Let's talk about the incident that occurred yesterday with you and Mike." Therapeutic Response: "Tell me what bothers you about going home…"	Minimizes importance of client concerns—discourages further exploration of feelings and thoughts May show the nurse's insecurity in talking about the issue
Agreeing or approving	Nurse: "You are absolutely correct." "I think that is a great idea." "You should do that." Therapeutic Response: "Tell me more about your idea…" "Let's look at that again…"	Can set the client up for failure if the idea doesn't work Can be seen as judgmental
Minimizing or belittling	Nurse: "That is how everyone feels when they are admitted." "We all resent being told what to do." Therapeutic Response: "I'm sure it is difficult for you to be told what to do…tell me what you are feeling."	Conveys an attitude that the client's feelings are common and devalues the uniqueness of the person
Focusing on the nurse	Client: "I just broke up with my boyfriend a few weeks ago." Nurse: "That has happened to me several times…" Therapeutic Response; "That must have been difficult…tell me about that time…"	Pulls focus from client problem and delays further exploration or information regarding the client's feelings
Stereotype Statements	Nurse: "Tomorrow will be a better day." "Hang in there." Therapeutic Response: "You seem rather low today; would you like to talk about it?"	Empty clichés that close the client to further response

valued, respected, and accepted by the nurse. Recognize that you may not always get the response or cooperation you anticipate. Used consistently however, these techniques can go a long way to accomplish the goal of initiating and maintaining a therapeutic nurse–client relationship.

> **Mind Jogger**
>
> In what way is therapeutic communication between the nurse and client a matter of trial and error?

Summary

- Clients with mental illness tend to demonstrate unusual speech patterns that reflect the distortion in their thoughts and processing of thought content into verbal transmission.
- Therapeutic communication includes both verbal and nonverbal techniques in the exchange of information between the nurse and the client.
- Communication techniques are as diversified as the situations themselves. No one approach will work in every circumstance or with all clients.
- Successful attempts are reliant on the willingness of the client to reveal personal information and the nature of their problem. The goal is then to use techniques that guide the client to express emotions and thoughts that surround the situation.
- It is important to recognize that the client is a mesh of many factors including age and gender, culture, beliefs and values, educational background, and experiences. Thoughts emerge through this picture album to form the basis for communication.
- The tone of our voice and manner in which we speak can convey either a message of caring and concern or one that is intimidating and condescending.

- Silence allows the client to regain composure or collect thoughts and is a way of showing respect and concern for what the client has to say.
- Active listening and open posture are vital to projecting a genuineness and willingness to help the client. Eye contact should be intermittent and attentive without staring or fixating to the point of intimidation.
- The nurse should maintain an awareness of mannerisms that could imply power that is nontherapeutic. Many clients do not trust anyone, especially those in authority.
- We can communicate in ways that do not evoke a therapeutic interaction with the client. Closed-ended questions, putting the client on the defensive, or disapproving of the client's statements can impede the communication exchange. Statements that devalue the client and interject the opinions or judgments of the nurse are nontherapeutic. Clichés that offer a stereotyped response usually close the client to further response.
- Communication used effectively will open the door for the therapeutic relationship to grow and produce an outcome that will aid clients in accomplishing their goals for improvement.

Bibliography

Browne, G., Cashin, A., & Graham, I. (2012). The therapeutic relationship and mental health nursing: it is time to articulate what we do! *Journal of Psychiatric & Mental Health Nursing, 19*(9), 839–843. Retrieved January 12, 2014.

Finfgeld-Connett, D. (2009). Model of therapeutic and non-therapeutic responses to patient aggression. *Issues in Mental Health Nursing, 30*(9), 530–537. Retrieved January 12, 2014.

Jahoda, A., Selkirk, M., Trower, P., Kroese, B. S., Dagnan, D., & Buford, B. (2009). The balance of power in therapeutic interactions with individuals who have intellectual disabilities. *British Journal of Clinical Psychology, 48*(1), 63–77. Retrieved January 11, 2014.

Jones, L. (2009). The healing relationship. *Nursing Standard, 24*(3), 64. Retrieved January 11, 2014.

Minardi, H. (2013). Emotion recognition by mental health professionals and students. *Nursing Standard, 27*(25), 41–48. Retrieved January 11, 2014.

Qureshi, A., & Collazos, F. (2011). The intercultural and interracial therapeutic relationship: Challenges and recommendations. *International Review of Psychiatry, 23*(1), 10–19. Retrieved January 11, 2014.

Varcolaris, E. M., & Halter, M. J. (2010). *Foundations of psychiatric mental health nursing* (6th ed.). Philadelphia, PA: Saunders/Elsevier.

Student Worksheet

Fill in the Blank

Fill in the blank with the correct answer.

1. It is important for the nurse to convey a _____ message through both verbal and nonverbal communication.

2. _____ eye contact will provide reassurance that you are interested and concentrating on what the client is saying.

3. _____ is an unconscious hindrance to thought processing that causes a person to stop speaking.

4. The coining of new words and definitions of words is referred to as _____.

5. _____ _____ describes continuous speech with shifting between loosely related topics.

6. Body movements or _____ such as hand gestures, facial expressions, arm placement, movement and other mannerisms can invite or block interaction with the client.

7. In most people, personal space is _____ which is about 2 to 4 ft.

Matching

Match the following terms to the most appropriate phrase.

1. _____ Blocking
2. _____ Neologism
3. _____ Loose association
4. _____ Verbigeration
5. _____ Flight of ideas
6. _____ Echolalia

a. "Your hair is red—I have a red dress—I like red apples—apples, oranges, pears—you are shaped like a pear..."

b. "And I need help—help—help—help—help..."

c. "Need a bath, need a bath, need a bath, need a bath..."

d. "'Whymothig' is used to describe a puzzle."

e. "I like to go camping—that book is old—my necklace is broke—the sky is cloudy—fish are lucky..."

f. "I have not seen my mother in 5 years...I need to go to the bathroom..."

Multiple Choice

Select the best answer from the multiple-choice items.

1. A client tells the nurse, "The voices say that I am evil and I am going to be punished." Which of the following would be the most therapeutic response?
   a. "The voices are not real so why are you worrying about it?"
   b. "I don't hear the voices, but the words must be frightening for you."
   c. "You are imagining the worst when nothing is going to happen."
   d. "How can you hear voices when you and I are the only ones in this room?"

2. The nurse is caring for a client who says, "I feel like I will never be able to leave this hospital." The nurse's most therapeutic reply would be:
   a. "You don't need to worry about that. We can only keep you for a certain length of time."
   b. "You keep working on your problem and you will be out of here before you know it."
   c. "Everyone feels like it is hopeless, but we will discharge you when you are better."
   d. "You feel as though you will not get better and leave the unit?"

3. During a conversation a client tells the nurse, "My husband left me 6 months ago." The nurse notes that the client is repeatedly twisting strands of her hair. The most appropriate technique for the nurse to utilize at this time would be:
   a. Silence
   b. Verification
   c. Restating
   d. Focusing

4. When initiating interaction with a client, which of the following would be most appropriate to open the communication?
   a. "How would you describe what you are feeling today?"
   b. "Tell me about your family."
   c. "Do you always look at things in such a negative way?"
   d. "You are sad today because no one is talking to you?"

5. A client who will be having several diagnostic tests the following day complains of being unable to sleep. When the client says, "I am so afraid something is really wrong with me," which of the following responses would be most therapeutic?
   a. "You seem worried about the results of your tests. Would you like to talk about it?"
   b. "It is important that you get some sleep. I will see what the doctor ordered to help you rest."
   c. "You really need to believe that everything will turn out okay."
   d. "Your doctor performs these tests every day. Everything will be fine."

6. A tall muscular client jokingly says, "You nurses are bossy just like my wife. In fact, every woman I know tries to put me in a dog chain." Which of the following would best clarify the nurse's perception of the client's statement?
   a. "Why do you think women try to push you around?"
   b. "I can't believe women can do that to someone like you!"
   c. "You don't have to put up with that kind of treatment."
   d. "You feel a lack of control in your life. Is that correct?"

7. A client with a history of alcohol abuse tells the nurse, "I haven't always drank this much, but lately my life has just gone to pot." The nurse notes the client is rubbing his hands together and squirming in his seat. Which of the following responses would be appropriate at this time?
   a. "Go on…"
   b. "Why do you think your life has gone to pot?"
   c. "Are you blaming someone else for your drinking?"
   d. "What could be so bad that you need to drink more?"

8. A client is talking about his family and suddenly changes the subject to what television show is his favorite. Which of the following strategies by the nurse would best elicit more information about the client's family situation?
   a. "Is there some connection between the TV show and your family?"
   b. "Why did you change the subject?"
   c. "Are you uncomfortable talking about your family?"
   d. "Let's get back to your family…"

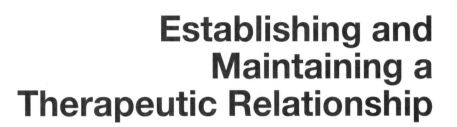

Chapter 8

Establishing and Maintaining a Therapeutic Relationship

◉ Learning Objectives

After learning the content of this chapter, the student will be able to:

1. Define what is meant by a therapeutic relationship.
2. Define phases of and important characteristics for establishing a therapeutic relationship.
3. Apply the concept of professional boundaries to the nurse–client relationship.
4. Describe what is meant by self-awareness and its influence on behavior.
5. Identify appropriate therapeutic responses to difficult client behaviors.

◉ Key Terms

acceptance
empathy
genuineness
orientation phase

professional boundaries
self-awareness
termination phase
working stage

The Therapeutic Relationship

The concept of a holistic being views a person as the totality of biological, psychological, social, and spiritual functioning that result in a unique person. Integral to this concept is that each person is influenced by a different combination of genetic and environmental issues. Each person views the environment subjectively as it relates to his or her past experiences and relationships. A person learns to adapt to life and the environment by observing the world in which he or she exists. This complex nature of each individual is a factor in the development of a therapeutic relationship. Because of the psychosocial differences between clients and nurses, there is no one effective model for establishing this association. Clients who have the same diagnosis may even have a different pattern of symptoms based on their past experiences, current situation, and individual needs. The external demands of the environment and the internal forces of each person will require an individual approach to the nurse–client interaction.

The therapeutic relationship is seen as a helping bond in which one person assists in the personal growth and improved well-being of the other. In this rapport, a series of interactions between the nurse and the client provide information about the client's needs and problems. The nurse works in collaboration with other members of the mental health team toward a common goal of assisting the client toward adaptive and improved functioning within society.

Important Characteristics for Establishing a Nurse–Client Relationship

The establishment of a therapeutic nurse–client relationship is dependent on certain consistent characteristics of the nurse. Box 8.1 lists components that are essential ingredients in this restorative rapport. One of the most important is that of **empathy** or the ability to hear what another person is saying, to have temporary access to that person's feelings, and to perceive the situation from that person's perspective. Empathy is vital to the establishment of trust. At the same time, it is important for the nurse to maintain enough distance from the situation to be objective and remain in touch with his or her own feelings. To become sympathetic and meld into the client's

problem is nontherapeutic. In order to reach an understanding of the client's view, the nurse must engage in active listening that attentively uses both the mind and the body. A seated distance of approximately 3 ft allows personal space but is close enough that interest is communicated and barriers can be avoided. Eye contact with a relaxed open posture facing the client shows a willingness to listen to what the other person is saying. This positioning allows the nurse to maintain a mental focus on meaningful interaction with the client.

Trust is vital in the nurse–client relationship related to the vulnerable position in which the client is placed. Because it can be easily broken, the establishment of trust comes slowly and without guarantee until it is proven. The client may perceive the nurse as an authority figure who is equated with power. Since many clients with mental problems do not trust those in authority, the nurse must earn their confidence by being consistent in following through with strategies that reinforce the security that is being shaped. **Genuineness** or realness is an attribute of concern that fosters an honest and caring foundation for the trust that is forming.

The nurse's **acceptance** of the client as a person with worth and dignity who is not judged or

---

BOX 8.1

A Tool for Self-Assessment/Awareness

- How do I respond to the world around me?
- How do I respond to other people?
- Am I able to discuss issues with others?
- Do I have close relationships? With whom?
- How do I respond when I disagree with others?
- How do others respond to me in this situation?
- What type of stressor is most recurrent in my life?
- How do I respond to stress?
- Do I usually think of myself first, or do I consider others?
- What type of personal space is my comfort zone?
- How do I explain problems to myself?
- If I am threatened or scared, how do I respond?
- Do I recognize my own anxiety? What symptoms do I have?
- What coping mechanisms do I use to adapt? Do I use them frequently or occasionally?
- How do I respond to others who are withdrawn, anxious, or aggressive?
- Do I blame others for my problems and anxiety?
- What thoughts are on my mind most often? Do they focus on myself or others?
- What changes can I make to improve my interactions with others?

labeled by the nurse's standards is also necessary for the establishment of a trusting climate. It is the nurse's willingness to recognize the emotionally ill person as one who deserves respect and needs approval that helps the client to accept the environment. The foundation of the relationship is based on dependable interactions that demonstrate honesty, integrity, and consistency. Involved in this honesty is the establishment of boundaries and limit setting with predetermined consequences. This assists the client in self-control and management of behavior. The client needs constant reassurance to develop a sense of emotional security within their surroundings.

Self-awareness is a consciousness of one's own individuality and personality, or looking at oneself in the mirror. A knowledge of self as a whole person can become a reality only with a gradual awakening to oneself. We cannot have an understanding of others unless we learn about ourselves, how our lives are held together, and how we respond to our own insecurities and anxiety. Box 8.2 provides a tool with questions to ask oneself in developing this insight into "who am I?" The awareness of oneself as a whole person comes with an attitude of openness and wanting to come to an honest evaluation of behavior with a desire to make changes. We must listen to our daily record of self-talk and be willing to change the recurrent negative scripts. When we move beyond ourselves and see the world from the perspective of others, we open the door for growth. Insight into the connection between our *thinking* and our *behavior* provides the opportunity for us to change our behavior. The key is in our thinking! It is this same honesty and openness we try to elicit in our

clients who have emotional and mental issues in order to help them view themselves and their behavior more realistically.

> ### Mind Jogger
> How can self-awareness assist the nurse to help clients view themselves and their behavior more realistically?

> ### Just the Facts
> Caring involves compassion, confidence in our own abilities, a desire to do the right thing, and the courage to intervene as indicated.

> ### Just the Facts
> Preserving oneself when caring for others requires recognizing and accepting our limitations, liking what you do, being knowledgeable, taking pride in accomplishments, and finding joy in the challenges of each day.

Phases of a Therapeutic Relationship

The therapeutic relationship is dependent on the situation and needs of the individual client. Interpersonal interaction in this relationship requires the nurse working with the mentally ill client to use observation and communication skills based on a knowledgeable understanding of human behavior. This is not a social interaction, but one that focuses on identifying the client's problems, developing goals for improvement, and promoting a return to independent living within societal norms.

The phases of this nurse–client association must center on the client's ability to function in the process. The relationship may vary in intensity, length, and focus depending on the particular client's needs. Basic to the therapeutic relationship are three phases of contact with the client: the orientation phase, the working stage, and termination.

Orientation Phase

The **orientation phase** involves getting to know the client. It involves an explanation of the purpose for the nurse–client interaction as a means of building trust, establishing roles, and identifying problems and expectations. The nurse and

---

BOX 8.2

Essential Components of a Therapeutic Relationship

- Empathy
- Caring
- Acceptance (unconditional positive regard)
- Mutual trust
- Honesty
- Integrity
- Consistency
- Genuineness
- Self-awareness
- Limit-setting
- Reassurance
- Explanations

client contract a time and place for a meeting, during which the focus is the client's problem; the nurse's role is to be a facilitator. Confidentiality is explained in terms of information that is shared only with members of the treatment team as it applies to the client's well-being. Rules and boundaries are explained to provide structure with guidelines for behavior. This gives the client an organized environment that is consistent with those in law and order for society. It is important to assess the content of any negative feelings the client may be experiencing while reinforcing the limits for behavior. The nurse can also use this time to assess other client behaviors, immediate concerns and needs, and perceived reason for treatment. These initial data provide a baseline for the next phase of the relationship. It is essential for the nurse to convey a caring and honest concern for the client and to send a congruent message through both verbal and nonverbal communication. By showing a genuine interest and supportive attitude, the nurse helps the client to feel worthwhile, and deserving of the nurse's time and respect.

> ### Just the Facts
> Establishing rules and setting limits for behavior are consistent with patterns of law and order in society.

Working Stage

The second phase is often referred to as the **working stage**. This is a period in which outcomes and interventions toward behavior change are planned and goals are developed to improve the client's well-being. This involves work by both the nurse and the client to develop an awareness of the problem and possible solutions to it. Through the use of problem-solving skills, the nurse assists the client to express feelings and thoughts about the present situation. It may be useful for the client to keep a journal of feelings and progress made between sessions. During this stage the nurse becomes a role model and teaches appropriate coping skills. The client is encouraged to practice adaptive responses and evaluate the effectiveness of changes. Every effort should be made to reinforce and support each small step of the client's progress toward change. Helping the client to set priorities provides a way of accomplishing short-term gains toward a bigger step or challenge.

Termination

The third phase or **termination** of the relationship is necessary to allow the client to depend on his or her own strengths while developing improved adaptive skills. The nurse should encourage the client to have increased social interaction and participate in all activities. This promotes independence in getting along with others in preparation for discharge and a return to the demands of society. It is important to discuss the termination with the client and respond to any feelings or concerns. It is not uncommon for nurses to feel like they are abandoning the client's trust as therapeutic closure occurs. However, when taken to extremes, traits found in good nurses such as commitment, selflessness, and responsibility can hinder progress toward client independence. The nurse should stress that the relationship has been valued and purposeful in helping the client toward relying on his or her own ability to deal with problems.

> ### Mind Jogger
> What behaviors might indicate the client's dependence on the nurse–client relationship?

Professional Boundaries

Nursing is a helping profession, one in which compassion and concern are integral to the care provided. However, for the mental health nurse, the emotional and psychological problems of the client are especially challenging. The desire to help the clients or ease their burden can easily draw the nurse into personal involvement that crosses the line of professionalism.

Within the therapeutic nurse–client relationship, it is the nurse's responsibility to initiate and maintain limits **or professional boundaries**. The guidelines for professional behavior are centered on a condition of helpfulness. Too much concern or not enough can both fall into the category of crossing this standard. According to the National Council of State Boards of Nursing, professional boundaries are the "spaces between the power of the nurse and the vulnerability of the client." The nurse can remediate these gaps by setting boundary standards that provide for safe interactions with the client.

It is important for the nurse to remember that the needs of the nurse are distinctly different from those of the client. Some interventions are helpful and promote independence, but others actually allow the client to develop a dependence on the relationship. An explanation is needed to help clients understand where the line of distinction lies in the nurse's response to their needs and requests. Clarification of the nurse's role may be necessary in situations in which the boundary may be violated. Situations such as involvement in personal relationships of the client, financial affairs unrelated to the treatment process, or a third-party liaison that is not treatment related are issues that must be clearly understood. The nurse must identify and reinforce explanations of where the boundaries lie with the client. For example, if a client asks the nurse to relay a personal message to his girlfriend who happens to live next-door to the nurse, the line must be clearly drawn and an explanation given to the client that the request is outside the professional role of the nurse. Events surrounding any situation that deviates from the baseline of helpfulness and involves professional boundaries should be clearly documented in the client's clinical record.

Just the Facts

When taken to extremes, qualities such as commitment, selflessness, and responsibility that are found in good nurses can hinder the client's progress toward independence.

Client-specific interactions and actions in which boundaries are clarified should be documented in the client medical record.

As clients improve, they are expected to function independently. When nurses allow a strong sense of commitment and need to help overshadow a focus on the client's needs, professional boundaries have been crossed. The nurse cannot let the relationship fulfill a personal need and remain objective about the client's needs at the same time. Anytime the nurse shows more concern for one client over another, he or she is at risk for becoming too involved. When focus on the client is maintained, it is less likely that the nurse will be manipulated into violating professional ethics. The nurse–client relationship must not extend beyond the therapeutic termination phase. Any further contact by phone, mail, e-mail, or socialization is in violation of the professional code of ethics. If former clients are seen outside of the mental health setting, it is important to avoid recognition or speaking to them unless they recognize and speak first. Detailed conversation or other interaction should be avoided.

BOX 8.3

The Nurse's Challenge

- Be aware
- Be cognizant of feelings and behavior
- Be observant of the behavior of other professionals
- Always act in the best interest of the client

National Council of State Boards of Nursing (NCSBN), "Professional Boundaries," www.ncsbn.org.

Mind Jogger

How might a nurse's strong sense of commitment lead to a violation of professional boundaries?

Violations of professional boundaries can occur when gray areas exist in the delivery of mental health care. The deviation from the standard is often an unintentional act that was intended to be helpful but crosses that line. Acts that may fall into this category of boundary violations include unnecessary personal disclosure by the nurse, secrecy, sexual misconduct, overhelping, controlling, and role reversal in the nurse–client relationship. Personal experiences and feelings associated with an issue can be transferred to the client situation and influence how the nurse responds. The nurse must maintain constant vigilance and mental review of feelings to separate self from the client. The nurse must also avoid flirtation in any manner or give specialized individual attention to any one client. A triangle in which the nurse becomes overinvolved in the client's problem to the exclusion of other team members clearly departs from the integrity of the professional role. Box 8.3 provides some guidelines for professional behavior from the National Council of State Boards of Nursing.

Response to Difficult Client Behaviors

The nurse–client relationship may involve situations in which the nurse is challenged with brief periods of inappropriate or difficult client behaviors, especially when working with clients who have mental illness. It is important for the nurse to observe and anticipate behaviors that may require an immediate or directed response. Most displays of excessive behavior response are the result of personality or character problems or in response to other issues such as illness or heightened anxiety levels. The basic dynamic at the root of these difficult situations is the individual response to anxiety created by environmental or internal stressors. Personality characteristics may be reflected in the reaction, or it may be totally out of character for the person. Under high levels of stress, a person may respond in a manner atypical of the normal expected behavior for that individual. Some of the more common difficult client situations include manipulation, violence or aggression, altered thought process (e.g., hallucinations, illusions, delusions), and sexually inappropriate behaviors or aggression.

Manipulation

Clients who are manipulative usually tend to be impulsive and are unable to tolerate frustration or inattention to their requests. There is a demand for instant gratification of their needs with a lack of self-control. The nursing approach is to recognize what the client is attempting to do and reinforce limits. It is important that limits are maintained by all the nursing staff in a consistent manner. A client who is manipulative can recognize when the boundaries are not firmly enforced. This leaves open the opportunity for the client to plot strategies that undermine the care plan.

Limits should be fair and explained thoroughly to the client. In response to manipulation, nurses should avoid reinforcing the negative behavior and focus on the feelings the client is experiencing at the present time. For example, a response to the client who is constantly asking the nurse to come to his or her room might be, "You seem to be uncomfortable being by yourself. Let's talk about what is frightening to you." Further interaction can then be aimed toward the client's thoughts and response.

Mind Jogger

How could limit setting be used to effectively establish behavior parameters in a way that is non punitive?

Violence or Aggression

It is not unusual for nurses to fear for their personal safety during an incident of client hostility or violence. If this should occur during a working session, it is important to take precautionary measures to protect both the client and yourself. For example:

- Maintain at least two-arm's-length distance between you and the client.
- Do not attempt to touch the client without his or her approval.
- Call for assistance—many units have a code for this situation.
- Do not provoke the behavior or threaten the client with action.
- Do not enter a room alone when a client is out of control.
- Offer the client time to regain control and stop the behavior.
- Change the subject from the topic that is threatening to the client.

It is most important to keep in mind the safety of the client and other persons in the immediate area. Clients usually communicate an increasing state of anxiety prior to any aggressive behavior. The nurse who recognizes these signs in the early stages can often de-escalate the behavior using communication and a calm approach that provides the time and space the client needs to regain control. In some situations, it may be best to ensure the safety of other clients and withdraw from the immediate location, thus allowing time for the client to defuse.

Altered Thought Process (hallucinations, illusions, delusions)

Clients with altered thought processes are often suspicious and guarded in their behavior. Because the basic feelings of the client are fear and mistrust, the nurse should be especially careful to provide explanations in a language and context the client can understand. During a therapeutic encounter it is important to impart a feeling of genuine concern for the discomfort that the client may be experiencing. All movement by the nurse should be purposeful and carefully executed to avoid actions that can be misinterpreted. Touch should be avoided and personal space maintained so that the client does not feel closed in or trapped.

Initially, if the client is seeing or hearing something that is not apparent to the nurse, the nurse should acknowledge and clarify the content. For example, if a client is seeing someone in the room who is not obviously present, the nurse can respond with, "I don't see anyone in the room except you and me. Tell me what the person is doing." If the client is hearing voices, a response such as, "I don't hear anyone talking. Tell me what they are saying to you" is appropriate. Once the nurse has insight into the content, the focus should be diverted from the hallucination or delusional thought. It is nontherapeutic to allow the client to continue the description. It is ineffective to argue or tell the person that what he or she is experiencing is not real. Remember that these are symptoms of the illness and are real to the person who is experiencing them. The nurse should reestablish the client's contact with reality and focus on the feelings the client is presently experiencing. For example, a client tells the nurse, "They are laughing at me and saying ugly things about me." Once the nurse has clarified the content, an appropriate reply might be, "I understand that is hard, but let's talk about the rejection you are feeling now." If the content of the altered thought process is threatening to the client, every effort should be made to protect the client and others from injury.

Sexually Inappropriate Behaviors or Aggression

Most clients will refrain from making suggestive or sexually oriented comments or advances once they are asked to do so. The nurse should be direct in letting the client know that the actions are disturbing and unacceptable. Once the limits have been established, the client has a choice to use self-control. The nurse can then proceed to discuss the underlying issue with the client. If the behavior continues, the nurse can terminate the session, citing the behavior as the reason (e.g., "I will not tolerate this behavior. I am going now. I will come back at a later time."). This will allow the client time to reflect on the actions and leave open the option of discussing the behavior at a later point. If the situation becomes unmanageable, the nurse should consult with a supervisor or colleague.

"Behavior in Overdrive"

Connie is a 35-year-old woman who is diagnosed with bipolar disorder. She is brought to the psychiatric unit after being detained in the county jail for disruptive behavior. In her present manic state, Connie is aggressive both verbally and physically. She has just removed all of her clothing in the hallway while loudly inviting male attention. She has not sat down in the 6 hours she has been on the unit nor has she eaten any food. She claims she is "Queen of the Nile in the body of a shark." Several of the other clients appear anxious and fearful as they observe her behavior.

What would be the best approach to this situation?

_____

_____

What is your responsibility to Connie? What is your responsibility to the other clients?

_____

_____

What critical thinking is needed to begin a therapeutic relationship with Connie?

_____

_____

How could limit setting be used to manage Connie's behavior?

_____

_____

Case Application 8.1

Summary

- The therapeutic relationship is a helping, interactive exchange between a client and a mental health professional. This compact is formed with the goal of improved functioning and well-being for the client.
- The nurse–client relationship is based on trust with honest communication that focuses on the client's feelings and problems. An empathetic and accepting approach is necessary to see the client as a unique person with individual needs and issues. Empathy allows the nurse to grasp and view the present situation from the client's perspective. Active listening engages the nurse attentively in both mind and body to capture what the client is conveying in both verbal and nonverbal messages.
- Self-awareness is a process of self-evaluation and an attempt to see oneself through the eyes of others. This provides insight into how we respond to our environment and how others react to our behavior.
- The willingness to see ourselves realistically can open the door for positive change and improved interpersonal relationships. This same awareness is encouraged in the client with mental health issues.
- Although it may be difficult for clients to identify problems related to their behavior, doing so can allow them to take ownership of the problem and commit to a plan for change.
- The therapeutic nurse–client relationship consists of an orientation phase, a working stage, and a termination point.
- The initial contact with the client identifies the purpose and guidelines for the interaction. In addition, it ensures a safe and trusting milieu designed to facilitate and encourage the client to express needs and problems without criticism or reprisal.
- A series of interactive sessions is conducted with therapeutic communication techniques designed to explore and identify client problems and possible options for resolution. These sessions maintain a client focus to help set priorities for short-term goals that lead to improved functioning.
- The relationship is terminated at a point when the client is seen as having adequate skills and emotional resources to function independently. This is an important step to helping the client move back into society in an adaptive manner.
- Professional boundaries are the gaps that exist between the indirect power of the nurse and the vulnerable state of the client. Because the nurse has the knowledge and control inherent in a professional role, it becomes vital that a perspective of helpfulness be maintained.
- The nurse must walk a fine line between what is too much and what is not enough. Client needs must be foremost and the focus of all therapeutic nursing interventions. The nurse must be cautious not to reverse these roles in the process of maintaining the relationship.
- To avoid an unintentional violation of the ethical standards of behavior, the nurse should maintain a constant vigilance and awareness of actions that might be perceived as overly involved in the client's situation.
- Some client situations may pose a threat or challenge to the nurse engaged in a given set of circumstances. It is important for the nurse to remain focused and anticipate behaviors that may demand an immediate or directed response. Manipulation, violence and aggression, altered thought processes, and sexually inappropriate behaviors can all require acute nursing observation and interventions.

Bibliography

Brown, G., Cashin, A., & Graham, I. (2012). The therapeutic relationship and mental health nursing: It is time to articulate what we do! *Journal of Psychiatric and Mental Health Nursing, 19*(9), 839–843. Retrieved January 18, 2014.

Cahill, J., Paley, G., & Hardy, G. (2013). What do patients find helpful in psychotherapy? Implications for the therapeutic relationship in mental health nursing. *Journal of Psychiatric and Mental Health Nursing, 20*(9), 782–791. Retrieved January 18, 2014.

Corey, G. (2008). *Theory and practice of counseling and psychotherapy* (8th ed.). Belmont, CA: Brooks/Cole Pub.

Dziopa, F., & Ahern, K. (2009). Three different ways mental health nurses develop quality therapeutic relationships. *Issues in Mental Health Nursing, 30*(1), 14–22. Retrieved January 18, 2014.

Milton, C. L. (2008). Boundaries: Ethical implications for what it means to be therapeutic in the nurse-person relationship. *Nursing Science Quarterly, 21*(1), 18–21. Retrieved January 18, 2014.

National Council of State Boards of Nursing. (n.d.) Professional boundaries: A nurse's guide to the importance of appropriate professional boundaries. Accessed January 18, 2014, from https://www.ncsbn.org/Professional_Boundaries_2007_Web.pdf

Varcarolis, E. M., & Halter, M.J. (2010). *Foundations of psychiatric mental health nursing* (6th ed.). Philadelphia, PA: W. B. Saunders.

Welch, M. (2005). Pivotal moments in the therapeutic relationship. *International Journal of Mental Health Nursing, 14*(3), 161–165. Retrieved January 18, 2014.

Student Worksheet

Fill in the Blank

Fill in the blank with the correct answer.

1. The ability to hear what another person says and to borrow those feelings to perceive a situation from that person's viewpoint is referred to as _____.

2. _____ is a consciousness of our own personality and behavior in response to the world around us.

3. Therapeutic relationships are dependent on the _____ and _____ of the individual client.

4. The termination phase of the therapeutic relationship promotes _____ for the client in getting along with others as preparation for discharge.

5. When nurses allow a need to "help" to overshadow a focus on the needs of the client, professional _____ have been crossed.

6. Clients usually demonstrate an increasing state of _____ prior to aggressive behavior.

Matching

Match the following terms to the most appropriate phrase.

1. _____ Self-awareness
2. _____ Holistic
3. _____ Orientation phase
4. _____ Working stage
5. _____ Active listening
6. _____ Professional boundaries

a. Listening attentively using both mind and body
b. Period of planning outcomes and interventions toward behavior change with improved client well-being
c. Consciousness of own individuality and personality
d. Totality of biological, psychological, social, and spiritual functioning of an individual
e. Gaps between the control of the nurse and the vulnerable state of the client
f. Time of building trust, establishing roles, and identifying problems and expectations

Multiple Choice

Select the best answer from the multiple-choice items.

1. When establishing a therapeutic environment, which of the following factors would be most important in forming the foundation for a trusting nurse–client relationship?
   a. Sympathetic attitude of the nurse
   b. Educational background of the client
   c. Amount of time spent with the client
   d. Honesty and consistent integrity of the nurse

2. The nurse is working with a client who says, "You are the only one who really cares about me. I feel like everyone else is giving me the shove just because I am getting out of here this week." Which of the following is indicated by the client's statement?
   a. Avoidance
   b. Withdrawal
   c. Ambivalence
   d. Manipulation

3. During a discussion between the nurse and a client, the client suddenly starts shouting and tightening his fists. Which of the following would be an appropriate action for the nurse at this time?
   a. Change the subject or topic of discussion
   b. Tell the client he will be secluded if he continues
   c. Touch the client's arm and ask him to calm down
   d. Walk away from the client without responding

4. Which of the following best prepares the nurse to assist the client in viewing themselves and their behavior more realistically?
   a. Developing an honest evaluation of oneself
   b. Psychosocial assessment of the client
   c. Knowledge of personality development theories
   d. Communication techniques

5. The nurse is explaining the content of a contract with guidelines for behavior to a client on the nursing unit. Which phase of the therapeutic relationship is the nurse facilitating?
   a. Orientation phase
   b. Working phase
   c. Termination phase
   d. Self-awareness

6. Which of the following statements best describes the role of the nurse in terminating the therapeutic relationship with the client?
   a. To reduce the amount of time spent with the client
   b. Encouraging independence and self-reliance of the client
   c. Reinforcing continued support following discharge
   d. Discussing possible solutions to the present problem

7. In which of the following situations has the nurse violated professional boundaries in the nurse–client relationship?
   a. Encouraged client to discuss feelings of remorse over rejection by another client
   b. Agreed to relay personal information about the client to the therapist
   c. Returned cell phone call received from a client discharged two weeks earlier
   d. Assisted a disabled client with physical hygiene and bathing

8. A client tells the nurse, "I feel so secure when I am with you. Don't tell the others, but you are the best nurse here." What is the most appropriate response for the nurse at this time?
   a. "I am glad you feel secure with me. I will try to spend more time with you."
   b. "You don't mean that. There are many good nurses here."
   c. "Why do you feel more secure with me than the others?"
   d. "It seems as though you are feeling anxious. Can you tell me about that?

9. Which of the following behaviors by the nurse would be considered a violation of professional boundaries in the nurse–client relationship?
   a. Accepting a gift from a client
   b. Showing genuine concern for the client
   c. Listening while client talks about a problem with intimacy
   d. Talking with client in privacy of client's room

Anxiety Disorders

⊙ Learning Objectives

After learning the content in this chapter, the student will be able to:

1. Distinguish between common anxiety and anxiety as a symptom.
2. Identify precipitating factors in uncontrolled anxiety attacks.
3. Describe signs and symptoms characteristic of each type of anxiety disorder.
4. Discuss psychotherapeutic use of anxiolytic drugs in treatment of anxiety disorders.
5. Describe other treatment methods for anxiety disorders.
6. Identify nursing diagnoses related to anxiety disorders.
7. Develop realistic anticipated outcomes for clients with anxiety disorders.
8. Plan appropriate nursing interventions toward client improvement.
9. Evaluate the effectiveness of planned nursing interventions toward goals.

⊙ Key Terms

agoraphobia
anticipatory anxiety
automatic relief behaviors
compulsion
cued
emotional numbing
free-floating anxiety

generalized anxiety
obsession
panic attack
social phobia
specific phobia
uncued

nxiety is a vague, uneasy emotional feeling experienced by a person in response to a perceived threat or danger. As the stimulus of a threatening situation is processed by the brain, the result is fear. Anxiety is felt as the fear is realized. When anxiety increases to the point of discomfort or distress, that the person senses something is wrong. Sometimes the person can identify the stimulus that is causing the uncomfortable feeling. In other cases, a cause cannot be identified. **Free-floating anxiety** occurs when the person is unable to connect the anxiety to a stimulus. This factor in itself can create additional anxiety.

The manifestations of anxiety can take many forms. Experiences range from vague discomfort to extreme panic. Increased levels of anxiety can be experienced continuously or periodically. Thoughts, feelings, and behavior are all affected as anxiety increases. A person may act "out of character" or in a bizarre manner, such as counting continuously or shouting. This is illustrated by a person who is late for an appointment and delayed in traffic. When a police officer approaches, telling him there is an accident scene that will be cleared in about 30 minutes, the man starts shouting at the officer.

In other situations, subtle manifestations of anxiety such as clenching the jaws, tapping fingers on a table, fidgeting, and other behaviors may be evident. These **automatic relief behaviors** are subtle unconscious behaviors that are aimed at relieving the anxiety. Although the person may be unaware of his or her actions, they may be annoying to other people. For example, the person sitting next to you at a conference is constantly clicking her ballpoint pen. After this continues for nearly 30 minutes, you ask her if she would mind laying her pen down as you cannot hear the speaker. Unaware of her behavior, she apologizes. She states that she is "very nervous in this room full of people." She goes on to say, "I was required to be here to keep my job." Both people in this example are experiencing anxiety, but the anxiety being experienced by the person who is uncomfortable in a crowded room will most likely continue to escalate unless she leaves the room. This situation illustrates how anxiety develops. Unless measures are taken to remove the cause, anxiety continues to grow. If it is unrelieved and continues over time, an underlying disorder may be identified.

Beyond the normal experiences of anxiety, *anxiety disorders are a group* of disorders characterized by uncontrolled anxiety that leads to impairment in social, interpersonal, and work functioning. Although signs and symptoms may vary from disorder to disorder, the common thread or feature of these conditions is overwhelming anxiety that is out of control. Unlike anxiety felt briefly during a thunderstorm, the level of anxiety that leads to a disorder is disabling and progressive unless treatment is obtained.

Types of Anxiety Disorders

Generalized Anxiety Disorder

In **generalized anxiety** disorder, the person experiences an increased level of anxiety and worry about various situations on most days over a period of at least 6 months. The person has difficulty controlling the anxiety, leading to considerable discomfort, lack of concentration, and impaired ability to function that cannot be attributed to the physiological effects of a substance or another medical condition. It is the most common anxiety disorder seen by primary care physicians in the United States and affects approximately 3% of the country's adult population.

Signs and Symptoms

In addition to the excessive worry and anxiety over several different activities or events, the person also experiences at least three other symptoms that include restlessness, irritability, muscle tension, difficulty falling or staying asleep, and fatigue. Other somatic complaints may also be reported such as chest pain, hyperventilation, headaches, tremors, increased urinary frequency, or gastrointestinal disturbances. The existence of continued tension and feeling on edge leads to a reduced quality of life and overall dissatisfaction with self and others. According to the DSM-5, in generalized anxiety disorder, the worries are excessive and usually interfere with his or her everyday psychosocial functioning. The occurrence of symptoms may be cyclical but tend to be chronic in nature. The signs and symptoms for generalized anxiety disorders are found in Box 9.1.

> **Mind Jogger**
>
> What physiological symptoms usually accompany an increase in anxiety?

> **Just the Facts**
>
> Typical fears of the person with generalized anxiety disorder include physical injury, major illness or death, mental illness, loss of control, and rejection.

Mind Jogger

What psychosocial factors might contribute to the familial tendency of generalized anxiety disorder?

Incidence and Etiology

Most people who are diagnosed with generalized anxiety disorder have felt excessive worry and anxiety all of their life, although most do not request treatment until their mid-30s. Onset is usually in childhood or early adolescence and is often associated with stressful life situations. Anxiety tends to run in families and is more common in females. The female-to-male ratio for anxiety disorders is about 3:2 and affects approximately 3% of the adults in the United States. A coexisting diagnosis of depression is commonly seen with generalized anxiety disorder.

Panic Disorder

A **panic attack** is described as an intense feeling of fear or terror that occurs suddenly and intermittently without warning. The person experiencing the panic is unable to determine when these attacks will occur or reoccur. When the person is unable to connect any particular stimulus with the panic attack, it is referred to as one that is **uncued**. It is said to be **cued** when an identified trigger can be associated with the attack. Some people may only experience a single attack, while others go on to develop a panic disorder.

Everything Is a Mess

Josephine is a 46-year-old female admitted with a diagnosis of generalized anxiety disorder and depression after the loss of her job has left her very despondent. She states, "I don't blame my boss—I could not concentrate or get anything done. I did not want to make any decisions because I was afraid any decision I made would hurt someone's feelings." Josephine is tearful, jumpy, and on edge during the assessment interview. She states, "I don't know what I'm going to do. I have to pay the bills because my husband can't work. The kids need clothes for school. I must be the most terrible mother and wife on earth. I can't sleep. Everything I try to do is a disaster. I'm such a failure. My family would be better off without me." You notice her speech is rapid and she has dark circles under her eyes. She is constantly fidgeting with a Kleenex in her hand.

What data will you need to collect related to Josephine's situation?

_____

_____

How can you help to lower her anxiety level?

_____

_____

What reassurance does she need at this time? What communication techniques will help the nurse in approaching her?

_____

_____

What outcomes would you expect Josephine to achieve?

_____

_____

How will you evaluate the outcome?

_____

_____

Case Application 9.1

BOX 9.1

Signs and Symptoms of Generalized Anxiety Disorder

- Chronic excessive worry and anxiety (no particular stimulus)
- Negative self-talk
- Fatigue
- Difficulty falling or staying asleep
- Increased startle reflex
- Feeling on edge, inability to relax
- Muscle tension
- Headaches
- Irritability
- Inability to control the anxiety
- Anticipating the "worst"
- Inability to concentrate
- Tremors
- Breathing difficulties
- Gastrointestinal disturbances and urinary frequency
- Teeth grinding (bruxism)

BOX 9.2

Signs and Symptoms of Panic Disorder

- Heartbeat rapid and pounding
- Increased perspiration
- Chilling or flushing
- Tingling or numbness of hands, shaking
- Nausea
- Chest pain, shortness of breath
- Feeling of being suffocated
- Fear of being out of control
- Fear of dying or having a heart attack
- Agoraphobia
- Depression

of having the "next attack" can cause significant impairment in the person's overall functioning. The signs and symptoms for panic disorder are found in Box 9.2.

Just the Facts

Persons who become aware of their anxiety learn to identify specific fears that overwhelm them during a panic attack.

Individuals with panic disorder often develop **agoraphobia**, or an avoidance of certain places or situations that tend to trigger the panic attacks. Because they fear a reoccurrence of the panic state, they often restrict their activities to avoid the possibility of this happening. Everyday activities such as shopping for groceries and attending church or family events may be avoided because of fear that escape from these situations might be difficult or embarrassing. They may have fears of being in a crowd or on a bridge, or traveling in a bus, airplane, or automobile. Should the person be entrapped in this situation, the anxiety experienced would lead to a feeling of helplessness and panic. By limiting the possibilities that this would happen, the person often becomes homebound or restricted to home surroundings.

Unemployment and school drop-out are common. Decreased work functioning is evidenced by the inability to complete tasks, repeated absences, and difficulty interacting with others. Up to two thirds of those with this disorder also experience depression or engage in substance abuse to cope with the anxiety.

A panic disorder is characterized by recurrent, unexpected panic attacks. The frequency and severity of these attacks may vary. Some people may be able to endure brief exposure to the situation that causes panic. Others may not be able to expose themselves to the situation at all. When this occurs, the consequences of the disorder are much greater, and the functional capacity of the person decreases significantly.

Mind Jogger

What type of life situations might trigger recurrent panic attacks?

Signs and Symptoms

A state of panic results in sympathetic nervous system symptoms of heart pounding, palpitations, shortness of breath, dizziness, sweating, weakness, and numbness. The person may also feel shaky and chilled with accompanying nausea, chest pain, tingling or numbness of the hands, feelings of suffocation, and being out of control. Attacks may occur daily, weekly, or monthly. Attacks may also occur during the night. Many last only a few minutes, but they may last longer. People experiencing panic attacks often have a fear of "going crazy" or "losing it." Self-esteem may also be affected in varying degrees. Many clients seek frequent medical attention because of their fear of having a life-threatening illness. Fear

Incidence and Etiology

Although they can occur at any age, panic disorders typically have an onset between late adolescence and the mid-30s. First-generation biological relatives are more likely to develop the disorder. Panic disorder affects approximately 6 million adults in the United States, with it being twice as common in females as males. More than 95% of those diagnosed with agoraphobia have an accompanying diagnosis of panic disorder.

 Mind Jogger

How would agoraphobia impact a person's lifestyle and day-to-day functioning?

Specific Phobia

A **specific phobia** is characterized by an excessive and persistent irrational fear of specific objects or situations that actually pose little threat or danger. The common categories of phobias include animals, height, water, storms, blood or needles, flying, elevators, or enclosed spaces. Others may have a fear of sensations such as choking or falling. Box 9.3 lists examples of specific phobias.

BOX 9.3

Examples of Specific Phobias

- Fear of animals—zoophobia
- Fear of fire—pyrophobia
- Fear of riding in a car—amaxophobia
- Fear of sleep—somniphobia
- Fear of confined spaces—claustrophobia
- Fear of spiders—arachnophobia
- Fear of yellow color—xanthophobia
- Fear of ghosts—phasmophobia
- Fear of blood—hematophobia
- Fear of the number 13—triskaidekaphobia
- Fear of heights—acrophobia
- Fear of crossing a bridge—gephyrophobia
- Fear of germs—microphobia
- Fear of pain—algophobia
- Fear of thunder—brontophobia
- Fear of being alone—autophobia
- Fear of open high places—aeroacrophobia
- Fear of flying—aviophobia
- Fear of a needle—aichmophobia

Just the Facts

Specific phobias usually cause little concern because the person can plan ahead to avoid the feared stimulus.

Case Application 9.2

Jack Goes to the Baseball Game

Jack is a 42-year-old male who loves baseball. However, Jack has a fear of crowded places from which there is no accessible exit. Jack usually has been able to secure a ticket for a seat close to the exit ramp. Once there, he discovers that his ticket is not for an aisle seat. He suddenly becomes very aware that the stadium is crowded and he will have to move between many people to get to his seat. He begins to feel his heart throb and has a general flushed feeling. Little beads of sweat begin to form on his scalp and down his back. Instead of going to his seat, he quickly goes back down the ramp toward the main entrance to the stadium. Thinking he will never get there, he has to weave around and in between people the entire trip. At this point, he panics and feels a sense of terror. He suddenly cannot think and feels nearly paralyzed. A stranger notices his distress and offers to drive him to the hospital. Jack manages to nod "yes" but is unable to verbalize which hospital. The stranger brings him to the emergency room of a local hospital where you are employed.

How does Jack's behavior support the presence of a panic disorder?

_____

_____

In what way is Jack's behavior different from free-floating anxiety?

_____

_____

How is this problem impairing his ability to function in a social setting?

_____

_____

Mind Jogger

How would fear of crossing a street or riding in an automobile affect the quality of a person's life?

Signs and Symptoms

When a person comes in contact with the object or situation that causes the fear, the person usually experiences an immediate severe anxiety or panic attack. The distance between the person and the feared object will affect the level of response. A person who fears dogs will experience the most anxiety while in close proximity to the animal. Whether there is a way to escape from the feared stimulus also plays a role in the intensity of the anxiety the person feels. A person who has a fear of going over bridges, for example, will have the most anxiety if there is no way to avoid crossing the bridge. Although children may not be aware of the stimulus causing the anxiety, adolescents and adults are usually aware that their response is extreme and unrealistic. Those with intense fears may experience anxiety symptoms when just thinking about the precipitating factor.

Some people avoid the activities of every-day life because they experience discomfort or increased anxiety when faced with the feared stimulus. During times when there is no exposure to the feared object or situation, however, their anxiety level is no higher than it would normally be. It is when this avoidance significantly impairs the person's ability to continue functioning in social and work settings that the diagnosis of specific phobia is made. The signs and symptoms for specific phobia disorder are listed in Box 9.4.

Incidence and Etiology

Specific phobias affect over 6 million adult Americans. They are twice as common in females as males. Although phobias are common, they are rarely severe enough to be diagnosed. Symptoms usually have an onset during childhood or adolescence and persist throughout adult life. The fear of a particular stimulus is usually present for some time before it is severe enough to be considered a disorder. Phobias following a traumatic event such as the fear of water after a near-drowning situation can develop at any age.

Social Anxiety Disorder (Social Phobia)

Social anxiety disorder, also known as **social phobia**, is characterized by an excessive fear of any social situation in which embarrassment is possible. The person with this disorder experiences intense discomfort when being watched or at risk of being judged or ridiculed by others. This experience typically occurs during social activities where the person will be speaking, dining, or writing in public. Although the person may recognize that the fear is extreme and unrealistic, he or she is helpless to stop it. Social anxiety may be related to one particular situation such as indoor activities or loud music, or it may be related to social occasions in general. Symptoms may be severe enough to interfere with the person's work or school functioning. Social isolation may result in which the person has few friends or contacts.

Mind Jogger

How might social phobia prevent or interfere with fulfillment of a person's goals in life?

Just the Facts

Persons with social anxiety disorder often try to decrease the overwhelming anxiety felt in the feared situation by using drugs and/or alcohol.

Signs and Symptoms

Physical symptoms of anxiety are usually experienced by the person with social anxiety disorder. These may include hyperventilation, palpitations, trembling hands or voice, inability to speak correctly, blushing, sweating, muscle tension, or diarrhea. The person may be embarrassed by the symptoms, which adds to their discomfort. Most people will avoid the difficult situation altogether,

---

BOX 9.4

Signs and Symptoms of Specific Phobia Disorder

- Irrational and persistent fear of an object or situation
- Immediate anxiety on contact with the feared object or situation
- Loss of control, fainting, or panic response
- Avoidance of activities involving feared stimulus
- Worry with anticipatory anxiety
- Possible impaired social or work functioning

BOX 9.5

Signs and Symptoms of Social Anxiety Disorder (Social Phobia)

- Hyperventilation, sweating, cold and clammy hands
- Blushing
- Palpitations
- Confusion
- Gastrointestinal symptoms
- Trembling hands and voice
- Urinary urgency
- Muscle tension
- Anticipatory anxiety
- Fear of embarrassment or ridicule

while others will tolerate the activity but with intense anxiety.

Anticipatory anxiety occurs well in advance of a particular situation such as a public speech or social event. This leads to thoughts of dread leading up to the event. The added anxiety results in actual or perceived failure in the situation, leading to embarrassment and further anxiety. This pattern sets up a vicious cycle of persistent discomfort that can be incapacitating. Many people who have social phobia are underachievers because of test anxiety, poor job performance, or poor communication skills. They may have few or no friends, a decreased support system, and poor interpersonal relationships. The signs and symptoms for social anxiety disorder are listed in Box 9.5.

Incidence and Etiology

The incidence of social phobia tends to be equally distributed between men and women. The disorder usually has an onset in childhood or early adolescence. Onset may be abrupt, following an embarrassing event, or may be insidious or slow in onset. There is a tendency for this condition to run in families.

Posttraumatic Stress Disorder (Trauma and Stressor-Related Disorders)

Posttraumatic stress disorder (PTSD) is characteristically seen when a person has been subjected to a situation that involves an actual death

Everyone Is Looking

JoAnn is a 28-year-old female who is admitted for treatment with a diagnosis of anxiety and social phobic disorder. She has difficulty participating in group activities with other clients. Her family reports that she has been very withdrawn for the past week prior to admission. She feels that everyone will laugh at her and criticize her for the way she looks and talks. Her family states she has not been eating well and seems to have no interest in anything she previously enjoyed. JoAnn is unable to maintain employment because of her fears. During your initial interaction with JoAnn, you note that her hands are trembling as you approach her. She is also hyperventilating and immediately asks to be excused to use the bathroom.

What approach would you use to establish a therapeutic relationship with JoAnn?

_____

_____

What objective symptoms support the diagnosis of social phobia disorder?

_____

_____

How can you help her decrease her level of anxiety?

_____

_____

How can the nurse support JoAnn in her attempts to interact with others?

_____

_____

Case ❸ Application 9.3

or threat of severe injury. The person with PTSD experiences an intense feeling of fear and dread with each recurring mental rerun of the event. The traumatic event may be directly experienced by the person, witnessing someone else's death or severe injury, or receiving word that a close relative has been seriously injured or has died.

> ### Just the Facts
> Traumatic events may include military combat, physical assault, robbery or mugging, sexual abuse, being kidnapped or taken hostage, murder, a terroist attack, natural or man-induced disasters, and fatal or severe motor vehicle accidents.

Signs and Symptoms

The person with PTSD is plagued with increased anxiety that was not present before the precipitating event. Some people may feel extreme guilt for surviving when others did not survive. People, activities, or places that may be connected to the situation are avoided because of the **emotional numbing** that accompanies the exposure. This numbness is shown by an expression of little or no emotion soon after the event as an attempt to prevent future mental pain. The person may continue to show a lack of affect for the remainder of his or her life. It is common for the person to reexperience the event mentally or to reencounter the trauma in dreams. This may lead to insomnia, inability to concentrate, and impaired social or work functioning. The duration of symptoms must be longer than 1 month to be given the diagnosis of PTSD. The signs and symptoms for PTSD are found in Box 9.6.

> ### BOX 9.6
>
> #### Signs and Symptoms of Posttraumatic Stress Disorder
>
> - Intense feeling or fear and dread following a traumatic event
> - Mental reruns of the event
> - Emotional numbness following the event
> - Avoidance of people, places, or things associated with the event
> - Insomnia
> - Increased vigilance or watchfulness
> - Startles easily
> - Irritability and aggressiveness
> - Depression
> - Impaired social or work functioning
> - Difficulty in interpersonal relationships

It is not uncommon for people experiencing the symptoms of PTSD to dissociate or depersonalize as a result of the mental anguish they experience. (For more information on dissociation, see Chapter 14). Persons with PTSD may experience a general lack of trust that impairs their ability to interact with others. Panic attacks, perceptual alterations or hallucinations, and depression may also result. Some people may resort to violence, drugs, or suicide to deal with the recurring disturbing mental pictures. Exposure to similar events can also impose flashbacks or mental images that increase the chances of these complications. This return to the trauma may increase the likelihood the person will resort to extreme means of dealing with the continued emotional pain.

> ### Just the Facts
> During a flashback, the person feels as though he or she is reliving the traumatic experience.

> ### Mind Jogger
> Why might an individual with PTSD tend to engage in aggressive verbal or physical behavior toward others, or reckless, self-destructive behavior?

> ### Just the Facts
> PTSD can disrupt a person's job performance, relationships, physical and mental health, and everyday life.

Incidence and Etiology

Not everyone who is exposed to a traumatic experience develops a posttraumatic disorder. Factors that contribute to the likelihood include the sudden occurrence of the event, such as a plane crash or fatal accident; the severity of the situation, such as the horror of the Sandy Hook school massacre, the terrorist attack of 9-11, or the devastation of Hurricane Sandy in New Jersey; and the time of exposure, such as that seen in a kidnapping or hostage situation. PTSD is more common in females and can be seen in any age group. When seen in children, the child may be unaware of the thoughts but demonstrates the trauma through repetitive play. There is evidence that PTSD is more common if there is a family history of the disorder.

TABLE 9.1   Common Types of Obsessive Thought Content

Contamination	Thoughts of being polluted with germ (e.g., by touching doorknobs or shaking hands with others)
Repeated doubts	Questioning thoughts as to whether one did or did not do something (e.g., turning off the stove or locking the door)
Orderliness	Thinking that one has to have everything in a particular order (e.g., placing things symmetrically on the desk or dresser, placing shoes in alphabetical order by color in a closet, or wearing clothes that always match perfectly with shoes and accessories)
Impulses that are aggressive or horrific in nature	Recurring thoughts about doing actions that could bring great distress to others (e.g., hurting someone who is completely defenseless such as a baby or a person who is physically impaired)
Sexual imagery	Thoughts about sexually revealing images or pornography (e.g., a person sees all people of the opposite sex as wearing see-through clothing or a monogamous married person thinks about sexual activity with multiple partners)

Obsessive-Compulsive Disorder

Obsessive-compulsive disorder (OCD) is characterized by **obsessions** or the reoccurrence of persistent unwanted thoughts or images that cause the person intense anxiety. Table 9.1 provides common types of obsessive thought content. **Compulsions** are the repetitive behaviors or rituals the person engages in to reduce the high level of anxiety. For diagnosis, the obsessions and compulsions have to be severe enough to cause a significant decline in the client's level of functioning with the actions consuming at least 1 hour of the person's day. In this category, the DSM-5 also addresses related disorders including hoarding disorder, or a persistent difficulty discarding possessions regardless of their actual value; disorders involving body-focused repetitive behaviors such as body dysmorphic disorder in which the person has a preoccupation with an imagined defect in appearance or an over-concern with an existing slight physical defect and experiences distress over the imagined or existing defect; trichotillomania (hair-pulling disorder); and excoriation (skin-picking) disorder.

Just the Facts

Hoarding may impose complications such as unsanitary living conditions, risk for falls and injury, fire hazards, and social isolation.

Signs and Symptoms

It is common for everyone to have some recurring uncomfortable thoughts or concern such as whether a car is locked or garage door closed. However, in OCD, the thoughts tend to be related to sexuality, violence, illness, death, or contamination. These thoughts are frequently invasive and inappropriate. The person may recognize the thoughts as unusual and self-generated but has no ability to control them. This lack of control leads to the extreme anxiety.

In an attempt to deal with the anxiety, the person performs repetitive acts that serve no purpose but to relieve the anxiety. The person who feels contaminated with sexual thoughts may wash his hair repeatedly until the scalp is bleeding. The person with violent thoughts of harming her family may check locks and gas knobs every few minutes. In the person with OCD, the symptoms severely interfere with social and occupational functioning. The ability to finish a task is impaired by lack of concentration, invasion of the obsessive thoughts, and need to perform the actions. Symptoms may be intermittent or get worse over time. Signs and symptoms for OCD are found in Box 9.7.

Incidence and Etiology

Occurrence of OCD is evenly distributed between males and females, although it tends to occur at an

BOX 9.7

Signs and Symptoms of Obsessive-Compulsive Disorder

- Recurrent unwanted thoughts referencing contamination, sexuality, aggression, need for perfection, or abnormal doubt
- Attempts to reduce the effect of the thoughts with other thoughts
- Repetitive acts, impulses, or rituals such as showering, washing hair or hands, checking, hoarding, rearranging things for perfect alignment, repeating words or phrases
- Recognition that the thoughts are produced in his or her own mind
- Lack of concentration and task completion
- Impaired social or work functioning

Not Good Enough

Meredith is a 25-year-old college student who has OCD. She has an older brother, Vince, who is a practicing lawyer. Meredith's parents have told her that she "can't hold a candle to Vince." No matter what she does or how well she does in her college courses, she never does as well as her brother. Recently, Meredith has begun having recurring thoughts that if her brother were not here, maybe she could be "somebody" to her parents. She finds herself wishing he would be killed in an accident or struck by lightning. She realizes the extreme and unreasonable nature of these thoughts, but cannot control their continuous intrusion in her mind or the anxiety they create. She has begun calling Vince 20 to 30 times night and day to make sure he is okay. He cannot convince her there is nothing wrong with him. Meredith is having difficulty maintaining her concentration and has been skipping classes to make the phone calls. Vince does not understand what is wrong with Meredith but is becoming annoyed by the phone calls. He has his mobile and home phone numbers changed and asks his secretary to screen calls at his office. This action increases Meredith's anxiety. She has decided to drop out of her college classes and moves to a location adjacent to Vince's home.

How is Meredith's behavior characteristic of OCD?

_____

_____

What impact is this behavior having on her functioning?

_____

_____

How does changing the phone numbers affect Meredith?

_____

_____

What psychological factors may be causing her obsessive-compulsive behavior?

_____

_____

earlier age in males. Prevalence within the general population is less than 5%. Onset is usually in childhood or adolescence. Most adults with the disorder have experienced the symptoms since childhood. There tends to be an occurrence of the behavior pattern in families.

Treatment of Anxiety Disorders

Treatment of anxiety disorders focuses on reducing the client's anxiety level. The two main approaches to the treatment of the anxiety disorders include medications and psychotherapy, either singly or in combination. The medications used are antianxiety drugs (anxiolytics), such as the benzodiazepines. The largest percentage of success is experienced when antianxiety drug agents are used in combination with psychotherapy sessions.

For the psychotherapy component of treatment, research demonstrates that cognitive-behavioral therapy is the most effective in helping the individual to replace negative thoughts and behaviors with more positive and productive ones. The basis for the outcome is that individuals have the ability to control and change their thinking and consequently, their actions. Anxiety support groups can also provide sharing of experiences and offer suggestions for coping.

Antianxiety Agents

Antianxiety agents (anxiolytics) are used to counteract or diminish anxiety. Current antianxiety medications were preceded by studies involving the calming effects of alcohol on the level of

TABLE 9.2 Half-Life of Benzodiazepine Drug Agents

Alprazolam (Xanax)	Short (7–15 h)
Lorazepam (Ativan)	Short (8–15 h)
Oxazepam (Serax)	Short (5–15 h)
Clonazepam (Klonopin)	Long (20–40 h)
Clorazepate (Tranxene)	Long (30–40 h)
Diazepam (Valium)	Long (20–50 h)
Chlordiazepoxide (Librium)	Long (5–30 h)
Prazepam (Centrax)	Long (30–100 h)

Senior Focus

Sensitivity to benzodiazepines is increased in older adults. Smaller doses may be effective as well as safer. The long-acting benzodiazepines have a long half-life (sometimes days) in the older adult, causing prolonged sedation and increased risk of falls and injury. Ambulation should be supervised for at least 8 hours after the administration of an injectable form to avoid injury. If needed, short- or intermediate-acting agents and decreased dosages are preferred (Table 9.2).

discomfort caused by anxiety. The effects of alcohol were limited by its rapid metabolism by the body, the tendency for tolerance to develop, and the tendency for rebound anxiety to occur. Researchers have attempted to find chemical agents that would produce the calming effects without the toxic and addictive qualities of alcohol. In the 1950s drugs chemically related to the barbiturates were developed and remain in existence. Their use, however, has been replaced by more effective drugs that are less addicting than the barbiturate drugs and produce lesser side effects. The earliest of these drugs were the benzodiazepines chlordiazepoxide (Librium) and diazepam (Valium); they were felt to be much safer and less addicting than the barbiturate drugs. Table 9.2 lists common long-acting and short-acting benzodiazepines that are available today.

Drugs in the benzodiazepine group are more useful in stopping severe anxiety symptoms, like those seen in panic disorders. It is important to note that tolerance is common and addictive tendencies are possible. Used continuously, and without adjunctive psychotherapy, their anxiety-reducing effects tend to diminish and tolerance develops. Their usefulness lies in the rapid onset of symptom relief because they enhance the binding of gamma-aminobutyric acid (GABA) receptors, which causes an inhibitory or calming effect on the excited response in the brain. Higher doses can create a more profound effect, inducing sleep or perhaps even coma, indicating their depressive action on the subcortical levels of the central nervous system (CNS). The benzodiazepines and other commonly used antianxiety agents, usual dosages, and their more common side effects are listed in Table 9.3.

TABLE 9.3   Antianxiety or Anxiolytic Drug Agents

CHEMICAL GROUP	GENERIC/BRAND NAME	USUAL DOSAGE (DAILY) (mg)	ADVERSE REACTIONS AND SIDE EFFECTS
Antihistamines	Hydroxyzine (Atarax, Vistaril)	100–400[a]	Dry mouth, drowsiness, pain at site of intramuscular injection
Benzodiazepines	Alprazolam (Xanax)	0.75–4[a]	Drowsiness, dizziness, ataxia, lethargy,
	Chlordiazepoxide (Librium)	15–100[a]	hypotension, blurred vision, nausea,
	Clonazepam (Klonopin)	1.5–20[a]	vomiting, anorexia, sleep disturbance,
	Clorazepate (Tranxene)	15–60[a]	tolerance, physical/psychological
	Diazepam (Valium)	8–40[a]	dependence
	Lorazepam (Ativan)	2–6[a]	
	Oxazepam (Serax)	30–120[a]	
	Prazepam (Centrax)	20–40[a]	
Propanediols	Meprobamate (Equanil, Miltown)	400–2,400 (not recommended for the elderly)	Drowsiness, dizziness, ataxia, reduced seizure threshold, tolerance, and dependence
Miscellaneous	Buspirone (BuSpar)	15–60	Drowsiness, dizziness, excitement, fatigue, headache, insomnia, nervousness, weakness, blurred vision, nasal congestion, palpitations, tachycardia, nausea, rashes, myalgia, incoordination

[a]Reduced dosages recommended for the elderly.

Other agents that may be used to treat anxiety disorders and neuropathic pain include the anticonvulsant medication gabapentin (Neurontin) and propranolol (Inderal, Inderide), a beta-blocker commonly used to treat heart conditions and hypertension. Propranolol is used to control heightened anxiety in social phobia, such as when a client has stage fright prior to a public appearance or speech.

Indications for Use

Antianxiety drugs are used in the treatment of anxiety disorders, anxiety symptoms, acute alcohol withdrawal, skeletal muscle spasms, convulsive and seizure disorders, status epilepticus, neuropathic pain, and preoperative sedation. Because these medications have a potential for abuse with the development of tolerance, dependence, and withdrawal, they are usually prescribed for short periods of time. Although some patients may require long-term treatment, most recommendations are for a time frame of several days or weeks. Discontinuance of long-term usage should be done with physician supervision and should occur gradually with tapered doses rather than abruptly ending treatment.

Contraindications

Antianxiety agents are contraindicated in clients with hypersensitivity, narrow-angle glaucoma, pre-existing CNS depression or psychosis, and in clients who are pregnant and lactating, younger than 12 years, or in shock or in a coma. Anxiolytics should not be taken in combination with other CNS depressants. They should be used with caution in older adults, those with hepatic or renal dysfunction, a history of drug dependence or abuse, and depression. Physical dependence is indicated by withdrawal symptoms if discontinued abruptly. Severe withdrawal symptoms are most likely in clients who have taken higher doses for a period of more than 4 months. The symptoms are caused by the acute separation of the drug molecules at the receptor site and the acute decrease in GABA neurotransmitters. These symptoms most commonly include increased anxiety, psychomotor agitation, insomnia, irritability, headache, tremors, and palpitations. In severe cases, psychotic manifestations and seizures may occur.

Mind Jogger

How do the effects of withdrawal from anti-anxiety agents resemble those experienced from alcohol withdrawal?

Nursing Diagnoses

Nursing diagnoses applicable to the client taking antianxiety medication may include the following:
- Risk for Injury, related to effects of the drug, seizures, increased anxiety, effects of medication toxicity or overdose
- Risk for Activity Intolerance, related to side effects of sedation, confusion, or lethargy
- Confusion, related to effects of drug on CNS
- Knowledge Deficit, related to medication regimen and drug effects

Nursing Interventions

Nursing interventions that may be used for the client taking antianxiety medications may include the following:
- Assess client mood and orientation daily.
- Monitor lying and standing blood pressure daily.
- Assess for paradoxical excitement—notify the physician if it occurs.
- Offer ice chips, hard candy, frequent sips of water, or sugarless gum to relieve dry mouth.
- Give medication with food or milk to prevent nausea and vomiting.
- Report any indications of blood dyscrasias (sore throat, fever, malaise, easy bruising, or unusual bleeding).
- Observe for side effects of antianxiety drug therapy.

Outcome Evaluation

Criteria that may be used to evaluate the effectiveness of antianxiety agents in the client include the following:
- Experiences no physical injury or seizure activity
- Demonstrates decreased anxiety and associated symptoms
- Is able to tolerate usual activity without excessive sedation
- Maintains cognition pattern free of confusion

Client and Family Teaching

Important information to teaching the client and family members about antianxiety agents includes the following:
- The most common side effects of antianxiety medication are drowsiness, fatigue, confusion, and loss of coordination.

- These medications should not be combined with alcohol or other medications such as anesthetics, muscle relaxants, CNS depressants, and other prescribed pain medications.
- Smoking decreases the sedative and antianxiety effects of the benzodiazepine drugs.
- Avoid driving or operating dangerous machinery while taking the drug.
- Do not discontinue taking drug abruptly. Abrupt withdrawal can be life-threatening. (Symptoms may include depression, anxiety, abdominal and muscle cramps, tremors, insomnia, vomiting, diaphoresis, convulsions, and delirium.)
- Rise slowly from a reclining position.
- Clients taking buspirone (BuSpar) may experience a lag time of 10 days to 2 weeks between onset of therapy and reduction of anxiety symptoms. Continue taking the medication during this time.
- Do not take over-the-counter (OTC) or nonprescription drugs without the permission of your physician.
- Report any symptoms of fever, sore throat, malaise, easy bruising, bleeding, or increased motor restlessness to the physician.
- Be aware of side effects and potential adverse effects.

Application of the Nursing Process to the Client with an Anxiety Disorder

When establishing a nurse–client relationship with the person experiencing excessive anxiety, it is important to initially take steps to lower the anxiety level. The person cannot identify the problem until this is accomplished. The nurse can best encourage trust by a calm and reassuring approach.

Nursing Assessment

When collecting data about clients with high levels of anxiety, observe basic characteristics such as thought processes, affect, communication, psychomotor and physiological responses, and ability to complete tasks (Box 9.8). Use directive questions to elicit subjective information about how the client is currently feeling and what happened before the onset of symptoms. Box 9.9 provides examples

---

BOX 9.8

Data Collection

- Thought processes
- Affect
- Communication ability
- Psychomotor and physiological response
- Ability to complete tasks

---

of leading statements to use to gain an understanding of the situation from the client's perspective. Ask the client about other somatic symptoms such as muscle aches, eating patterns, bowel habits, sleeping patterns, and fatigue that might further indicate a psychological origin for the complaints.

Observe the client during activities of daily living and interaction with others to determine when symptoms are most obvious. Assessing the client during usual activities can also provide clues about the client's thought processes. Even though something may not mean much to others, it may be very meaningful to the client. For example, while sitting in the dayroom with peers watching a movie, a client leaves the room quietly and does not return. When assessing what just happened, the nurse finds out that part of the movie took place in a circus, similar to the circus where the client had been raped as a child. Although seeing

---

BOX 9.9

Leading Statements That Encourage Client Participation in Providing Information

- Tell me what happened.
- Tell me details of what happened.
- How did you feel at that time?
- What were you thinking when that happened?
- What emotion were you feeling at that particular time?
- Give me a specific example of what that was like for you.
- Tell me more about that.
- Go on…And…
- Who were you there with?
- What year did this occur?
- What did friends and family say to you?
- Can you describe your feeling?
- How do you feel right now?
- What emotion do you feel?
- What are you doing to decrease that feeling?
- What can you do to decrease that feeling when this situation happens outside this room?

a circus in a movie was insignificant to the other clients, it was very significant to that particular client. Withdrawing from the stimulus was an attempt to lower anxiety.

When questioning a client, consider that your questioning may increase the client's anxiety and interfere with his or her ability to answer. When faced with a frightening situation, a person's anxiety levels increase and his or her thoughts can become more disorganized or extremely focused. The client may complain of not being able to collect his or her thoughts or not being able to control the thoughts. Either way, the client is unable to think, speak, or perform tasks as effectively as before. While taking a test, for example, a student knows the answer to a question but cannot recall it; the student can remember what page the answer is on and which paragraph it is in but still cannot recall it. This is an example of increased anxiety affecting thought processes of memory. Thought blocking or inability to recall information is a common response when suddenly faced with increased anxiety. After relaxing at home later that evening, the student may be able to recall the answer without difficulty. Similarly, when questioning clients, remember that thought blocking may occur and further increase the client's anxiety. The clients may approach the staff at a later time stating the information asked of them earlier.

It is important to note the client's affect. Facial expressions are not easily disguised and may provide more meaningful insight into the client's feelings. A client may report that he is fine but has a facial grimace. The facial expression usually reflects true feelings before behavior does. You may note a flat affect several times during the day when the client is unaware that he or she is being observed. Observe for congruence of nonverbal and verbal messages during each observation or contact with the client.

Determine how well the client is able to communicate. When assessing for interactive skills, take into consideration the client's level of education. For example, a client who has been in the hospital for 4 days consistently complains about the food and asks the staff to order something different for him. While observing the client selecting food for the next day from the menu, a nurse notices that the client is very anxious and unable to make decisions or direct thought processes long enough to mark the menu. Using a sensitive approach, the nurse determines that the client is illiterate and is unable to understand what food choices are available. Determining how well the client is able to communicate thoughts is also relevant. If the speech is choppy and pressured, the client may be experiencing anxiety and subsequent distress from impaired communication skills. During interaction with the client, be aware of your own verbal and nonverbal message. Anxiety is contagious and can contribute to the client's difficulty in communicating.

Also observe the client's ability to perform and complete tasks. Psychomotor responses can reach a hyperactive level and be counterproductive when anxiety is high. On the other hand, when anxiety is extremely high, psychomotor responses can become slowed and also decrease functional ability. Collecting observations helps to determine if the client's inability to perform tasks is the result of impaired thought processes or impaired motor responses. For example, when observing a depressed client attempting to get dressed, a nurse notes several articles of clothing lying on the bed. The client is across the room crying and wringing her fingers. At this point, the nurse concludes the client may be experiencing increased anxiety about making a decision between choices of what to wear; this would be an impaired thought process.

Observation of the client with particular attention to specific anxiety-reducing behaviors should be part of the initial and ongoing assessment for each client. Sometimes symptoms are expressed in subtle ways, such as leaving group therapy to go to the bathroom or avoiding an activity where several clients are participating. It is important to note if behaviors are improving with the administration of antianxiety medications or if the client is experiencing any side effects from the drug.

Nursing Diagnosis

Once the assessment is made and data are collected, the information is reviewed and sorted into meaningful clusters. From this data, problems are identified to determine applicable nursing diagnoses. Relevant nursing diagnoses for the client with an anxiety disorder may include the following:

- Anxiety, related to a feeling of actual or perceived threat
- Anxiety, related to intrusive thought processes
- Ineffective Coping, related to unmet needs
- Fear, related to extreme and unrealistic perceptions

- Powerlessness, related to lack of control over anxiety
- Risk for Self- or Other-Directed violence, related to reoccurring intrusive thoughts
- Disturbed Sleep Pattern, related to excessive worry and anxiety
- Social Isolation, related to feelings of guilt or emotional numbness
- Altered Family Processes, related to situation crisis
- Skin Integrity Impaired, related to compulsive repetitive behaviors
- Situational or Chronic Low Self-Esteem, related to feelings of inadequacy

Expected Outcomes

Once the nursing diagnosis is made, appropriate outcomes for clients can be determined. Careful consideration should be given to a realistic time frame in which the outcomes can be achieved. Outcomes are always client-centered and time-limited. Examples of outcomes may include that within 7 days, the client will:

- Identify initial signs and symptoms of anxiety
- Identify effective coping methods to use when anxiety begins to occur
- Demonstrate effective strategies to lower anxiety
- Experience increased energy
- Identify alternative methods of coping that decrease social isolation
- Demonstrate decreased cleaning rituals
- Participate in small group discussions with decreased anxiety
- Look at pictures of a phobic stimulus without excessive anxiety
- Ventilate anxiety appropriately and safely to others
- Experience improved sleep pattern
- Demonstrate improved impulse control

Nursing Interventions

When dealing with anxiety in others, the nurse should take into consideration your own anxiety level and how it may affect nursing care. Subtle behaviors such as a change in the tone of voice, rushed movements, or spending less time with the client can communicate your anxiety to the client. This in turn can generate increased anxiety in the client resulting in a decreased ability to function.

Establishing a sense of trust includes maintaining a calm and supportive environment in which the client feels a sense of safety and security. It is important to use caution when touching or approaching the person having a panic attack. Doing so may pose an additional threat to the client or an invasion of his or her personal space.

Nursing interventions should be timely, client-centered, and realistic. Interventions should include only what the client is able to do at that time. It may be difficult for the client to take more than small steps toward reaching expected outcomes. Overwhelming the client with unrealistic expectations may indicate anxiety on the nurse's part and lead to counterproductive results in the client. Assessing the client's tolerance for change is essential for planning appropriate client-centered nursing interventions. Reassessment should occur to ensure the continuing relevance of the interventions. Every effort should be made to assist the client in identifying the issues that precipitate the feelings of anxiety. Linking the behavior exhibited by the client to a particular situation can help the client to develop an awareness of feelings that precede the anxiety attacks. As the nurse, you can also model and help the client to try new, more adaptive coping strategies.

Additional nursing interventions include the following:

- Encourage participation in social interaction and exercise activities.
- Give positive reinforcement for the client's efforts to participate.
- Teach stress-management techniques (progressive relaxation, music therapy, deep breathing).
- Assist the client with compulsive behaviors to find ways to set limits on the rituals.
- Acknowledge the behaviors but do not focus on them—it is important to express an empathetic response rather than criticize the behavior. For example, in response to a client who has shampooed her hair four times in 2 hours, the nurse might say, "I am sure your scalp is getting sore from washing your hair so much," rather than, "You only need to wash your hair once a day."
- Observe for automatic relief behaviors.
- Encourage open discussion of feelings and thoughts.
- Monitor for indications of escalating anxiety.
- Encourage time-out for impulsive clients to regain self-control.

Evaluation

Evaluation of the plan of care occurs at the end of the time frame that was set to reach client outcomes. Success is determined based on whether the outcome criteria were achieved. The plan of care is revised if outcomes were not met, the problem persists, or if a new problem has developed.

Effectiveness of planned interventions will be demonstrated in the client's ability to recognize and deal with the anxiety-producing factors. Once the client identifies the relationship between unreasonable thoughts and subsequent behaviors, it is more realistic to anticipate the use of more effective coping strategies to reduce his or her anxiety. It is important for the client to express openly feelings and thoughts related to the situation. The effectiveness of active listening by the nurse and learned coping skills are shown when the client reports that anxiety has been reduced to a manageable level. This can also be demonstrated as the client shows relaxed participation in activities and reports longer periods of restful sleep. Further indication of learned skills is shown as the impulsive client resolves conflict situations using improved self-control. It is anticipated that through learning what precipitating factors can be changed and steps that can be taken to lower anxiety for those that cannot be changed, the client will demonstrate more effective problem-solving methods to improve overall functioning and well-being.

CLIENT TEACHING NOTE 9.1

Sources of Information on Anxiety Disorders

- National Institute of Mental Health (NIMH) 6001 Executive Blvd., Room 8184, MSC 9663 Bethesda, MD 208922-9663 Phone: 301-443-4513 or 1-866-615-NIMH (6464), toll-free (www.nimh.nih.gov)
- Anxiety Disorders Association of America 8730 Georgia Ave., Suite 600 Silver Springs, MD 20910 (www.adaa.org)
- Obsessive Compulsive (OC) Foundation 227 Notch Hill Road North Branford, CT 06471 (www.ocfoundation.org)
- National Mental Health Association (NMHA) 2001 N. Beauregard St., 12th Floor
- Alexandria, VA 22311 Phone: 1-800-969-6642 (www.nmha.org)
- American Psychological Association 750 1st St., NE Washington, DC 20002-4242 Phone: 1-888-357-7924 (www.psych.org/index.cfm)

- Provide explanations regarding medications and side effects to client and family.
- Avoid giving advice to client.
- Provide client education regarding anxiety and precipitating factors.
- Administer antianxiety medications
- Provide sources of information about anxiety disorders such as those found in Client Teaching Note 9.1

Summary

- Anxiety is an unconscious uneasy feeling that everyone experiences at some time. Although often unaware of the cause, we manage to cope and manage everyday life.
- When anxiety perceived as threatening increases to high levels, some individuals are unable to find an effective coping strategy.
- Inability to associate a precipitating factor with the uncontrolled behavior is common to all anxiety disorders.
- The level of anxiety that results in a disorder is intense and disabling.
- Generalized anxiety disorder involves an increased level of anxiety and worry about various situations on most days over a period of at least 6 months.

- Panic disorder results in a sense of terror and fear that is exhausting and emotionally draining. Some with panic attacks develop agoraphobia and avoid triggering events or places.
- Specific phobias are demonstrated in those who experience intense anxiety when exposed to certain objects of situations.
- Social phobia (social anxiety disorder) occurs in situations when embarrassment may result from the exposure and the individual is unable to control the symptoms.
- OCD is characterized by *obsessions* (recurring, persistent, unwanted thoughts or images that cause intense anxiety), coupled with *compulsions* (repetitive behaviors or rituals the person engages in to reduce the high level of anxiety).

- Actions in OCD are repetitive and ritualistic in nature and have a crippling effect on work, social, and interpersonal relationships. Although aware that the thoughts are psychological, the person is unable to control them.
- Experiencing or witnessing a horrific event can result in a PTSD that leaves a reaction of emotional numbing and continued mental images that intermittently plague the unconscious mind.
- Treatment of anxiety focuses on reducing the anxiety level to a point at which the person can identify the precipitating factors and their connection to the resulting behaviors.
- Antianxiety medications used in combination with psychotherapy have proven to be the most beneficial treatment approach.
- Antianxiety agents (anxiolytics) are used in the treatment of anxiety disorders, anxiety symptoms, acute alcohol withdrawal, and convulsive or seizure disorders.
- Once ineffective skills are identified, improved adaptation methods can be taught and implemented.
- The nurse's role is to assess symptoms and client response to therapeutic treatment. A calm, reassuring approach is necessary to provide the client a sense of a safe and supportive environment.

Bibliography

American Psychiatric Association. (2013). *Diagnostic and statistical manual of mental disorders text revision* (5th ed.). Washington, DC: American Psychiatric Association.

Beck, A. T., & Emery, G. (with Greenberg, R. L.). (Rev. ed. 2005). *Anxiety disorders and phobias: A cognitive perspective*. New York, NY: Basic Books.

Dubenetzky, S. (2013). Differential diagnosis of anxiety disorders. *Annals of Psychotherapy and Integrative Health, 16*(2), 40–46. Retrieved January 25, 2014.

Guiterrez, M. A., Roper, J. M., & Hahn, P. (2001). Paradoxical reactions to benzodiazepines. *American Journal of Nursing, 7*(101), 34–39.

Herdman, T. H. (Ed.) (2012). *NANDA International-nursing diagnoses 2012–2014*. Oxford, UK: Wiley-Blackwell Publishers.

Jacob, M. L., Morelan, D., Suveg, C., Brown Jacobsen, A. M., & Whiteside, S. P. (2012). Emotional, behavioral, and cognitive factors that differentiate obsessive-sompulsive disorder and other anxiety disorders in youth. *Anxiety, Stress & Coping, 25*(2), 229–237. Retrieved January 31, 2014.

Lippincott. (2013). *Nursing 2014 drug handbook*. Philadelphia, PA: Springhouse Publishing Co.

Low, N. C., Dugas, E., Constatin, E., Karp, I., Rodriguez, D., O'Loughlin, J. (2012). The association between parental history of diagnosed mood/anxiety disorders and psychiatric symptoms and disorders in young adult offspring. *BMC Psychiatry, 12*(1), 188–195. Retrieved January 25, 2014.

Naeem, A. (2012). Management of panic anxiety with agoraphobia by using cognitive behavior therapy. *Indian Journal of Psychological Medicine, 34*(1), 79–81. Retrieved 25, 2014.

National Institute of Mental Health. (2009). Anxiety Disorders. NIH Publication. Retrieved 31, 2014, from http://www.nimh.nih.gov/health/publications/anxiety-disorders/index.shtml.

Patel, G., Fancher, T. L. (2013). In the clinic: Generalized anxiety disorder. *Annals of Internal Medicine, 159*(11), 1–12. Retrieved January 31, 2014.

Townsend, M. C. (2011). *Nursing diagnoses in psychiatric nursing* (8th ed.) Philadelphia, PA: F. A. Davis Co.

Varcolaris, E. M. (2011). *Manual of psychiatric nursing care planning*. (4th ed.) St. Louis, MO: Saunders Elsevier.

Student Worksheet

Fill in the Blank

Fill in the blank with the correct answer.

1. Free-floating anxiety occurs when the person is unable to _____ the anxiety to a _____.
2. _____ are behaviors of which the person is unaware that are aimed at relieving anxiety.
3. An excessive and persistent irrational fear of objects or situations that actually pose little threat of danger is referred to as a _____ _____.
4. Social phobia is characterized by excessive fear of any social situation in which _____ is possible.
5. _____ are recurrent persistent and unwanted thoughts or images that cause intense anxiety for the person experiencing them.
6. The usefulness of the anxiolytic (antianxiety) drugs lies in their _____ of symptom relief that causes an inhibitory or calming effect on the excited response in the brain.

Matching

Match the following terms to the most appropriate phrase.

1. _____ Microphobia
2. _____ Hematophobia
3. _____ Amaxophobia
4. _____ Zoophobia
5. _____ Claustrophobia
6. _____ Arachnophobia
7. _____ Gephyrophobia
8. _____ Acrophobia

a. Fear of heights
b. Fear of crossing a bridge
c. Fear of spiders
d. Fear of confined spaces
e. Fear of riding in a car
f. Fear of germs
g. Fear of blood
h. Fear of animals

Multiple Choice

Select the best answer from the choices provided.

1. Initially, which of the following nursing interventions would be the most important to implement when a client is experiencing a panic attack?
   a. Administer a prn dose of antianxiety medication
   b. Provide a detailed explanation of what causes panic attacks
   c. Assure the client you will remain until the panic attack subsides
   d. Hug the client to show empathy for the distress he or she is experiencing

2. A client with generalized anxiety disorder approaches the nurse and states he feels dizzy. Which of the following would be the best response for the nurse to make?
   a. Don't worry, it is just one of the symptoms you can expect."
   b. "Stay right here. I will be back with some medication to help you."
   c. "I'll help you to your room so you can lie down and rest until you feel better."
   d. "Can you tell me what happened about the time you started feeling this way?"

3. A client has just been diagnosed with panic disorder. Which of the following symptoms would the nurse expect to observe?
   a. Hypotension
   b. Feelings of suffocation
   c. Constipation
   d. Logical thought processes

4. A college student with known social phobia or social anxiety disorder receives an assignment that requires a class presentation. The student is so distraught over the assignment that he drops the class, even though it is required for his degree plan. What term would be applied to the dread felt by this student that leads to his actions?
   a. Free-floating anxiety
   b. Automatic relief behavior
   c. Uncued anxiety
   d. Anticipatory anxiety

5. Which of the following is the most appropriate initial outcome for the nurse to set for the client experiencing a panic level of anxiety?
   a. Will develop a trusting relationship with the nurse
   b. Will demonstrate insight into cause of anxiety
   c. Will identify alternate methods of coping
   d. Will reduce anxiety at least one level

6. Which of the following chart entries by the nurse would demonstrate progress in the client who experiences agoraphobia?
   a. Attends group therapy sessions four out of five times a week
   b. Conversing with two other clients during mealtime
   c. Participated in outing to park this afternoon
   d. Has showered and shampooed hair once today

7. Initially, which nursing intervention would receive the highest priority for the client with OCD?
   a. Confront the client about the ridiculous nature of the behavior
   b. Isolate the client to reduce proximity to others
   c. Set limits for client to conform to unit schedule
   d. Allow extra time for client to perform rituals

8. Which of the following clients would require additional health teaching regarding the effects of a prescribed benzodiazepine drug agent?
   a. 32-year-old who smokes two packs of cigarrettes a day
   b. 50-year-old who drinks three cups of coffee each morning
   c. 28-year-old client who is an internet stock broker
   d. 47-year-old company CEO who works an average 50-hour week

9. A client is being seen for increasing symptoms of panic attacks. The client asks the physician for "something for my nerves." Which of the following comments by the client should the nurse report to the physician?
   a. "The panic attacks happen most when I am in a room full of people."
   b. "None of my family seems to understand just how bad this feeling is."
   c. "I am happiest when I am breast-feeding my 2-month-old daughter."
   d. "Sometimes I feel like I am going crazy and have to leave the room."

10. The nurse is doing patient teaching for a client taking a newly prescribed antianxiety medication. Which statement by the client would alert the nurse to the need for further teaching?
    a. "I will continue taking the drug even if it makes me sleepy."
    b. "Maybe now I can enjoy an evening of wine and dinner with my wife."
    c. "I guess I won't feel better right away from taking this drug."
    d. "Hopefully, I will only need to take this for a short period of time."

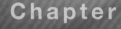

Chapter 10

Mood Disorders

⊙ Learning Objectives

After learning the content in this chapter, the student will be able to:

1. Define mood and affect as they relate to an abnormal state.
2. Describe signs and symptoms of common depressive disorders.
3. Describe the identifying criteria for bipolar and related disorders.
4. Identify treatment methods for individuals with depressive and bipolar disorders.
5. Discuss the use of mood-stabilizing agents in the treatment of bipolar disorder.
6. Describe the nursing process related to antidepressant and mood-stabilizing drug therapy.
7. Describe nursing assessment of clients with a mood disorder.
8. Develop appropriate nursing diagnoses related to mood disorders.
9. Plan expected outcomes for categories of mood disorders.
10. Identify appropriate nursing interventions for clients with mood disorders.
11. Evaluate the effectiveness of planned nursing strategies toward outcomes.

⊙ Key Terms

affect
anergia
anhedonia
antidepressant
bipolar disorder
clang association
depression
euphoria
grandiosity
hypomania
labile

mania
monoamine oxidase inhibitor (MAOI)
mood
mood disorder
negativism
persecution
rapid cycling
serotonin-specific reuptake inhibitors (SSRIs)
unipolar

Life involves everyday situations that trigger our emotions. On one end of the emotional spectrum are feelings of sadness and loss. Most people feel a sense of sadness in response to disappointments such as not winning a ballgame or not receiving an anticipated job promotion. Some people also feel sadness during holidays or occasions on which a loss has occurred. Sadness is seen as a normal state of depression, often referred to as feeling "down" or "blue." In most people, this sadness is limited, and they are able to return to a normal state of functioning. On the other end of the emotional spectrum are the feelings of happiness and joy. Elation is a normal feeling of well-being experienced with success and momentous occasions. The variance between happiness and sadness in most people is mild and congruent with the situation that triggers the feeling. The prolonged inability to regain a sense of emotional balance, however, is considered abnormal.

Mood and Affect Defined

Mood is an emotion that is prolonged to the point that it colors an individual's entire psychological thinking. The feelings are changeable depending on the person's perception of sensory stimuli. For example, one individual might respond to a separation or divorce with deep feelings of sadness, regret, and failure, while another might feel a more contented feeling of relief and freedom. **Affect** describes the facial expression an individual displays in association with the mood (e.g., smiling when happy, grimacing when angry).

Alterations in mood can range from mild to severe. When the mood alterations are mild, the person may experience minor changes in daily routine with minimal impairment in functioning. For example, one might be disappointed after the cancellation of a much anticipated lunch date but view it as a simple change in plans, or a person may feel sad for a time after the death of a pet but decide to replace the loss with another pet. Severe mood alterations, however, can result in significant impairment of the person's ability to function. For example, the cancelled lunch date might be seen as personal rejection and a reason to become socially reclusive, and the loss of a pet could be followed by despair and depression.

The prolonged inability to regain a sense of emotional balance is considered abnormal. A *depressed mood* is one in which sadness is intensified

and continues longer than would normally be expected in a particular situation. In contrast, an excessive feeling of happiness or elation is seen in **euphoria**. This euphoric state can escalate to a frenzied unstable mood of **mania** in which the person may be out of touch with reality.

In the DSM-5, the depressive disorders and bipolar related disorders have been separated with bipolar and related disorders being placed between the psychotic disorders and depressive disorders to reflect a link between the two disorders with reference to symptoms, family, and genetic history. In the depressive disorders, a common symptom of a sad and empty mood along with psychosomatic changes is present, whereas in bipolar and related disorders, there is a pattern of mood swings between mania or euphoria and depression which often include a psychotic component.

Depressive Disorders

Depression is described as a persistent and prolonged mood of sadness that extends beyond 2 weeks' duration or longer. In the depressive disorders, there is a distinctive change in the affect and cognition, with the sadness being severe enough to interfere with the individual's functional activity. This state can occur in a single episode or in a recurring pattern over time. Depressive disorders are often referred to as **unipolar**, indicating that the person does not experience episodes of mania or hypomania. Specific types of depressive disorders include major depressive disorder and persistent depressive or dysthymic disorder.

Major Depressive Disorder

Major depressive disorder occurs when a person experiences a depressed mood or loss of interest in most activities for most of each day for a period of 2 weeks. This can occur as a single episode or recurrent depressive episodes. The persistence and severity of the symptoms during the major depressive episode help to differentiate it from that seen in other psychotic or delusional disorders. The depressive episode may have a precipitating circumstance, such as chronic pain, loss of a job, lack of a support system, financial difficulties, or conflict with a friend or loved one. People who are timid and anxious tend to have more difficulty adapting to loss and the increased pressures of life than people who are bold, confident, and easygoing.

Recovery from the impact of these situations may precipitate depression in those with inadequate coping skills.

Depression that occurs without a precipitating event is often associated with decreased neurotransmitter availability in the brain and usually responds to antidepressant medication. Seasonal depression is associated with decreased daylight hours during the winter months. An episode of major depression is usually severe enough to require treatment.

> ### Just the Facts
> The average person with major depressive disorder experiences four episodes over a lifetime.

Signs and Symptoms

Indications of depression include feelings of hopelessness, guilt and self-blame, melancholy, fatigue, loss of appetite, weight changes, and a decreased libido or sex drive. In addition, a person who suffers from major depression may experience crying episodes, irritability, excessive worry, anxiety, and increased somatic complaints (e.g., headaches, body pains, gastrointestinal disturbances). The person may have lapses of memory, a lack of concentration, and difficulty making decisions. Even small tasks may seem overwhelming, leading to decreased efficiency and productivity. For example, a mother who previously had no problem shopping for groceries to feed her family now is unable to make decisions in the supermarket. Instead of selecting items, she feels defeated and leaves the store with nothing. **Anergia**, or a marked decrease in energy level, may make the person depend on others for even basic needs.

Many individuals with depression experience sleep disturbances such as waking too early or having difficulty falling asleep. Others may wake in the middle of the night and be unable to return to sleep, while others may sleep for prolonged periods. The person may require a longer time to complete basic tasks such as bathing and dressing. Hygiene is often neglected in response to the poor self-image and worthlessness felt by the person. Often **anhedonia**, or a lack of pleasure in things an individual previously enjoyed, accompanies the depressed state. This is illustrated by a person who previously had enjoyed reading to children at the library and now avoids the sessions

---

BOX 10.1

Signs and Symptoms of Major Depressive Disorder

- Mood of worry, anxiety, hopelessness, and worthlessness
- Guilt and self-blame
- Crying episodes
- Fatigue, anergia
- Sleep disturbances
- Weight and appetite changes
- Decreased sex drive
- Poor concentration and memory lapse
- Difficulty making decisions
- Decreased productivity
- Irritability
- Extreme sadness with sad affect
- Physical complaints
- Anhedonia or decreased pleasure in things previously enjoyed
- Thoughts of death and suicide

---

because he no longer feels worthy of the children's attention. The affect of the depressed person is one of sadness and misery, with a lack of eye contact and apathy. Dwelling on exaggerated and perceived failures, the person is unable to see strengths and successes. Recurring thoughts of death and suicide are common. Signs and symptoms for major depressive disorder are found in Box 10.1.

Incidence and Etiology

Depression is more common in females and those who have a familial tendency for the disorder. Adolescents between the ages of 14 and 16 and adults older than age 65 have a higher incidence of major depression. At least one-fourth of the population will experience depression in their lifetime. Approximately 15% of those with major depressive disorder will attempt suicide. A major depressive episode may develop over days or weeks and last for several months. Some may experience a single episode, while others have a recurrent pattern of symptoms. A major episode can occur at any age although the average age of onset is the mid-20s. Studies show that approximately half of those experiencing a major depressive episode will have another.

There are various theories about the cause of depression. Perhaps the most common is related to functional deficits of neurotransmitters in the brain that lead to a chemical imbalance. This theory supports the successful use of antidepressant drugs in the treatment process. In addition, genetic and biologic predisposition, substance/medication effects, premenstrual dysphoria, viruses, thyroid and other endocrine disturbances, and psychosocial factors are all cited as possible causes.

Mind Jogger

What impact would the symptoms of major depression have on the person's family, work environment, and social life?

Persistent Depressive Disorder (Dysthymia) Disorder

The person with persistent depressive disorder or dysthymia experiences a recurrent state of depression over a period of at least 2 years. Depressive symptoms become a part of the person's day-to-day experience, never disappearing for more than 2 months at a time. The client with persistent depressive disorder has never had a major depressive episode and does not exhibit any symptoms of manic behavior. The symptoms of persistent depressive disorder are less severe than those of major depression, but the disorder tends to be more chronic.

Common Signs and Symptoms

People with persistent depressive disorder tend to struggle with the symptoms of depression over a lifetime. Life experiences have taught the person that he or she is ineffective and inadequate at coping with loss. The feelings of inadequacy, failure, and emptiness often result in a pessimistic attitude toward most aspects of the person's existence. **Negativism** is a learned sense of helplessness. Ill-equipped to cope with these continued feelings of despair, people with persistent depressive disorder may resort to substance use, spending sprees, sexual promiscuity, or acting-out behaviors to escape the mental pain. The person may experience sleep difficulties, changes in eating habits, fatigue, low self-esteem, loss of sexual desire, feelings of hopelessness, decreased concentration, and decision-making ability. Persons with persistent depressive disorder tend to abuse alcohol, nicotine, or other drugs in an attempt to treat insomnia or anxiety. Signs and symptoms for persistent depressive disorder are found in Box 10.2.

BOX 10.2

Signs and Symptoms of Persistent Depressive Disorder (Dysthymia)

- Chronic depression symptoms
- Feelings of inadequacy, failure, emptiness
- Hopelessness
- Negativism
- Maladaptive coping skills
- Sleep difficulties
- Increased or decreased appetite
- Fatigue
- Low self-esteem
- Difficulty concentrating
- Decreased decision-making ability

Just the Facts

The depressed person feels an on-going sense that something considered essential for happiness is missing from their life.

Mind Jogger

What life situations might cause an individual with dysthymia to be vulnerable? What might have happened for the client's defenses to fail?

Incidence and Etiology

Dysthymia occurs two to three times more frequently in women than men. The disorder is more likely to occur in first-degree biologic relatives with depressive disorders. There is usually an early-onset beginning anytime from childhood through early adulthood. Some of those who first experience depressive episodes will eventually develop bipolar disorder. In most cases where this occurs, there is a family history of bipolar illness.

Mind Jogger

Why do you think dysthymia and depression are more common in women?

Bipolar and Related Disorders

In **bipolar disorders**, formerly known as manic depression, there is a brain dysfunction that causes abnormal and erratic shifts in mood, energy, and functional ability. The episodes of alternate changes between extreme moods, ranging from high manic episodes (euphoric, excessively happy, high energy) to low depressive periods may occur rapidly, may be intermixed with periods of normal functioning, or these can occur simultaneously in a mixed episode. The rapid shifts in mood in a short period of time are referred to by the DSM-5 as **labile**, or alternating from euphoria to dysphoria and irritability. In the DSM-5 criteria for bipolar disorder, the mood change must be accompanied by persistently increased activity or energy levels that are obvious to those observing the person. The frequency of the mood swings between the two states is unpredictable and varies from person to person. The severity of the symptoms may vary from mild to severe. Based on the severity of the episodes and duration, individuals may be diagnosed with bipolar II disorder or cyclothymic disorder. If the person has four or more mood shifts within a year, the person is said to be **rapid cycling**. This feature is more common in later stages of the illness.

Just the Facts

Bipolar disorder typically begins with depression accompanied by at least one manic episode.

Signs and Symptoms

Although the disorder may not be recognized in its early onset, the first indications may be a state of mild to moderate mania called **hypomania** that lasts for a period of at least 4 days. The person is unusually cheerful with excessive energy and the ability to keep going long after others are exhausted. The need for sleep may decrease to 3 or 4 hours. This level of acceleration may feel good to the person, who may deny anything is wrong. There is an obvious inflated self-esteem or feeling of **grandiosity** during which time the person may experience hallucinations or delusional thinking. The person may demonstrate an increase in goal-directed activity but with increased irritability and moodiness. The person usually talks incessantly with a flight of ideas or jumping from one subject to another, and may describe thoughts as racing or pressured. Attention is easily distracted to things in the environment that are insignificant.

Irresponsible and impulsive behavior may accompany the increased moodiness and irritability. It is common for the person to spend large amounts of money on unneeded items or make senseless business deals. A preoccupation with

seductive thoughts often leads to sexual promiscuity. The changes in mood are obvious to others, but not usually severe enough to require hospitalization. The person in hypomania does not experience psychotic symptoms of delusions or hallucinations.

Mind Jogger

There are artists and actors who have created some of their best work while in a state of hypomania. What characteristics of the mood might account for this?

When the person experiences periods of severe highs, or full-blown manic episodes, the symptoms are more extreme and pronounced. The elevated mood lasts for at least a week and causes disruption in the person's ability to function. The person's lack of insight and excessive level of activity predispose him or her to a dangerous and volatile psychotic state. The person may be offensive and violate the rights of others. When his or her wishes are not fulfilled, the mood may shift from extreme euphoria to extreme aggressive irritability. During these interpersonal conflicts, the person may perceive injustice and have delusional thoughts of **persecution** that a threat of harm exists. The constant shift in attention from one thought to another is seen in flight of ideas. Words may be strung together in rhyming phrases or **clang associations** that have no connected meaning (i.e., "Hair is bare and bear is a scare, scare is a fair, fair is there, you are a pear…"). The person projects an expansive thought pattern of grandiosity with false beliefs of wealth, power, and identity. Auditory and visual hallucinations may occur during the height of the manic episode. The female may dress bizarrely with bright flamboyant colors, excessive jewelry, and inappropriate makeup. Hygiene is often neglected as the thought processes escalate and activity accelerates. Items such as magazine pictures, containers, and food may be collected and stockpiled as the hyperactivity absorbs the person's time. Signs and symptoms for bipolar I disorder and bipolar II disorder are listed in Box 10.3.

Just the Facts

During a state of mania, the person has continued mental flood of overly confident self-expectations that lead to frenzied psychomotor activity.

BOX 10.3

Signs and Symptoms of Bipolar I/ Bipolar II Disorders

Hypomania/Mania:
- Extreme euphoria
- Inflated self-esteem or grandiosity
- Talkative with rapid, racing speech
- Flight of ideas
- Excessive energy
- Decreased need for sleep
- Easily distracted
- Extreme irritability and moodiness
- Reckless and impulsive behaviors
- Lack of judgment
- Increased motor activity
- Irresponsible buying sprees or business deals
- Sexual indiscretions
- Delusions of grandeur or persecution (mania)
- Auditory and visual hallucinations (mania)
- Bizarre dress and accessories
- Poor hygiene

Incidence and Etiology

In many cases of bipolar disorder, there seems to be a genetic factor that is shown by the familial pattern of the illness. There are studies that show an increase in the severity in future generations. Environmental factors are also cited as a cause since not all cases have a family history of the disorder. Despite these theories, we do not know exactly what causes this condition. Evidence has linked bipolar symptoms to changes in the chemical neurotransmitters in the brain. Substance abuse and stressful life events have also been linked to the episodes.

Women are at greater risk than men for developing manic episodes, which can occur at any time. The average age of onset for a first manic episode is in the early 20s, but it can be as early as adolescence and as late as age 50. Manic episodes that occur in adolescence may lead to school failure, behavioral problems, and substance abuse. Manic episodes can also occur during postpartum periods in women.

Just the Facts

Bipolar disorders have a younger age of onset and shorter cycles than major depressive disorders.

Mind Jogger

What factors related to the postpartum period might contribute to a psychotic state of mania or depression? How might this lead to a dangerous situation?

BOX 10.4

Signs and Symptoms of Cyclothymic Disorder

- Recurrent episodes of hypomania and dysthymia
- States not as severe as in bipolar disorders
- Short periods or normalcy
- No psychotic symptoms
- Functioning not severely impaired

Cyclothymic Disorder

Cyclothymic disorder is a chronic mood disturbance characterized by fluctuating periods of hypomanic symptoms and periods of depression. The symptoms of cyclothymic disorder are insufficient in number, severity, or duration to meet the criteria for a hypomanic or major depressive episode.

Common Signs and Symptoms

The symptoms of cyclothymia include recurrent episodes of hypomania and dysthymia. The signs and symptoms for cyclothymic disorder are found in Box 10.4. These alternating periods are recurrent with short periods of normalcy that usually do not last longer than 2 months. Delusional thinking and hallucinations are not present. The person's functioning is not severely impaired and hospitalization is usually not necessary.

Incidence and Etiology

Cyclothymic disorder occurs equally in men and women and begins in adolescence or early adulthood. It is usually chronic with an insidious onset. Most people do not realize the disorder is present until many symptoms have existed over years. There is a greater risk for the person with this disorder to develop bipolar disorder.

Treatment of Depressive Disorders

Treatment of depressive disorders may include pharmacologic, psychotherapeutic, psychosocial, and electroconvulsive therapy (ECT) approaches. Psychotherapeutic drug agents are used very successfully in managing depression. Drug therapy includes the antidepressants and mood-stabilizing drugs. As the medication becomes effective in restoring levels of neurotransmitters, the client's mood and energy level usually will improve as well. It is generally felt that drugs help make the client more accepting of other interventions, but used alone, prove ineffective for long-term treatment. Although drug therapy can level out the brain chemistry to minimize the symptoms of the disorder, many clients fail to reap the benefits due to noncompliance with treatment.

Depending on the situation, the two most common psychotherapies are interpersonal and cognitive behavior therapy. Both have been demonstrated to be effective in the treatment of depression and dysthymia. Psychotherapy for the depressed client involves assisting the client in exploring how negative thoughts and feelings are affecting his or her behavior. Once the underlying thoughts and feelings are understood, the client can identify more effective ways of coping. The client must be willing to explore and discuss painful thoughts for improvement to occur. Individual, group, and family psychotherapies may be needed. The type of psychotherapy depends on the circumstances and severity of the client's illness. Support or self-help groups are very useful for long-term management of depression.

ECT involves passing an electric current through the brain (see Chapter 5). The actual mechanism by which ECT works is not known. It is thought that changes in neurotransmitter systems lead to the expected mood elevation. Unfortunately, because of the many changes in the brain, memory deficits occur. Depending on whether unilateral or bilateral ECT is used, the person may have either short-term or long-term memory deficits. ECT is used in cases where the client has experienced several episodes of severe depression and nothing else has worked. This type of depression is usually the result of a long period of events and losses that eventually lead to depression. When there is one incident that leads to depression, it is usually a more acute type of depression.

Psychotherapeutic drug agents are used very successfully in managing depression. As the medication becomes effective in restoring levels of neurotransmitters, the client's mood and energy level usually improve as well.

Antidepressants

Antidepressants are used in the treatment of depression to elevate mood, increase physical activity and mental alertness, improve appetite and sleep, and restore interest or pleasure in usual activities and things previously enjoyed. Because the neurotransmitters involved in depression also affect these other body functions, they can be used to treat other types of disorders such as eating disorders and sleep dysfunction. Most medications used to treat depression increase the amount of chemicals in the brain that help balance moods. Depression results from a decrease in monoamine neurotransmitter (norepinephrine, serotonin, and dopamine) concentration to a level insufficient to stimulate the receptors. The effects of these neurotransmitters last longer than those of GABA chemicals. Research has demonstrated that by inhibiting the breakdown of the monoamines or promoting their reuptake to increase their presence in the brain, mood can be effectively elevated.

Antidepressants generally fall into three types: **monoamine oxidase inhibitors (MAOIs)**, tricyclic antidepressants (TCAs), and **serotonin-specific reuptake inhibitors (SSRIs)**. Early pharmacologic studies led to the development of a group of drugs called MAOIs. Monoamine oxidase is an enzyme that metabolizes or inactivates the monoamine neurotransmitters. Specifically, MAOIs work by releasing monoamine neurotransmitters in the brain, blocking their reuptake into the presynaptic compartments, or mimicking the effects of the monoamines at the receptors. These drugs can interact with numerous foods and drugs (Box 10.5) to produce a hypertensive crisis. Foods to avoid contain tyramine, a precursor of norepinephrine.

The TCAs, named for their three-ring chemical structure, were developed in the 1950s. These

---

BOX 10.5

Foods and Drugs to Avoid When Taking an MAOI Drug Agent

- **Foods:** Aged cheese (cheddar, swiss, blue cheese, parmesan, provolone, romano), alcoholic beverages (beer, red wines), avocados, bananas, caffeine-containing beverages, smoked and processed meats (salami, pepperoni, bologna, summer sausage), caviar, corned beef, chicken livers, chocolate, fava bean pods, figs, meat tenderizers, pickled herring, raisins, sour cream, soy sauce, yogurt.
- **Drugs:** Amphetamines, antihistamines containing ephedrine derivatives, antidepressants (tricyclic and SSRIs), antiallergy or antiasthmatic agents containing ephedrine derivatives, antihypertensive drugs, levodopa, meperidine.

drugs work to correct the chemical imbalance of neurotransmitter concentrations in the synaptic cleft of CNS nerve cells. They effectively inhibit the reuptake of the neurotransmitters back into the cells, promoting a higher concentration of the neurotransmitters within the brain. TCAs also affect other body chemicals and characteristically produce a number of adverse and potentially dangerous side effects, including cardiac arrhythmias. This factor requires that all clients taking these agents be monitored closely.

The 1980s brought a new class of antidepressants that were designed to block the reuptake of serotonin, rather than norepinephrine. **Serotonin** is a potent vasoconstrictor thought to be involved in neural mechanisms related to arousal, sleep, dreams, mood, appetite, and sensitivity to pain. The SSRIs are all chemically related and have relatively fewer side effects than the TCAs, making them a safer and more desirable alternative. Figure 10.1 demonstrates the action of SSRIs to selectively block the reuptake of serotonin into the presynaptic compartment of the nerve cell.

This causes increased concentration of serotonin at nerve endings in the CNS. These drugs have little or no effect on the cardiovascular system and fewer anticholinergic side effects. Since the advent of the SSRIs, physicians have readily prescribed them, and more people are being treated and benefiting from treatment.

The effect of antidepressant drugs on the state of depression is not immediate. Antidepressants must be taken continuously for several weeks before therapeutic effects are evident and the client begins to feel better. This is because a continuous presence of the drug is needed in the brain for the level of the neurotransmitters to balance the deficit causing the depression. It is important that the client continues taking the medication, even if it does not seem to be helping. All of these drugs are effective, but some drugs work better for certain types of depression. A withdrawn client, for example, may benefit from a drug with stimulating effects, whereas another client may benefit from a drug that has a calming effect. Dosage and type of drug used will depend

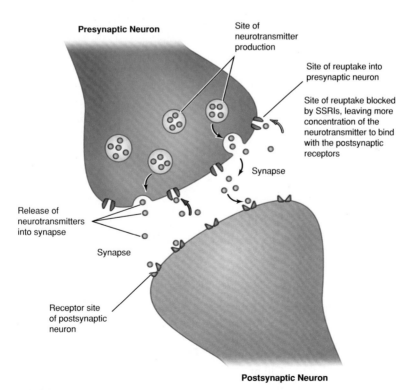

FIGURE 10.1

The release of serotonin from the presynaptic nerve ending into the synaptic cleft where the neurotransmitter is free to connect with the receptors of the next neuron. The neurotransmitter may be deactivated by chemical processes or be taken back into the presynaptic compartment (reuptake). SSRIs block the site of reuptake so that more of the neurotransmitter is available at the receptor sites.

TABLE 10.1   Antidepressant Drug Agents

CHEMICAL GROUP	GENERIC/BRAND NAME	USUAL DOSAGE (DAILY)[a]	ADVERSE REACTIONS AND SIDE EFFECTS
Tricyclic antidepressants	Amitriptyline (Elavil,[b] Endep)	50–100 mg	Lethargy, sedation, blurred vision, dry eyes, dry mouth, cardiac arrhythmias, hypotension, ECG changes, constipation, urinary retention, photosensitivity, blood dyscrasias, nausea and vomiting, increased appetite and weight gain, changes in blood glucose
	Amoxapine (Asendin)	50–100 mg	
	Desipramine (Norpramin, Pertofrane)	75–300 mg in divided doses	
	Doxepin (Sinequan, Adapin)	75–300 mg	
	Imipramine (Tofranil)	75–150 mg	
	Nortriptyline (Aventyl, Pamelor)	40–150 mg	
	Protriptyline (Vivactil)	15–60 mg	
	Trimipramine (Surmontil)	75–300 mg	
Heterocyclics	Bupropion (Wellbutrin, Zyban)	100 mg (1–3 times) (Wellbutrin XL—daily)	Agitation, headache, dry mouth, nausea, vomiting, change in appetite, weight gain or loss, photosensitivity, tremors, changes in blood sugar, seizures are possible, priapism, hypotension, tachycardia
	Maprotiline (Ludiomil)	75–300 mg	
	Mirtazapine (Remeron)	15 mg	
	Trazodone (Desyrel)	100–600 mg	
Serotonin-specific reuptake inhibitors (SSRIs)	Citalopram (Celexa)	20–40 mg	Apathy, confusion, drowsiness, insomnia, weakness, agitation, anxiety, increased depression, cough, orthostatic hypotension, tachycardia, dry mouth, nausea, altered taste, ejaculatory delay, impotence, amenorrhea, photosensitivity, rash, pruritus, weight changes, tremors
	Fluoxetine (Prozac)	20–80 mg	
	Fluvoxamine (Luvox)	50–300 mg	
	Paroxetine (Paxil)	20–50 mg	
	Sertraline (Zoloft)	50–200 mg	
	Escitalopram (Lexapro)	5–20 mg	
Nonselective reuptake inhibitors (serotonin and norepinephrine) (SNRIs)	Venlafaxine (Effexor)	75–225 mg	Abnormal dreams, anxiety, dizziness, headache, insomnia, nervousness, weakness, dry mouth, parasthesia, rhinitis, visual disturbances, altered taste, abdominal pain, nausea, vomiting, constipation, diarrhea, tachycardia, palpitations
	Desvenlafaxine (Pristiq)	50–100 mg	
	Duloxetine (Cymbalta)	40–60 mg	
Monoamine oxidase inhibitors	Isocarboxazid (Marplan)	20–40 mg	Dizziness, headache, orthostatic hypotension, constipation, nausea, arrhythmias, tachycardia. May interact with numerous foods and drugs to produce hypertensive crisis (severe hypertension, severe headache, fever, possible myocardial infarction or intracranial hemorrhage). See Box 10.5
	Phenelzine (Nardil)	60–90 mg	
	Tranylcypromine (Parnate)	20–30 mg	

[a]Decreased dosages recommended for the elderly.
[b]Brand name no longer available in the United States.

on the type and severity of the condition and the age of the client.

It is important to remember that these drugs are not curative and cannot solve the problems underlying the client's mental state. Clients with suicidal tendencies must be closely observed, because therapeutic levels of these drugs can energize their ability to carry out a suicide plan. Antidepressant medication combined with therapy and counseling is usually the preferred approach to treating clients with depression.

Antidepressant agents, their usual dosages, and common side effects are listed in Table 10.1.

Indications for Use

Antidepressant drugs are used in the treatment of major depression, dysthymic and bipolar disorders, depression accompanied by anxiety, childhood enuresis, depression associated with organic disease (alcoholism, schizophrenia, intellectual disability), obsessive–compulsive disorder, ADHD in children, panic disorder, chronic pain, and bulimia. Bupropion (Zyban) is indicated for use with smoking cessation.

Contraindications

Antidepressants are contraindicated in clients who are hypersensitive to the drug class and those who are pregnant or lactating. TCAs are also contraindicated in the acute recovery period following a myocardial infarction. They should be used with caution in clients with a history of urinary retention or benign prostatic hypertrophy, glaucoma, asthma, or hepatic or renal disease.

Concomitant use with MAOIs is contraindicated for all classes of antidepressants. MAOIs are further contraindicated in clients with hepatic or renal insufficiency, a history of or existing cardiovascular disease, hypertension, or severe headaches, or children younger than 16 years. They should be used cautiously in clients with a history of seizures, diabetes mellitus, suicidal tendencies, angina pectoris, or hyperthyroidism. There are many drug–drug interactions that may occur with antidepressant medications. A physician or pharmacist should be consulted before combining these drugs with any other prescription or non-prescription (OTC) drugs.

Nursing Diagnoses

Nursing diagnoses applicable to the client receiving antidepressants may include the following:
- Risk for Injury, related to side effects of sedation, orthostatic hypotension, photosensitivity, lowered seizure threshold, priapism, arrhythmias, or hypertensive crisis
- Risk for Self-Directed Violence, related to mood dysphoria
- Social Isolation, related to depression
- Constipation or Urinary Retention, related to side effects of the medication
- Self-Care Deficit, related to fatigue and low self-esteem
- Ineffective Coping, related to depressed mood
- Anxiety, related to situational crisis
- Sleep Pattern Disturbance, related to psychological factors
- Sexual Dysfunction, related to effects of medication or decreased libido
- Situational Low Self-Esteem, related to mood disturbance
- Risk for Suicide, related to feelings of worthlessness and hopelessness

Nursing Interventions

Nursing interventions applicable to the client taking antidepressants may include the following:
- Provide explanations of drug action and side effects
- Monitor vital signs
- Observe for orthostatic hypotension/advise to change positions slowly
- Administer with food or milk to avoid gastrointestinal upset
- Assist with ambulation or activity requiring mental alertness
- Encourage increase in fluid intake
- Offer hard candy or sugarless gum for dry mouth
- Assess for suicidal ideation
- Monitor mood at frequent intervals
- Monitor for hoarding of drugs, cheeking, or other overdosing cues
- Ensure use of protective sunscreen when outdoors (TCAs)
- Discourage caffeinated beverages

Outcome Evaluation

Criteria that may be used to evaluate the effectiveness of antidepressants in the client may include the following:
- Is free of injury or adverse effects of drug
- Has not harmed self
- Interacts and communicates with staff and others
- Demonstrates more positive view of self
- Performs activities of daily living (ADLs)
- Communicates feelings about present situation
- Experiences normal sleep patterns and appetite
- Reports decreased feelings of anxiety
- Participates in unit activities
- Client and family acknowledge need for ongoing therapy
- Client and family demonstrate knowledge of medication and side effects

Client and Family Teaching

Important information to teach the client and family members about antidepressant drug therapy includes the following:
- Take medication exactly as directed by the physician
- Do not use more of the drug, do not use it more often, or do not use it for a longer period than ordered by the physician

- Take the drug as directed consistently for several weeks to see a therapeutic effect
- Take the medication with food or milk to avoid stomach upset
- Keep regular doctor appointments
- Use caution when driving, operating dangerous equipment, or engaging in activities that require mental alertness and coordination
- Do not mix the drug with alcohol or other CNS depressants
- Report any side effects to your physician
- Do not suddenly stop taking the medication—it must be withdrawn gradually
- Take a missed dose as soon as possible—if several hours have lapsed or it is nearing time

for the next dose, the dose should not be doubled to catch up
- Avoid smoking when taking TCAs—smoking enhances the metabolism and increased dosage may be required
- Wear protective sunscreen when outdoors (TCAs)
- Rise slowly from a reclining position

Treatment of Bipolar and Related Disorders

Mood-stabilizing agents are the drugs of choice to treat clients with bipolar disorders. These drugs may be used alone or in combination with selected atypical antipsychotics, and are used along with

Case Application 10.1

"Sad and Lonely"

Doris is being admitted to the inpatient psychiatric unit. The nurse first notes a flat affect slumped posture and an unkempt appearance. During the admission intake, Doris cries frequently and does not provide eye contact. She states, "My husband not only left me alone in this world, but left me all of the bills too." She begins to sob and states, "I just don't think it is worth it anymore."

What is the nurse's best response at this point?

_____

_____

Doris is in the day room talking to her family and saying her good-byes. The physician has given an order to implement suicide precautions for her. What are some objects that should be removed from her room?

_____

_____

Once her room is made as safe as possible, Doris is introduced to her temporary environment. The nurse plans to implement a no-harm contract with her before leaving the room. What is the rationale for this intervention?

_____

_____

After 3 weeks of psychotherapy and antidepressant drug treatment, Doris is anticipating discharge. She has been participating in all unit activities and socializes with everyone on the unit and seems eager to go home. Discharge plans are being discussed with her and her family. She tells the nurse, "Maybe now I can do the things that I had planned to do before I came in here." How should the nurse respond to this statement?

_____

_____

Why is the post-discharge period a particularly vulnerable time for the client?

_____

_____

psychotherapy to stabilize and control the initial extreme mood swings.

Lithium carbonate was the first to be named a mood-stabilizer drug because of its combined antimanic and antidepressant properties. Today, the term *mood stabilizer* is currently used to describe psychotropic drugs that reduce mood swings and the likelihood of subsequent episodes. In addition to lithium, anticonvulsants and second-generation antipsychotic drugs are included in this category. It is important to note that lithium carbonate is used to treat both spectrums of mood shifts, whereas other drugs in this category are primarily agents that keep the manic episodes under control.

Lithium carbonate is a naturally occurring metallic salt, much like sodium carbonate. It is used in the management of bipolar illness, both to treat manic episodes and to prevent the recurrence of these episodes. Lithium is more effective in treating highs or manic periods than in preventing lows or depressive periods. Lithium is well absorbed from the gastrointestinal tract and may be given by capsule or concentrate. It has a peak blood level of 1 to 3 hours with a half-life of about 24 hours. Lithium is not metabolized by the body and is entirely excreted by the kidneys unchanged, so adequate renal functioning is necessary for its use. Most of a lithium dose is reabsorbed in the proximal renal tubules. The reabsorption of sodium and lithium is closely related, with any increase or decrease in dietary sodium intake affecting the levels of lithium in the blood plasma. A decrease in dietary sodium or loss through perspiration, vomiting, or diarrhea causes more lithium to be reabsorbed and increases the risk of lithium toxicity. Excessive intake of sodium causes an increase in the excretion of lithium and may lower the serum level to a nontherapeutic level. Therapeutic serum levels are 0.6 to 1.2 mEq/L and severe toxic reactions possible when levels reach 2 to 2.5 mEq/L. It is important to note that the therapeutic serum level of lithium is not much lower than a toxic serum level. Lithium dosage is determined based on both the clinical response and serum levels of the drug. Lithium blood levels should be monitored closely for therapeutic range. Acute lithium toxicity is manifested by increased tremors, headache, vomiting, and confusion.

In recent years, more drugs have become available for the treatment of bipolar illness. The wide use of anticonvulsants over lithium in treating acute mania and mood cycling is due to a wider therapeutic range and lack of renal toxicity. The choice of drug is difficult because of the adverse side effects and because no drug is effective for all individuals with symptoms of bipolar disorders. Mood-stabilizing agents, their usual dosages, and side effects are listed in Table 10.2.

Indications for Use

Mood-stabilizing agents are indicated for manic episodes associated with bipolar disorder and maintenance therapy to prevent or diminish future episodes. Lithium is also used in the treatment of migraine headaches and schizoaffective disorders. The action of anticonvulsants and calcium-channel blockers in the treatment of bipolar disorders is not clear; however, they have been used effectively to stabilize the manic episodes in bipolar disorders.

Contraindications

Mood stabilizers are contraindicated in clients with hypersensitivity to the drug, cardiac or renal disease, and sodium imbalance and in clients who are pregnant or lactating. These agents should be used cautiously in older people and those with metabolic disorders, urinary retention, or seizure disorders.

Anticonvulsants and calcium-channel blockers should not be used in those who are hypersensitive to these drugs, have a history of bone marrow suppression, or have taken an MAOI within 14 days of therapy. They should be used with caution in older people, women who are pregnant or lactating, and those with hepatic or cardiac disease.

Nursing Diagnoses

Nursing diagnoses applicable to the client taking mood-stabilizing drug agents may include the following:

- Risk for Injury, related to side effects of drowsiness and dizziness
- Risk for Poisoning, related to lithium toxicity
- Risk for Injury, related to sodium imbalance
- Risk for Violence, Self-Directed or Other-Directed, related to manic excitement, impulsive behavior
- Risk for Deficient Fluid Volume, related to side effects of medication (nausea, vomiting, diarrhea)
- Sensory Perception, Disturbed, related to chemical alterations
- Self-Esteem, Chronic Low, related to perceived lack of control
- Deficient Knowledge, related to prescribed drug and side effects

TABLE 10.2   Mood-Stabilizing Drug Agents

CHEMICAL GROUP	GENERIC/BRAND NAME	USUAL DOSAGE (DAILY)[a]	ADVERSE REACTIONS AND SIDE EFFECTS
Antimanic	Lithium carbonate (Eskalith, Lithane)	900–1,200 mg (maintenance) 1,800–2,400 mg (acute mania)	Lethargy, drowsiness, headache, fatigue, dry mouth, metallic taste, nausea, vomiting, diarrhea, thirst, polyuria, leukocytosis, muscle weakness, fine tremors **Life-threatening:** Arrhythmias, bradycardia, renal toxicity, epileptiform seizures, coma
Anticonvulsants	Carbamazepine (Tegretol)[b] Clonazepam (Klonopin) Divalproex, valproic acid (Depakote, Depakene, Epival) Oxcarbazepine (Trileptal) Lamotrigine (Lamictal) Gabapentin (Neurontin)[b]	800–1,200 mg 3–20 mg 500–1,500 mg 600–2,400 mg 25–200 mg 300–1,200 mg	Sedation, headache, nausea, vomiting, indigestion, diarrhea, diplopia, elevated liver enzymes, drowsiness, sore gums, increased appetite with weight gain, vertigo, ataxia, dry mouth, confusion, hallucinations, prolonged bleeding **Life-threatening:** Heart failure, arrhythmias, worsening of seizures, blood dyscrasias, toxic hepatitis, respiratory depression
Calcium-channel blocker	Verapamil (Calan, Isoptin)	240–320 mg	Dizziness, headache, transient hypotension, constipation, nausea, elevated liver enzymes, prolonged bleeding time **Life-threatening:** Heart failure, bradycardia, ventricular arrhythmias, AV block
Second-generation psychotropics (atypical antipsychotics)	Clozapine (Clozaril, Fazaclo) Olanzapine (Zyprexa) Quetiapine (Seroquel) Risperidone (Risperdal) Ziprasidone (Geodon) Aripiprazole (Abilify)	75–900 mg 10–20 mg 500–800 mg 2–6 mg 120–160 mg 10–30 mg	Sedation, weight gain, dry mouth, constipation, potential mental confusion, orthostatic hypotension, tachycardia, hypersalivation, nausea and vomiting, agranulocytosis, seizures, Parkinson-like symptoms (flat affect, stiff muscles, slowed movements), or internal feelings of restlessness or agitation (**akathisia**), photosensitivity, rhinitis

[a]Decreased dosages recommended for the elderly.
[b]Not FDA approved for bipolar disorder but is used by many psychiatrists.

Nursing Interventions

Nursing interventions applicable to the client taking mood-stabilizing agents may include the following:

- Administer medication with food to avoid dyspepsia and nausea
- Increase fluid intake to 2,000 or 3,000 mL daily
- Maintain consistent dietary intake of sodium, and increase sodium if activity results in heavy perspiration
- Assess for signs of toxicity in the client taking lithium carbonate (muscle weakness, diplopia or blurred vision, severe diarrhea, persistent nausea and vomiting, tinnitus, and vertigo)
- Report any indication of lithium toxicity
- Monitor for changes in mood

- Educate client to look for expected side effects of the drug without causing anxiety
- Teach client that side effects such as nausea, dry mouth, flatulence, dizziness, mild tremors, and insomnia should subside with continued treatment

Outcome Evaluation

Criteria that may be used to evaluate the effectiveness of mood-stabilizing agents in the client may include the following:

- Experiences no physical injury while on medication therapy
- Maintains consistent therapeutic levels of lithium
- Is able to participate in normal day-to-day activities

- Maintains consistent dietary intake of sodium and fluid intake
- Does not experience extreme mood swings
- Has not harmed self or others
- The client and family verbalize importance of continuing drug therapy even if feeling well
- The client and family verbalize importance of keeping regular appointments with physician and having drug levels drawn regularly
- The client and family verbalize understanding of medication side effects and which symptoms to report to the physician

Client and Family Teaching
Important information to teach the client and family members about mood-stabilizing agents includes the following:
- Use caution when operating a motor vehicle or dangerous machinery
- Do not stop taking the drug abruptly—serious withdrawal symptoms can occur
- Take medication regularly, even when feeling well
- Report any symptoms of drug side effects to your physician
- Keep your physician appointments
- Have regular blood samples taken (usually drawn 8 to 12 hours after last dose taken) if taking lithium carbonate
- Take medication at the same time each day. If you miss a dose, do not double the dose the next time (toxicity could occur)
- Consult with physician or pharmacist before taking any prescription or nonprescription medication with lithium
- Report any extreme mood swings to your physician
- If you take lithium, increase your fluid intake to eight to ten 8-oz glasses of water each day. Maintain a consistent intake of dietary sodium each day, and increase your intake if activity results in heavy perspiration
- If you take a calcium-channel blocker, rise slowly from a sitting or reclining position

Application of the Nursing Process

Assessment
During the assessment of a person with a mood disorder, collect data about mood and affect, thinking and perceptual ability, somatic complaints, sleep disturbances, changes in energy level, and the character of speech patterns. Mood and affect should be assessed for congruency. For example, when observed crying, a client should report feeling sad or down. A client who says he is sad but is laughing is not showing this consistency. Because mood is a subjective experience, it is important to ask the client what feeling or emotion he or she is experiencing. Clients experiencing a manic episode will likely display a bright or happy affect, while a person with depression will usually display a flat affect with a lack of eye contact.

During mania, thought processes become faster and may become fragmented, leading to disorganized patterns of speech. The person may not be able to complete one thought process before the next one begins. Complaints of racing thoughts are common in people experiencing a manic episode, or there may be a preoccupation with delusional thinking.

Some guidelines for collecting data in the person with a mood disorder include the following:
- Determine whether the client can understand what is being said
- Note whether the client is able to verbalize thoughts and feelings
- Observe behavioral clues for what the client may be thinking if the client does not respond verbally
- Determine the client's level of orientation. In depressive states, thought processes are retarded or slowed; concentration may be difficult for either the manic or depressed client
- Assess for any suicidal ideation and whether a plan has been devised
- Monitor patterns of verbal speech. The tone of voice, pace at which thoughts are processed and communicated, and the rate at which words are spoken are all relevant. Changes in the tone and rate can provide clues to mood and energy level. Clients in a manic state have very pressured or loud and forceful speech. Some clients may be unable to verbally communicate feelings, but may do so in drawings or written text
- Ask the client about any somatic complaints. During depression, the tolerance for pain may decrease, giving rise to generalized body aches, headaches, and gastrointestinal disturbances
- Assess for clues that indicate increased or decreased sleep patterns. People going into a

manic episode often go 2 to 3 days without sleep. Depressed people often have insomnia with difficulty falling asleep and staying asleep. Others may have hypersomnia and sleep for prolonged periods of time

- Assess the client's energy level. Those with mania will usually report a drastic increase in energy, while the depressed client usually reports anergia or decreased energy levels
- Assess appetite, recent eating patterns, and weight changes. Clients with depression may have little appetite or overeat as a coping tool. A loss of weight may be seen during a manic phase as the excessive activity minimizes the perceived need for food. The person does not take time to eat or is unable to remain seated long enough to eat.
- Determine the amount of assistance required for personal hygiene, dressing, and elimination needs. Both the manic and depressed person may lack attention to hygiene and bowel habits.

Selected Nursing Diagnoses

Once data have been collected, identify the individual needs of the client. The needs of the depressed person may be very different from those of one experiencing a manic episode. To differentiate the planning process for the individual client, nursing diagnoses are written to address the problems for each state.

Nursing diagnoses for the *client in a state of depression* may include the following:

- Activity Intolerance, related to fatigue and anhedonia
- Anxiety, related to psychological conflict
- Ineffective Coping, related to situational crisis and ineffective skills
- Hopelessness, related to stress or lack of support system
- Risk for Self-Directed Violence, related to suicidal thoughts
- Powerlessness, related to negativism and past failures
- Social Isolation, related to feelings of worthlessness
- Disturbed Sleep Pattern, related to insomnia or hypersomnia
- Chronic Low Self-Esteem, related to perceived unmet needs
- Ineffective Sexuality Pattern, related to decreased sex drive
- Dysfunctional Family Processes, related to changes in role

- Imbalanced Nutrition: less than body requirements, related to loss of appetite and feelings of worthlessness
- Self-Care Deficit, related to feelings of hopelessness and helplessness

Nursing diagnoses for the *client in a state of hypomania or mania* may include the following:

- Anxiety, related to threats to self-concept
- Impaired Verbal Communication, related to pressured speech
- Ineffective Coping, related to delusional ideas
- Acute Confusion, related to delusions of grandiosity or persecution
- Disturbed Sensory Perception, related to bizarre thinking and overload
- Dysfunctional Family Processes, related to manipulation and irresponsibility of family member
- Imbalanced Nutrition: less than body requirements, related to inadequate food intake and excessive activity
- Disturbed Personal Identity, related to delusional thinking
- Disturbed Sleep Pattern, related to inability to recognize fatigue and hyperactivity
- Risk for Self-Directed or Other-Directed Violence, related to irritability and delusional thinking
- Risk for injury, related to increased substance use
- Self-care deficit, related to hyperactivity and delusional thoughts

Expected Outcomes

Once problems have been identified, anticipated outcomes that are realistic in terms of the individual client should be formulated. Clients are often in a severe mood state when admitted to a psychiatric facility. Stabilization is necessary before the person is able to recognize and deal with the underlying issues. Outcomes should be determined as related to the type and level of mood alteration that is exhibited.

Expected outcomes for the *client in a depressed state* may include the following:

- Has increased energy level
- Identifies personal strengths
- Demonstrates improved skills to deal with loss
- Experiences decreased feelings of self-blame and doubt
- Openly expresses feelings
- Resumes sexual functioning with partner
- Demonstrates increased interaction with others

- Participates in at least two unit activities per day
- Consumes at least 75% of each meal
- Reports feeling well rested with 4 to 6 hours of sleep before awakening
- Reframes thoughts into positive statements
- Performs ADLs independently

Expected outcomes for the *client in a state of hypomania or mania* may include the following:
- Demonstrates self-control with decreased agitation
- Verbalizes feelings in an appropriate manner
- Demonstrates decreased activity level
- Consumes at least 75% of each meal and nutritional supplements
- Performs ADLs independently within level of ability
- Receives 4 to 6 hours of uninterrupted sleep
- Demonstrates ability to complete simple tasks to completion
- Participates appropriately in unit activities
- Interacts appropriately with others
- Verbalizes realistic expectations of self
- Experiences family participation in planning process
- Channels psychological energy into productive activity
- Maintains accurate perception of reality

Nursing Interventions

Nursing interventions should be planned individually for each client. All clients with an alteration in mood states may be very sensitive to behaviors and verbal statements of others. It is important for the nurse to plan actions that allow the person to make progress toward improved functioning and a sense of well-being. Interventions should be implemented according to priority of need. Interventions will differ depending on the mood state the client is experiencing. The client with depression is often withdrawn and avoidant, making interaction more challenging. The nurse should employ methods that assist the client in meeting needs until he or she is psychologically and physically able to do so independently.

Nursing interventions for the *client in a state of depression* may include the following:
- Establish and maintain a therapeutic relationship with the client
- Monitor for changes in current depressive symptoms or development of new ones
- Ask the client about any suicidal thoughts indicating a plan of how, when, or where the client might harm or kill self

- Assess the client's energy level—as energy increases, the ability to carry out a plan for suicide increases
- Encourage the client to participate in unit activities
- Provide positive feedback when the client makes efforts toward goals
- Assess the client's ability to perform ADLs, and assist as needed
- Provide a safe environment by removing potentially dangerous items
- Educate client regarding depression and treatment
- Stress the importance of taking medications as ordered
- Assist in request for referral for spiritual needs
- Encourage the client to explore feelings and communicate them in a safe manner
- Assist the client to express anger and other negative feelings appropriately
- Help client to recognize situations he or she can control and explore alternatives for those that cannot be controlled
- Encourage the client to recognize negative thoughts and teach reframing techniques
- Teach alternative methods of coping that are constructive and safe
- Focus on client's strengths and positive attributes
- Assist the client in establishing realistic goals

It is important to remember that because of the nature of mania, implementing nursing interventions may be difficult. Refrain from becoming emotionally reactive to the client's acting-out behaviors. Treatment modalities during the manic episode include various types of psychotherapies and the use of psychopharmacologic drugs. The most common drug used to treat mania is lithium carbonate, which assists in stabilizing the mood swings.

Nursing interventions for *the client in a state of mania or hypomania* may include the following:
- Create a safe environment
- Decrease environmental stimuli
- Observe the client frequently
- Assess risk for accidents to self or others
- Monitor own anxiety level and convey messages with a soothing tone of voice
- Refrain from becoming angry with clients who are hostile or behaving in an inappropriate manner
- Avoid arguing with or being charmed by clients
- Convey a "matter-of-fact" or nonreactive attitude when the client displays bizarre or sexually inappropriate behavior

- Educate client regarding medications and other treatment methods
- Encourage noncompetitive activities to prevent escalating anxiety and anger
- Provide nutritional finger foods when the client is unable to sit long enough to eat
- Monitor intake and output—prevent dehydration by providing water and juices in containers client can carry
- Monitor for escalating anxiety that may lead to explosive behavior
- Set and maintain limits such as unit rules and policies
- Spend time with the client—if the client is unable to sit, walk with him or her
- Provide positive feedback when appropriate
- Encourage client to dress appropriately and redirect the client when acting out in a sexual manner

Specific Interventions for a Suicidal Client

On admission, the client should be assessed for current risk factors that indicate suicide may be a possibility. Determine the content of any suicidal thoughts or ideations. If the client has a plan, this usually indicates that the client is more serious about committing suicide. Determine the lethality of the method. A more lethal method usually indicates increased likelihood of an attempt. It is also important to ask when the client intends to carry out the plan. The longer a client takes to carry out an attempt, the more time the client is willing to take to find another solution. If the client has decided on a location to do the act, determine how easy or difficult it will be to access this location.

Suicide precautions are usually initiated on admission to a psychiatric unit for those who

Case Application 10.2

"Out of Control"

Byron was admitted to the hospital while experiencing a manic episode of bipolar I disorder. Over the past 4 days, he has become increasingly loud and animated. He describes himself as a diplomat assigned to gather information. He carries a number of calling cards in his shirt pocket, all of which, he states, are his contacts. Today, the nurse is preparing to administer medication to another client and hears Byron asking very personal sexually oriented questions of a female client sitting next to him. As the nurse approaches them, Byron says the conversation is private and he is collecting classified information.

What actions should the nurse take at this point?

_____
_____

What other symptoms can be anticipated in Byron's behavior?

_____
_____

Two days later, Byron approaches the nurse and says he has to leave because he has a meeting with other national leaders from around the world that evening. He goes on to say that since he has been elected head of the CIA, he has little time for trivial issues anymore.

_____
_____

How should the nurse respond to this grandiose delusional thinking?

_____
_____

What is the nurse's responsibility to the other clients?

_____
_____

are at risk of self-harm. These precautions may vary from one unit to another and are often implemented by levels. If the client has recently attempted suicide, continuous monitoring of the client with one-to-one observation may be indicated. Sharp and potentially dangerous items (e.g., scarves, belts, shoelaces, nail files, scissors, electric appliance cords) are removed from the client's room and personal effects. A "no-harm" contract may be established with the client every shift and renewed at a specific time. The contract should include a statement that the client will not kill or injure himself or herself and will notify the staff when suicidal thoughts first occur. Random client checks are done to avoid possible anticipation of time intervals that the checks are done. Clients often carry out incidents of self-harm during times when nurses are busiest, such as shift changes.

Watch for "cheeking" behaviors in which the client holds medication in the pouch of the cheek to avoid swallowing it. The client can stockpile medication for use to overdose at a later time.

It is especially important to spend time with the client who is considering suicide as the only option. By using active listening and being present, the nurse conveys a sense of caring and appreciation for the worth of the client who is unable to find that feeling within his or her own self.

Evaluation

Evaluation will focus on determining whether improvement has occurred in the client's thought processes, behavior, and overall functioning. The effectiveness of interventions related to anxiety and coping ability will be demonstrated as the

---

"Life on the Edge"

Bianca is a 32-year-old who has been managing a local department store for the past 4 years. She has been divorced for 2 years and has two daughters, 6 and 9 years of age. She is admitted to the psychiatric unit after being brought to the emergency room by her mother who states that her 9-year-old granddaughter called and said, "My Mom won't wake up!" The grandmother hands the nurse an empty bottle containing a label for alprazolam (Xanax). She tells the nurse that her daughter was also drinking alcohol. She states, "Bianca has been drinking more since her divorce. She doesn't seem to care about herself anymore."

What is the nursing priority for Bianca at this time?

_____

_____

Why is it dangerous to mix a psychotropic drug with alcohol?

_____

_____

The physician prescribes the antidepressant citalopram (Celexa) for Bianca. What patient teaching should the nurse do concerning this drug?

_____

_____

What side effects may occur with an SSRI drug?

_____

_____

How will the nurse evaluate the effectiveness of the drug?

_____

_____

Case Application 10.3

client appropriately verbalizes feelings and thoughts. Behavior changes indicate an improvement in self-control and application of more effective coping skills. Interest and participation in self-care and hygiene show an elevation in self-appreciation. Increased hope and worth relieves the acute need for self-destruction, although an increased risk may exist for those who are energized enough to carry out a preconceived plan.

As anxiety and excessive mood states are reduced, the client is able to eat and sleep with less disturbance. Improved communication and social interaction will result as thought processes become more rational and reality oriented. Hopefully, the client can return to a state of productivity and independent living. The maintenance of a continued state of mood stability will depend on compliance with the medication and follow-up treatment plan.

Summary

- Alterations in mood levels have a ripple effect to every aspect of the person's life, resulting in problems and behaviors that are devastating to the individual and those around them.
- Mood disorders involve an array of emotions and can significantly impair a person's ability to function.
- Depression can occur as a single episode or in a recurring pattern. There may be a precipitating cause such as a loss, or it may occur without an identified reason.
- Clients with major depression do not exhibit any signs of euphoric states. Sadness and melancholy permeate all areas of the person's life with impaired functioning in personal, social, and work activities. Some people are unaware that the signs of depression are present in themselves or others.
- A client with dysthymia exhibits a lower level of depression and demonstrates a recurring cycle of the depressed state over a 2-year period. The person has feelings of hopelessness and despair combined with a negativistic attitude and indulgence in self-pity.
- Most medications used to treat depression increase the amount of chemicals or neurotransmitters in the brain that help to balance the moods.
- Antidepressant medications must be taken continuously for several weeks before therapeutic effects are evident and the client begins to feel better. A continuous presence of the drug is needed in the brain for the level of the neurotransmitters to balance the deficit causing the depression.
- Bipolar disorders are characterized by shifts between mania and depression that produce dramatic behavior changes. During the manic phase, the person's irrational thought processes and unrealistic inflated self-image lead to actions that bring regret and hurt to those around him or her.
- Cyclothymic disorder is characterized by mood disturbances, which involve periods of hypomanic symptoms that are not as severe as those seen in a manic episode and periods of depression that are not
- as severe as those seen in a manic episode and the depressive symptoms are not as severe as in a major depressive episode.
- Mood-stabilizing drugs are used to reduce the mood swings and the likelihood of subsequent episodes.
- Although drug therapy can level out the brain chemistry to minimize the highs and lows, many clients do not comply with treatment. This is in part related to the grandiose thinking in hypomania that they are fine and do not need medication. Once blood levels of the drug decline, a vicious cycle is begun. Maintenance of a continued state of mood stability will depend on compliance with the medication and follow-up treatment plan.
- During the plunge of the depressive state in the person with bipolar disorder, the statistics of suicide attempts and lives ended are alarming.
- Treatment of the mood disorders may include pharmacologic, psychotherapeutic, psychosocial, and ECT.
- Psychotherapy for the depressed client involves assisting the client in exploring how negative thoughts and feelings are affecting his or her behavior, and identifying more effective ways of coping.
- Assessment of the person with a mood disorder should include mood and affect, thinking and perceptual ability, somatic complaints, sleep disturbances, changes in energy level, and the character of speech patterns. Mood and affect should be monitored for congruency.
- Assess client for current risk factors that indicate suicide may be a possibility. Determine the content of any suicidal thoughts or ideations. If the client has a plan, determine the lethality of the method.
- Clients with suicidal tendencies must be closely observed, because therapeutic levels of antidepressants can energize their ability to carry out a suicide plan.
- As anxiety and excessive mood states are reduced, the client is able to eat and sleep with

less disturbance. Improved communication and social interaction result as thought processes become more rational and reality oriented.

- As anxiety and excessive mood states are reduced, the client is able to eat and sleep with less distur-

bance. Improved communication and social interaction result as thought processes become more rational and reality oriented.

- It is anticipated the client can return to a state of productivity and independent living.

Bibliography

American Psychiatric Association. (2013). *Diagnostic and statistical manual of mental disorders* (5th ed.). Washington, DC: Author.

Bauer, M. S., & Mitchner, L. (2004). What is a 'mood-stabilizer'? An evidence-based response. *The American Journal of Psychiatry, 161*(1), 3–18. Retrieved February 16, 2014.

Blake, T. (2012). Three medication pathways for bipolar disorder. *Nursing, 42*(5), 28–36. Retrieved February 16, 2014.

Coryell, W. (2013). Depressive disorders. *Merck Manual Professional.* Retrieved February 2, 2014 from http://www.merckmanuals.com/professional/psychiatric_disorders/mood_disorders/depressive_disorders.html

Coryell, W. (2013). Bipolar disorders. *Merck Manual Professional.* Retrieved February 15, 2014 from http://www.merckmanuals.com/professional/psychiatric_disorders/mood_disorders/bipolar_disorders.html

Crowe, M., Whitehead, L., Wilson, L., Carlyle, D., O'Brien, A., Inder, M., & Joyce, P. (2010). Disorder-specific psychosocial interventions for bipolar disorder – A systematic review of the evidence for mental health nursing practice. *International Journal of Nursing Studies, 47*(7), 896–908. Retrieved February 16, 2014.

Cavies, M. A., McBride, L., & Sajatovic, M. (2008). The collaborative care practice model in the long-term care of individuals with bipolar disorder: A case study. *Journal of Psychiatric & Mental Health Nursing, 15*(8), 649–653. Retrieved February 16, 2014.

Fountoulakis, K. N., Gonda, X., Vieta, E., & Rihmer, Z. (2011). Class effect of pharmacotherapy in bipolar disorder: Fact or misbelief? *Annals of General Psychiatry, 10*, 8. Retrieved February 16, 2014 from http://www.ncbi.nlm.nih.gov/pmc/articles/PMC3078905/

Gao, K., Tolliver, B. K., Kemp, D. E., Ganocy, S. J., Bilali, S., Brady, K. L, Findling, RL, Calabrese, J. R. (2009). Correlates of historical suicide attempt in rapid-cycling bipolar disorder: A cross-sectional assessment. *Journal of Clinical Psychiatry, 70*(7), 1032–1040. Retrieved February 16, 2014.

Guiterrez, M. A., Roper, J. M., & Hahn, P. (2001). Paradoxical reactions to benzodiazepines. *The American Journal of Nursing, 101*(7), 34–39. Retrieved February 16, 2014.

Herdman, T. H. (Ed.). (2012). *NANDA International – nursing diagnoses: Definition & classification 2012–2014.* Oxford, UK: Wiley-Blackwell Publishers.

Karch, A. M. (2013). *Nursing 2014 drug handbook.* Philadelphia, PA: Wolters Kluwer/Lippincott Williams & Wilkins.

Kaye, N. S. (2005). Is your depressed patient bipolar? *The Journal of the American Board of Family Practice, 18*, 271–281. Retrieved February 16, 2014 from www.jabfm.org/cgi/content/full/18/4/271

Keating, C., Dawood, T., Barton, D. A., Lambert, G. W., & Tilbrook, A. J. (2013). Effects of selective serotonin reuptake inhibitor treatment on plasma oxytocin and cortisol in major depressive disorder. *BMC Psychiatry, 13*(1), 1–7. Retrieved February 16, 2014.

Koukopoulos, A., Sani, G., Koukopoulos, A. E., Minnai, G. P., Girardi, P., Pani, L., Albert, M. J., & Reginaldi, D. (2003). Duration and stability of the rapid-cycling course: A long-term personal follow-up of 109 patients. *Journal of Affective Disorders, 73*, 75–85. Retrieved February 16, 2014.

Mitchell, P., Parker, G. B., Gladstone, G. L., Wilhelm, K., Austin, M. P. (2003). Severity of stressful life events in first and subsequent episodes of depression: The relevance of depressive subtype. *Journal of Affective Disorders, 73*, 245–252. Retrieved February 16, 2014.

National Institute of Mental Health. (2008). Bipolar disorder. NIH Publication No. 08-3679. Retrieved February 16, 2014 from http://www.niml.nih.gov/publicat/bipolar.cfm

Spijker, J., van Straten, A., Bockting, C. L., Meeuwissen, J. A., & van Balkom, A. J. (2013). Psychotherapy, antidepressants, and their combination for chronic major depressive disorder: A systematic review. *Canadian Journal of Psychiatry, 58*(7), 386–392. Retrieved February 16, 2014.

Townsend, M. C. (2011). *Nursing diagnoses in psychiatric nursing* (8th ed.). Philadelphia, PA: F.A. Davis Co.

Varcolaris, E. M. (2011). *Manual of psychiatric nursing care planning* (4th ed.). St. Louis, MO: Saunders Elsevier.

Wilson, B. A., Shannon, M. T., & Shields, K. M. (2013). *Prentice hall nurse's drug guide 2014.* Upper Saddle River, NJ: Pearson Prentice Hall.

Student Worksheet

Fill in the Blank

Fill in the blank with the correct answer.

1. The average person with major depressive disorder experiences _____ episodes over a lifetime.

2. _____ disorder is a milder form of bipolar-related disorder characterized by recurrent symptoms of hypomania and dysthymia.

3. _____ is a recurrent state of depression over a period of at least 2 years.

4. Delusions of _____ occur during interpersonal conflicts where a perceived injustice is viewed as a threat of harm.

5. _____ is the most common mood-stabilizing drug agent used in the treatment of bipolar illness.

6. Antidepressant drug agents require _____ weeks of continuous blood levels to produce significant mood elevation.

7. Clients on suicide precautions should be monitored at _____ time intervals to prevent anticipated checks.

Matching

Match the following terms to the most appropriate phrase.

1. _____ Euphoria
2. _____ Anhedonia
3. _____ Clang association
4. _____ Cheeking
5. _____ Anergia
6. _____ Negativism
7. _____ Rapid cycling
8. _____ Grandiosity
9. _____ Labile
10. _____ Unipolar

a. Being tired with decreased energy
b. Learned sense of helplessness
c. Depressive episode without hypomania or mania
d. Strings of words in rhyming phrases
e. Alternating from euphoria to dysphoria and irritability
f. Lack of pleasure in previously enjoyed activities
g. Holding medication in the mouth without swallowing
h. Four or more mood shifts within 1 year
i. Thinking of self as excessively important
j. Excessive feelings of happiness

Multiple Choice

Select the best answer from the multiple-choice items.

1. The nurse is monitoring a client with mania who is constantly pacing the hallway and unable to be seated when the other clients are eating. Which of the following nursing interventions would best meet the needs of the client at this time?
   a. Keep food at the nurse's station until the client asks for something to eat
   b. Allow the client to eat in a separate area to avoid distraction
   c. Provide finger sandwiches and juice for client during the activity
   d. Teach client the importance of nutrition in providing energy

2. The nurse is documenting observations of a client experiencing a manic episode who is very talkative, extremely happy, and laughing. Which of the following would be most appropriate to include regarding this client?
   a. Euphoric with appropriate affect
   b. Dysthymic with inappropriate affect
   c. Bright affect with dysphoric mood
   d. Flat affect with elated mood

3. When caring for a client with a manic episode, which of the following nursing interventions would convey a therapeutic attitude of acceptance?
   a. Tell the client to remain isolated until impulsive actions are controlled
   b. Allow the client to describe delusional thoughts as long as needed
   c. Walk alongside the client at intervals as long as pacing continues
   d. Reprimand the client for inappropriate sexual hand gestures

4. The plan of care for a client with a diagnosis of major depressive disorder should include which of the following interventions?
   a. Group physical activity that will provide exercise and socialization
   b. Provide a structured schedule of activities that offers client participation
   c. No socializing activities unless the client asks to be included
   d. Encourage participation in competitive games of chess or ping pong

5. The nurse is caring for a client whose serum lithium carbonate level is 1.5 mEq/L. The nurse would expect the physician to:
   a. Order an additional dose to be given one time only
   b. Increase the daily dosage of the medication
   c. Order the next dose of the drug to be held
   d. Stop the medication

6. It is important for the nurse to include which of the following instructions when doing client teaching for the client taking a tricyclic antidepressant medication:
   a. Take the medication with coffee or tea to enhance its effect
   b. The medication can be discontinued after a few weeks of therapy
   c. You can omit the morning dose of your medication if it makes you too sleepy
   d. Wear a hat and long-sleeve shirt when you are outdoors in the sun

7. The client for whom an MAOI is prescribed should be taught to avoid which of the following dietary items?
   a. Milk or milk products
   b. Smoked or processed meat
   c. Foods high in sodium
   d. Legumes and nuts

8. A client tells the nurse how difficult recent weeks have been. She states she used to enjoy taking her grandchildren to the park but this is no longer pleasurable for her. The client is describing feelings related to which of the following symptoms?
   a. Anhedonia
   b. Anergia
   c. Euphoria
   d. Negativism

9. A client who has been admitted after a suicide attempt from an overdose of antidepressant medication tells the nurse, "Why couldn't I just die. There is nothing left here for me." The most therapeutic response for the nurse is:
   a. "Why did you want to die?"
   b. "There is always a reason things happen as they do."
   c. "What do you mean there is nothing here for you?"
   d. "You are feeling as though life is meaningless right now?"

10. The nurse planning interventions for a client with major depressive disorder would give first priority to which of the following individual needs?
    a. Social isolation
    b. Self-care deficit
    c. Low self-esteem
    d. Ineffective individual coping

Chapter 11

Psychotic Disorders

⊙ Learning Objectives

After learning the content in this chapter, the student will be able to:

1. Define psychosis.
2. Describe common characteristics of psychotic disorders.
3. Describe treatment methods for clients with psychotic disorders.
4. Describe the relationship of antipsychotic drug agents to the treatment of psychosis.
5. Identify extrapyramidal side effects and their effect on compliance with drug therapy.
6. Describe components of a nursing assessment of the client with a psychotic disorder.
7. Select appropriate nursing diagnoses for the client with a psychotic disorder.
8. Identify expected outcomes for problems seen in the client with a psychotic disorder.
9. Implement appropriate nursing interventions for the client with a psychotic disorder.
10. Evaluate effectiveness of nursing care delivered to clients with a psychotic disorder.

⊙ Key Terms

akathisia
alogia
antipsychotic agents
avolition
catalepsy
catatonic
delusion of reference
delusion
derailment
dystonia
echolalia
echopraxia
extrapyramidal
hallucinations
illusions
loose associations

mannerisms
neuroleptic malignant
  syndrome
posturing
poverty of speech
prodromal phase
psychosis
schizoaffective
stupor
tardive dyskinesia
thought broadcasting
thought insertion
thought withdrawal
water intoxication
waxy flexibility
word salad

Introduction to Psychotic Disorders

There are a number of different situations in which the symptoms of psychosis are manifested. They may be evidenced in some medical conditions, delirium, drug toxicity, dementia, mood disorders, and other delusional disorders (Box 11.1). In most situations, the symptoms are not present at all times. Psychotic disorders affect the mind and affect a person's ability to think clearly and respond effectively to the world around him or her.

The most common and severe form of psychotic disorders is schizophrenia—a form of psychosis in which there are disorganized thoughts, perceptions, and bizarre behaviors. The occurrence of schizophrenia worldwide is about 1%. About half of the people admitted to mental units are diagnosed with schizophrenia. The cost of mental health care and social services related to schizophrenia in all age groups is significantly higher than that of other mental disorders.

Before discussing schizophrenia in depth and touching on the other types of psychotic disorders, it is important to discuss psychosis and the characteristic symptoms that define this disturbance.

Psychosis

The term **psychosis** is linked with a variety of meanings. Most often it makes reference to a set of symptoms, including perceptual disturbances, disorganized thinking, and behavior alterations, that demonstrate disorganization in the mental processes. These symptoms reflect the behavior, emotional response, and thought processes of the person who has lost contact with reality. Most people associate the disturbances of "hearing voices" or other strange behaviors with this psychosis. Those who experience these symptoms also tend to withdraw from society and retreat into their own unreal world.

BOX 11.1

Associated Causes of Psychosis

- Depression
- Bipolar disorder
- Epilepsy
- Brain tumor
- Dementia
- Stroke
- Alcohol and other drug use

Perceptual Disturbances

Hallucinations are false sensory perceptions that have no relation to reality and are not supported by actual environmental stimuli. When a hallucination occurs, the person has the perception of seeing (visual), hearing (auditory), smelling (olfactory), feeling (tactile), or tasting (gustatory), although there is no stimulus present.

Although all of these may occur, auditory hallucinations are the most common. Most of these are in the form of voices or sounds that can only be heard by the person experiencing them. The voices may originate inside or outside the person's head and may be talking to the person or commenting on his or her behavior. Many of the voices are commanding, telling the person to harm himself or others and are very frightening to the person. Studies show that those who experience the command hallucinations may react in panic or demonstrate violence toward themselves or others.

⚡ Mind Jogger

Considering that the client hearing commanding voices is not in touch with reality, what is the best approach to communicating with this individual?

Visual hallucinations are less common but may involve seeing people or images that are not actually present. Feeling that something is crawling on the skin or moving inside the body parts are typical of tactile hallucinations. Olfactory (smell) and gustatory (taste) misperceptions account for a small percentage of perceptual disturbances.

Illusions are experienced when sensory stimuli actually exist but are misinterpreted by the person. For example, the person may refer to spots on the floor as insects or to an electric cord as a snake.

Disorganized Thinking

In psychosis, the thought processes become confused and disrupted, leaving the person with an inability to carry on a logical conversation. A **delusion** consists of fixed, false ideas or beliefs without appropriate external stimuli that are inconsistent with reality and that cannot be changed by reasoning. These thoughts usually involve a theme that is dominant in the mind. For example, the client who thinks someone is trying to kill him will demonstrate this both verbally and behaviorally. The client might say, "I'm not taking this medication because you are trying to poison me," or "I'm not eating my supper because the FBI put poison in my food."

The content or theme of the delusions can include depressive (they have committed terrible deeds), somatic (their body is disintegrating into another substance or infested with insects), grandiose (they are very important and powerful), and persecution (others are out to get them). Others may be **delusions of reference**, a false belief that the behavior of others in the environment refers to oneself. For example, the person may believe that something such as a newspaper article or television commercial is sending a special message to them. Content can also include a belief that **thought broadcasting** occurs, in which the person's thoughts can be heard by others (e.g., "I have a direct wire attached to the commander of intelligence to rule the underground"). **Thought insertion** may also be claimed in which the person believes the thoughts of others can be inserted into his or her mind (e.g., "Men from Mars are implanting seeds of destruction into the layers of my mental dirt"). **Thought withdrawal** indicates a belief that others are robbing thoughts from one's brain (e.g., "Those who steal the knots of my wisdom are employed in drawers of the intelligence bureau").

> ## Just the Facts
> The most common delusional themes tend to be related to thoughts of persecution, religious ideas, or somatic reference.

As a typical brain organizes and directs thought processes into spoken words, associations or connections give meaning or logic to the content. *Content* refers to the meaning of the words or conversation that is spoken. People with disorganized thinking convey the fragmented content in the way they speak. They may be talking and suddenly change the course of the conversation to something with no logical connection to the original topic. The inability to organize and connect sudden changes in thought processes that are vague, unfocused, and illogical is referred to as **loose associations** or **derailment**, meaning that the content is offtrack (e.g., "This meat is tough, but I saw meat in the store and nails are keeping it together until the cows get home."). **Alogia or poverty of speech**—a decrease in the amount or

speed of speech—may occur, in which the person may not answer questions or may stop in the middle of a thought.

Word salad refers to a jumble of unconnected and disorganized thoughts that indicate severe impairment (e.g., "You see I am living in the sky where it snowed yesterday with thunderous wires darting in and out of the highway...brilliant colors keep the orchestra moving the ball down the railroad track toward the divine intellect of my intestines"). The person may make up new words that have special personal meaning such as, "The malitars are coming to get me." These new words or neologisms are indicative of disconnected thought processes. Clang associations may also be demonstrated with insignificant rhyming of words (e.g., "The sky is blue, so are you... two plus two, much to do so to fear, far and near, let's have a beer...").

Behavior Alterations

Psychotic behavior may be described as agitated, aggressive, childlike, inappropriate, silly, and unpredictable. Wild, purposeless, agitated movements are described as frenzied motor activity. Disorganized behavior can lead to an inability to perform activities of daily living or carry out goal-directed activity. The person may appear very unkempt and dress inappropriately for the situation. Many times the person will wear multiple layers of clothing regardless of the environmental temperature. Because the person with psychosis has poor impulse control, behavior may also be sexually inappropriate, unpredictable, and include sudden explosive outbursts. The person is unable to recognize what is considered by most as a norm of society. For example, most people refrain from going without clothes or masturbating in public because this is not acceptable. In psychosis, however, the person displays behavior that reflects his or her own personal thought process and is oblivious to moral boundaries.

Catatonic behaviors involve a decreased reaction to environmental surroundings. Movements may be severely decreased or absent and accompanied by a **stupor** or lack of awareness and orientation. **Posturing** is seen when the person in a trance-like state assumes a rigid bizarre posture often held against gravity, and resists efforts to be moved for extended periods of time (e.g., "crucifix position"). An extreme form of posturing is termed **catalepsy**. **Waxy flexibility** occurs when the person remains in one position until someone changes it. An arm, leg, or other body part can be moved by another person and it will remain in that position until moved.

During an excitement phase, the person may have stereotyped repetitive, purposeless movements (e.g., rocking), or **mannerisms** that are repetitive and more goal-directed movements (e.g., saluting or bowing). This behavior involves excessive motor activity that is not triggered by any external stimulus. **Echolalia** in which the person repeats another's speech, and **echopraxia** where another's movements are imitated are also seen.

Types of Psychotic Disorders

The major symptoms of psychotic disorders are the occurrence of delusions and hallucinations. Some individuals may experience this as a single psychotic event, such as that seen after an extremely stressful event or trauma. The episode may last a few days but usually resolves within several weeks. In other situations, such as in schizoaffective disorder (discussed later in the chapter), there is a combined presence of schizophrenic symptoms and those of a mood disorder.

Schizophrenia

Schizophrenia is a form of psychosis in which there are disorganized thoughts, perceptual alterations, inappropriate affect, and decreased emotional response as the links to reality are lost. It is a chronic and disabling mental illness that causes the person to withdraw into a world of delusional thoughts and misperceptions. The word *schizophrenia* derives from Greek, meaning "split mind." The person's ability to distinguish real from unreal becomes painfully disordered. This does not mean, however, that the personality is disintegrated as in multiple personality disorder. Although not all people suffering from schizophrenia experience all the symptoms, the impact to their personal, family, and social life is severe.

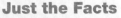

Just the Facts

The cost of mental health care and social services related to schizophrenia in all age groups is significantly higher than that of other mental disorders.

Just the Facts

About half of the people admitted to mental units are diagnosed with schizophrenia.

Signs and Symptoms

In most cases, the onset of symptoms is insidious, with the person experiencing them for some time before the first full-blown psychotic episode occurs. This period is often referred to as the **prodromal phase** and actually indicates the beginning of the illness (Box 11.2).

The person may have increasing anxiety with inability to concentrate or complete goal-oriented tasks. In the case of the student, there is a loss of connections, which destroys the ability to think and learn. There may be an alternation between hyperactivity and inactivity. As the deterioration continues, the person becomes more distracted and feels that something is happening or expresses fear of "losing my mind." The person may misread things that are happening in the environment, often becoming paranoid about being followed or poisoned. Delusions may center on imaginary people who appear and harass or ridicule the person. Gradually the delusions and hallucinations become a part of each day with jumbled speech patterns and bizarre behaviors. Social relationships deteriorate to the point that the person is unable to function in a romantic, peer, or work relationship. Interest is lost in any type of competition or planning for the future. There tends to be an increase in the deterioration and dysfunction with each acute episode or relapse. This is often

---

BOX 11.2

Behavior Associated with Schizophrenia

- Easily distracted and inattentive to environment
- Memory impairment
- Depressive, hopeless feelings
- Poor judgment or inability to interpret the environment correctly
- Lack of insight or understanding of the illness and need for consistent treatment and management
- Illogical thought processing
- Impaired decision-making ability
- Ideas of reference or lack of ego boundaries and self-concept
- Inability to distinguish clear distinction between self and other objects or their body and that of another
- Difficulty in relating to others

the point at which many individuals turn to drug use to compensate for a loss of self-confidence and self-esteem.

> ## Mind Jogger
> Homeless people without shelter or housing have a sense of isolation and rejection. What might contribute to the fact that many people with psychotic disorders become part of this population?

Associated with psychotic disorders such as schizophrenia is the potential for clients to over-hydrate by drinking excessive liquids, sometimes as much as 10 to 15 L a day. The client is seen constantly carrying a cup or container with frequent trips to the water fountain or requests for something to drink. Some have been observed drinking from the toilet bowl or sink. The continued intake of fluid may result in **water intoxication** or a psychosis-induced metabolic state of fluid overload that can lead to cerebral edema and other potentially lethal situations. It is thought that a possible cause of this overload is related to the effects of antipsychotic drugs on the pituitary gland, which produces antidiuretic hormone (ADH) and thus inhibits the excretion of water.

The symptoms of schizophrenia are primarily categorized as positive and negative (Box 11.3).

Positive Symptoms

Positive symptoms are evidenced early in the progress of the disorder. These are usually demonstrated in the initial contact that the person has with the health care system which is usually a hospitalization for what is called *acute schizophrenia*. These symptoms include alterations in thinking, perception, and behavior.

The delusional patterns seen in schizophrenia are distorted and often bizarre with no logical connections. These thoughts often indicate an underlying feeling of worthlessness and low self-esteem. In the case of psychosis, the behavior that occurs while thoughts are processed and spoken actually provides more information than the content of what is said. The fragmented and disorganized thought processes are demonstrated in speech patterns of word salad and derailed loose associations. These jumbled words can reflect the theme of what the person is experiencing within his or her head. However, the theme reference and feelings can also be reflected in behavior. For

---

> ### BOX 11.3
> #### Symptoms of Schizophrenia
> **Positive Symptoms**
> - Delusions
> - Word salad
> - Clang associations
> - Thought broadcasting
> - Thought insertion
> - Loose associations
> - Neologism
> - Hallucinations
> - Illusions
> - Depersonalization
> - Bizarre behavior
> - Agitation
> - Catatonia
> - Autism
>
> **Negative Symptoms**
> - Blunt or flat affect
> - Lack of energy
> - Failure to find pleasure in activities
> - Lack of motivation
> - Inability to initiate self-care skills
> - Inability to interact with others
> - Impoverished speech
> - Substance use
> - Depression and suicidal acts
> - Violent behavior

example, the person who has recurring delusions of persecution may demonstrate fear by constantly looking to the side or over a shoulder as if someone is lurking behind or following him or her.

Themes of persecution are the most commonly experienced delusions in individuals with schizophrenia. Clients experiencing delusions of persecution hold the false belief that someone is plotting to harm them. Often the person believes this is being devised by very important people or alien powers (e.g., a client believes the CIA is sending signals through telephone wires or Internet lines that will electrocute him). Beliefs such as these may hold some resemblance to life experiences such as a young man who was abused as a child and believes his father will electrocute him using the light switches. Others are more bizarre and have no realistic theme. For example, a client thinks there is a machine in her stomach that is timed to explode on New Year's Eve. The delusional thinking persists regardless of evidence that proves it inaccurate. Delusions of grandeur centralize on false beliefs that one is a very powerful and important person. These delusions often tend to have religious or governmental themes. For instance, a client may believe that he is a disciple sent by God to lead the world through the Internet.

> **Just the Facts**
> Delusional thinking often indicates an underlying feeling of worthlessness and low self-esteem.

Perceptual alterations may include all sensory types of hallucinations. Auditory and visual hallucinations are perhaps the most common in people with schizophrenia. Hearing voices or sounds, both within the confines of the mind or externally, is perhaps the most familiar of these alterations. These individuals may respond to the voices, which often talk directly to them or make remarks about their actions. This is illustrated by the young man who thought his girlfriend was talking to him from his shirt pocket. He would face the wall as if wanting privacy, open the flap of the pocket, and answer the voice.

Misperceptions of personal identity are also seen, with the inability to distinguish oneself from the realness of another. They are often confused about their sexual identity, feeling that parts of others are meshing with their own body parts. They may feel disconnected to their own body or depersonalize themselves. For example, a woman views her blood vessels as worms floating through the air.

Patterns of strange, bizarre, and unusual behavior can occur in many forms. The person may dress oddly, assume strange positions, or demonstrate restless physical movements. The person may have stereotyped behavior without purpose such as picking up trash items but not depositing them in a trashcan. Many clients with schizophrenia demonstrate a negative response to directions or instructions by doing the opposite of what is asked of them. The person who is told to sit down and eat may get up and start pacing in the hall. Agitation is often relieved by pacing, with some clients walking great distances without realizing how far they have gone.

Negative Symptoms

Negative symptoms develop slowly over time. They are reflected in the person's inability to deal with the way their illness affects their life. The

"Out of Touch"

Antonia is a client in the psychiatric unit with a diagnosis of paranoid schizophrenia. She has a history of noncompliance with medications. Today she is very delusional and refuses her breakfast. She approaches the nurse and states, "God told me to warn you that meteors are descending toward the earth. They will get into the brains of all women to prevent the overpopulation of the outer planets." Antonia paces frantically and finally crawls under the coffee table in the day room holding her arms over her head.

What type of theme does Antonia's delusional thought process indicate?

What is the speech pattern of this client?

How can the nurse best approach Antonia regarding her behavior?

Case Application 11.1

devastating effects result in isolation and withdrawal from the uncomfortable inability to interact with others in a meaningful way.

Affect is perhaps the most noticeable of these symptoms. The person with schizophrenia typically has a blunted or flat affect that is expressionless and blank. The affect can also be inappropriate, such as smiling when the situation is sad. Other times, the person may exhibit bizarre expressions such as giggling while mumbling to a water faucet in the bathroom. The behavior is often described as autistic, referring to a focus on an inner fantasy world while excluding the external environment.

As the disorder takes over the person's life, interrelating with others and maintaining relationships becomes impossible. The person experiences **avolition:** lacking motivation to make decisions or initiate self-care such as hygiene and grooming. Dress becomes unkempt and inappropriate. Anergia or decreased energy and a passive lack of ambition are evident. Anhedonia is seen as little interest is shown in activities that were previously enjoyed. Speech may regress to brief phrases, a one-word response, or mutism.

Substance abuse, suicide, and violence are common associated symptoms that accompany the devastating effects of schizophrenia. Depression with a suicidal end to the helpless and isolated pattern of living is not uncommon. Both psychoactive drugs and illegal substances are abused by people with schizophrenia. Alcohol, marijuana, cocaine, and other drugs are used to offset the haunting symptoms of the illness. And often, the use of these drugs contributes to violence and severe acts of cruelty toward others.

Mind Jogger

It is said that most people with schizophrenia who attempt suicide are also in major depression. What factors might be contributing to this state?

Incidence and Etiology

Schizophrenia affects approximately 1% of the world's population. The onset typically occurs between late adolescence and mid-30s. There are instances where schizophrenia begins in childhood, and there is a late-onset type that occurs after age 45. There is evidence that indicates that this disorder manifests differently in

men than in women. For men, the average age of onset is between 18 and 25 years, and that of women occurring between 25 and 30 years. Late onset is more common in women than in men. Women tend to experience less severe symptoms with fewer hospitalizations than men. This disorder is prevalent in all populations without bias as to race, gender, culture, or socioeconomic groups. There is a higher risk in those who have first-degree biological relatives with the disorder. Most people who develop schizophrenia have the symptoms for the remainder of their lives.

Just the Facts

Approximately 20% of people with schizophrenia attempt suicide, while about 5% actually do commit a fatal attempt.

There is no particular single cause of schizophrenia. It has long been known that a genetic factor exists, but the hereditary mechanism is not clear. Research regarding a connection to brain chemistry is providing possible links to an imbalance in the neurotransmitters dopamine and glutamate. Other studies show abnormalities in the brain structure of those with schizophrenia. All research efforts are being made to identify the genes and contributing factors for the development of this debilitating illness. Environmental stressors can trigger recurrence of symptoms but are not considered causative of the disorder.

Subtypes of Schizophrenia

Along with the diagnosis of schizophrenia, a further distinction is usually made based on the symptoms that are exhibited.

Paranoid Type

People with paranoid type schizophrenia experience prominent hallucinations and delusions. The hallucinations are often auditory in nature with delusions of being persecuted or followed. The delusions are usually very organized and focus on the theme. For example, one person may think that everyone who wears black is sent by the devil to harm him. Everything the person does is centered on this theme. Because this is threatening to the person, he or she assumes a defensive behavior toward anyone who is wearing black. This can endanger others if the delusion is severe.

Disorganized Type
Those with disorganized type schizophrenia exhibit disorganized and unintelligible speech, bizarre behavior, and a flat affect. Delusions do not center on any particular theme but tend to be fragmented and varied in focus. Unusual mannerisms and posturing may prevent these individuals from eating, toileting, or attending to personal hygiene. They may demonstrate inappropriate laughter or be strangely silly. It is not unusual to see these individuals sitting in an empty room laughing and acting theatrical.

Catatonic Type
The catatonic type of schizophrenia is characterized by a severe decrease in motor activity and responsiveness to the environment. The person may be mute and suddenly start repeating words heard at an earlier time. These individuals may make strange motions with their arms while walking with rigid posture or make stereotyped movements that mimic the actions of others. When assuming a rigid, fixed posture for extended periods, these individuals usually have waxy flexibility and can be repositioned without a return to the previous pose. This type is rarely seen as a single diagnosed condition.

Undifferentiated Type
The person with schizophrenia of the undifferentiated type exhibits a number of classic symptoms such as delusions, hallucinations, disorganized speech, strange behavior, and blunted affect. The symptoms are not defined to meet the criteria for any other subtype. The person may exhibit the prominent symptoms but none that are specific to any one type of the disorder.

Residual Type
The person with residual type of schizophrenia has experienced prominent psychotic symptoms with a previous diagnosis of schizophrenia but no longer has them. There is lingering evidence of unusual behavior, a blunted affect, some unrealistic thinking, or social withdrawal.

Mind Jogger
Many people with schizophrenia are caught in a cycle that takes them from acute care management to a supervised milieu, and back to the community only to be readmitted with an acute exacerbation of the illness. Why do you think this pattern exists?

Disorders Related to Schizophrenia
In addition to schizophrenia, the DSM-5 includes seven other disorders in the schizophrenia spectrum and related psychotic disorders (Table 11.1).

Schizoaffective disorder is considered to be primarily a form of schizophrenia as the person must have primary symptoms such as delusions, hallucinations, and disorganized behaviors. To be given the diagnosis of schizoaffective, the individual must also at some time have demonstrated symptoms of major depression or mania. The variance from a mood disorder lies in the presence of the primary symptoms of schizophrenia for at least 2 weeks without any mood symptoms. The disorder tends to be chronic and disabling with

TABLE 11.1 Schizophrenia Spectrum and Related Psychotic Disorders

Schizoaffective disorder	Mood episode and active symptoms of schizophrenia occur together preceded by at least 2 weeks of delusions and hallucinations
Schizophreniform disorder	Schizophrenic symptoms that last at least 1 month but less than 6 months (typically used as a preliminary diagnosis for schizophrenia)
Brief psychotic disorder	Short periods of psychotic behavior, usually in response to a crisis or severely stressful event, with quick recovery (i.e., catastrophic loss such as tornado or hurricane, plane crash)
Delusional disorder	Delusional thoughts coinciding with life situations that could be true and last for at least 1 month (i.e., feeling of being followed or stalked)
Catatonia	Marked psychomotor disturbance with 3 or more of 12 psychomotor features (stupor, catalepsy, waxy flexibility, mutism, negativism, posturing, mannerism, stereotypy, agitation, grimacing, echolalia, echopraxia)
Psychotic disorder due to another medical condition	Result of a condition that compromises brain function such as dementia, delirium, trauma, or brain tumor
Substance-induced psychotic disorder	Result of use of or withdrawal of a drug or substance such as alcohol, cocaine, or methamphetamine

some vacillating between a diagnosis of schizoaffective illness and schizophrenia.

Treatment of Psychotic Disorders

Most types of psychotic disorders are treated with a combined approach of medications and psychotherapy. The most common type of psychotropic agents used is the antipsychotic drugs. These medications do not provide a cure for the disorders, but are used in various levels of effectiveness in managing the problematic symptoms. Various types of psychotherapy including individual, group, and family therapy may be used in conjunction with the administration of the drugs. Some clients may require hospitalization for stabilization of their conditions, while many can be managed as outpatients. Each person responds to treatment differently with some improving quickly, and others taking weeks or months to receive symptom relief. In those whose symptoms are severe and disabling, the treatment may be needed indefinitely. Most people with schizophrenia need to take some type of medication along with supportive therapy for the rest of their lives.

Studies show that compliance with treatment in those with diagnosed schizophrenia and other psychotic disorders is improved when psychosocial treatment is afforded to them. Having a good relationship with a therapist or case manager provides the support needed to deal with their illness on a day-to-day basis. Although clients may not take their medication, because they do not believe they need it, many may not remember to take the medication at each scheduled time or stop taking the drug because they do not like the side effects. Difficulty in communication and developing relationships with the outside world adds to their isolation. A trained professional can often be the reminder and link to the person's ability to manage their own illness in a more effective way.

Antipsychotic Drug Agents

People with psychosis rarely have insight into the pathological complexity of their symptoms, often not realizing they are ill. This unusual lack of insight in many with psychosis during both periods of wellness and acute exacerbations of the symptoms is another dimension of the disabling and bizarre nature of the disorders. People with psychosis often have the mistaken belief that because they are feeling better when taking medications that control the symptoms, they can stop taking them. This leads to acute exacerbations and hospitalization to restabilize the client.

Antipsychotic agents, also referred to as neuroleptics, are used to treat serious mental illness such as bipolar affective disorder, depressive and drug-induced psychosis, schizophrenia, and autism. Because the symptoms of the psychoses are extremely uncomfortable for most people, the effects of antipsychotic drugs are one of the most dramatic in modern medicine. Today, these drugs can reverse most or all symptoms in many with psychotic illness. Early agents, such as Thorazine (chlorpromazine), a typical antipsychotic agent developed in 1950, produced remarkable reversal in symptoms and resulted in a dramatic decrease in the number of clients confined to institutions and hospitals for the mentally ill. This trend continues today, with shortened hospital stays and longer periods of functional community living for many whose symptoms are controlled with antipsychotic medication. However, since many lack insight into the complexity of their illness and need for continued treatment, compliance is generally inconsistent. This inconsistent adherence to treatment largely accounts for relapse and hospitalization to restabilize the individual drug regimens.

Typical or traditional antipsychotics block various dopamine receptors in the brain. Due to their varied chemical structures and strength, these agents are grouped into high-, moderate-, and low-potency classes, as shown in Box 11.4. The term *potency* indicates how much of the drug is required for it to be effective. The potency of the drug also influences the level and frequency of side effects experienced by the client. This accounts for the need for some clients to receive higher dosages to achieve optimum clinical results. For example, a much larger dose of a low-potency drug such as thioridazine (Mellaril) may be needed to produce the same level of symptom control that a lower dose of haloperidol (Haldol), a high-potency drug, offers. There is, however, a significant difference in the side effects they produce. Low-potency agents cause more anticholinergic effects, whereas high-potency drugs cause more extrapyramidal effects (discussed on page 173). Knowledge of the side effects enables the nurse to prepare the client for both the therapeutic benefits and potential adverse effects of the drug.

BOX 11.4

Grouping of Typical Neuroleptics (Antipsychotic) Drugs by Chemical Potency

High Potency	Moderate Potency	Low Potency
Haloperidol (Haldol)	Loxapine (Loxitane)	Thioridazine (Mellaril)
Thiothixene (Navane)	Molindone (Moban)	Mesoridazine (Serentil)
Trifluoperazine (Stelazine)	Perphenazine (Trilafon)	Chlorprothixene (Taractan)
Fluphenazine (Prolixin)	Droperidol (Inapsine)	Chlorpromazine (Thorazine)
Pimozide (Orap)	Acetophenazine (Tindal)	Promazine (Sparine)
		Triflupromazine (Vesprin)

Later generation antipsychotic drugs are classified as atypical, not falling into any particular chemical class. The newer agents have had a major impact on the reduction of negative symptoms of psychoses (those developed over a prolonged period of time such as flattened affect, verbal deficits, and diminished drive) with a reduced risk of extrapyramidal side effects. The reduction of negative symptoms is ultimately the desired outcome of antipsychotic therapy and is a tool used to measure progress of treatment. As a rule, the typical or positive psychotic symptoms (hallucinations and delusions) are those that lead to the most bizarre behavior. These symptoms are quite responsive to the typical antipsychotic agents. Along with reduced symptoms, these agents improve reasoning and decrease the ambivalent feelings and delusional thought processes that are both frustrating and frightening to the person experiencing them. By reducing the inner turmoil the person is

"Easy Way Out"

Missy is a 20-year-old client with a diagnosis of paranoid schizophrenia who was discharged 3 weeks ago from the acute care psychiatric unit. Today, her mother brings her to the clinic where you are working, stating that Missy doesn't want to take her medication because she isn't sick anymore and doesn't need "that poison." Her mother states Missy believes she has a "scientific machine in her colon that clips off pieces of her internal organs to ship to the FBI. The spies are in the medication and will make the machine interrogate faster."

Missy tells you that she is fine and that her mother is "wacko." She agreed to come with her mother today so she will quit nagging her about the medicine. She also states, "That stuff makes me dizzy and my mouth dries up like a bone...I can feel them clipping in my colon and then I have diarrhea big time!" Missy's mother shows you the bottle of Haldol 5 mg that was prescribed at the time of discharge.

How would you describe Missy's present behavior?

_____

_____

What is the best nursing approach to begin a therapeutic relationship with Missy?

_____

_____

What might Missy's complaints be related to her medication?

_____

_____

What nursing interventions might be planned to help Missy?

_____

_____

Case @ Application 11.2

TABLE 11.2   Typical or Traditional Antipsychotic Drug Agents

CHEMICAL GROUP	GENERIC NAME (BRAND NAME)	USUAL DOSAGE (DAILY[a])	ADVERSE REACTIONS AND SIDE EFFECTS
Phenothiazines	Chlorpromazine (Thorazine) Fluphenazine (Prolixin) Mesoridazine (Serentil) Perphenazine (Trilafon) Prochlorperazine (Compazine) Promazine (Sparine) Thioridazine (Mellaril) Trifluoperazine (Stelazine) Triflupromazine (Vesprin)[b]	40–800 mg 1–40 mg 30–400 mg 12–64 mg 15–150 mg 40–1,200 mg 150–800 mg 4–40 mg 60–150 mg	Extrapyramidal reactions, tardive dyskinesia, sedation, pseudoparkinsonism, EEG changes, drowsiness, dizziness, blurred vision, dry mouth, constipation, increased appetite, urine retention, weight gain, mild photosensitivity **Life-threatening:** seizures, neuroleptic malignant syndrome, blood dyscrasias
Butyrophenone	Haloperidol (Haldol) Pimozide (Orap)[c]	1–15 mg (Maximum 100 mg) 1–2 mg	Severe extrapyramidal reactions, tardive dyskinesia, sedation, drowsiness, lethargy, headache, insomnia, confusion, vertigo, tachycardia, hypotension, blurred vision, dry mouth, anorexia, nausea, constipation, diarrhea, dyspepsia, urine retention, rash
Dibenzoxazepine Dihydroindolone Thioxanthene	Loxapane (Loxitane) Molindone (Moban) Thiothixene (Navane) Chlorprothixene (Taractan)	60–100 mg 15–225 mg 20–60 mg 30–200 mg	Extrapyramidal reactions, sedation, drowsiness, numbness, tardive dyskinesia, pseudoparkinsonism, dizziness, tachycardia, orthostatic hypotension, blurred vision, dry mouth, constipation, urine retention, weight gain, rash **Life-threatening:** neuroleptic malignant syndrome, blood dyscrasias
Atypical Antipsychotic Drug Agents			
Benzisoxazole Partial dopamine agonist	Risperidone (Risperdal) Aripiprazole (Abilify, Aripiprex)[d]	2–6 mg 10–30 mg	Somnolence, extrapyramidal symptoms, headache, insomnia, agitation, anxiety, tardive dyskinesia, arthralgia, aggressiveness, tachycardia, rhinitis, constipation, nausea, vomiting, dyspepsia, cough, rash, dry skin, photosensitivity **Life-threatening:** neuroleptic malignant syndrome, prolonged QT interval
Dibenzodiazepine Dibenzothiazepine Thienobenzodiazepine	Clozapine (Clozaril) Quetiapine (Seroquel) Olanzapine (Zyprexa) Ziprasidone (Geodon) Paliperidone palmitate (Invega)[e]	25–450 mg 25–50 mg 10–15 mg 20–80 mg 3, 6, and 9 mg tabs	Extrapyramidal symptoms, dystonia, orthostatic hypotension, increased QT intervals, tachycardia, increased risk of myocarditis, abdominal pain, nausea, dry mouth, constipation, hypersalivation, urinary retention, face edema, myalgia, photosensitivity, agitation, dyspnea, fungal dermatitis, weight gain **Life-threatening:** agranulocytosis, neuroleptic malignant syndrome, cardiomyopathy, heart failure

[a]Total daily dosage.
[b]Available in LAI—Fluphenazine (Prolixin)
[c]Available in LAI—Haloperidol (Haldol)
[d]Available in LAI—Risperidone (Risperdal), Aripiprazole (Abilify Maintena—once monthly)
[e]Available in LAI—Olanzapine (Zyprexa), Paliperidone palmitate (Invega, Sustenna)

feeling, these agents allow the person to devote more energy to external activity and interpersonal relationships.

There have been few advances in adjuvant therapies to the antipsychotic agents. Latest trials have found that allopurinol (Zyloprim) may be a promising adjuvant with antipsychotic agents to reduce the positive and negative symptoms of schizophrenia in clients having little improvement with long-term use of antipsychotic agents. Studies continue to determine the effectiveness of allopurinol in the treatment of schizophrenia.

Antipsychotic drug agents are listed in Table 11.2, including categories, usual dosages, side effects, and adverse reactions. Several long-acting injectable (LAI) antipsychotics are now available in the United States, primarily used as a strategy for treating patients with schizophrenia who are noncompliant with taking their antipsychotic medication. The LAI are administered by injection at 2- to 4-week intervals. In addition to inhibition of postsynaptic receptors of the neurotransmitters, these drugs also have properties that affect the cholinergic, alpha-1-adrenergic, and histamine receptors. This allows them to be used as antiemetics and in treating neurological conditions such as intractable hiccups and tics (Tourette's disorder).

Extrapyramidal Side Effects

Antipsychotic agents are capable of producing numerous side effects. The lower-potency drugs tend to produce the anticholinergic (dry mouth, urine retention, constipation, blurred vision) and antiadrenergic (hypotension) actions, whereas the higher potency drugs can produce severe **extrapyramidal side effects**. These side effects block the neurotransmitter dopamine causing irritation of the pyramidal tracts of the CNS that coordinate involuntary movements. These reactions are much more devastating than anticholinergic and antiadrenergic side effects and contribute to the noncompliance exhibited by many clients for whom these drugs are prescribed. The resistance to treatment leads to relapse and return of symptoms with readmission to acute hospitalization. The physician can make dosage adjustments or prescribe medications to counteract these effects if they occur and are recognized early. Extrapyramidal side effects include the following:

- **Akathisia**—motor restlessness, inability to sit still
- **Dystonias**—rigidity in muscles that control posture, gait, or eye movement

- **Tardive dyskinesia**—late-appearing and irreversible movements of the mouth and face that include lip-smacking and grinding of teeth, protruding tongue movements. A mask-like facial appearance, tremors, shuffling gait, cogwheel rigidity, pill-rolling, and stooped posture are common indications that long-term use of these drugs has occurred.
- **Drug-induced parkinsonism**—symptoms that mimic parkinsonism such as tremors, rigidity, akinesia, or absence of movement with diminished mental state
- **Neuroleptic malignant syndrome**—a potentially fatal reaction most often seen with the high-potency antipsychotic agents. This response typically has an onset from 3 to 9 days after treatment is initiated. Symptoms include muscular rigidity, tremors, inability to speak, altered level of consciousness, hyperthermia, autonomic dysfunction (hypertension, tachycardia, tachypnea, diaphoresis), and elevated white blood cell count. Although neuroleptic malignant syndrome occurs in a very low percentage of clients taking these medications, the need for early recognition and immediate medical intervention is imperative.

Indications for Use

All antipsychotic drugs are used in the treatment of acute and chronic psychoses, mania, and dementia-induced psychosis. The phenothiazines and haloperidol are also indicated in the treatment of intractable hiccups and control of tics and vocal disturbances. In addition, the phenothiazines may be used as antiemetics.

Contraindications

Antipsychotic agents are contraindicated in clients with hypersensitivity; coma or severe depression; liver, renal, or cardiac insufficiency; blood dyscrasias; and Parkinson's disease. They should be used with caution in older clients; those with diabetes mellitus, chronic pulmonary disease, or prostatic hypertrophy; and in clients who are pregnant or lactating.

Nursing Diagnoses

Nursing diagnoses applicable to the client taking antipsychotic agents may include the following:

- Noncompliance with Medication Regimen, related to suspiciousness and lack of trust in health care workers
- Deficient Knowledge, related to drug therapy

- Activity Intolerance, related to medication side effects
- Risk for Injury, related to medication side effects
- Ineffective Coping, individual, related to medication compliance and medication side effects

Nursing interventions to include in caring for the client taking antipsychotic medications are as follows:

- Monitor for extrapyramidal side effects of antipsychotic drug therapy using AIMS assessment scale. (The AIMS assessment tool and procedure are found in Box 11.5.)
- Reinforce importance of consistent compliance with medication therapy.
- Reassure the client that interventions for behavior control will be initiated.
- Monitor for decreased symptoms of psychosis.
- Maintain a calm attitude with matter-of-fact response to reinforce reality.
- Provide sugarless candy, gum, or frequent sips of liquid to combat dry mouth.
- Encourage frequent oral hygiene.
- Observe elimination pattern for difficulty urinating or constipation.
- Monitor intake and output.

Outcome Evaluation

Criteria that may be used to evaluate the effectiveness of antipsychotic agents in the client may include the following:

- Symptoms are reduced to minimal occurrence
- Controls and refrains from violent behaviors
- Learns to use appropriate outlets for anger and frustration
- Identifies and seeks help when symptoms are overwhelming
- Takes medications as directed

Client and Family Teaching

It is essential that the client and responsible family members receive information about antipsychotic medications and the potential for adverse effects. At the same time, the importance of continuous adherence to the treatment must be stressed. Important information to teach the client and family members about antipsychotic agents includes the following:

- Take medication only as directed—discuss effects of noncompliance and the return of symptoms when medications are discontinued.
- Side effects may occur—discuss interventions to help relieve them.

- Report any signs and symptoms of tardive dyskinesia to the physician.
- Take medication with food or milk to decrease stomach irritation.
- Avoid taking antipsychotic medication within 1 hour of taking antacids or antidiarrheals (may decrease effectiveness of antipsychotic drug).
- Several days to several weeks of drug therapy may be needed before full effects of treatment are achieved.
- Keep scheduled appointments with the physician and follow through with laboratory testing.
- Use caution when operating motor vehicles or machines that require coordination and mental alertness as drowsiness may occur with medication.
- Avoid direct exposure to sunlight, or use a sunscreen when in the sun.
- Avoid vigorous exercise and overheating while taking the medication.
- Phenothiazines may possibly turn urine pinkish red, red, or reddish brown (is harmless and may be expected).
- Do not stop taking medication abruptly without checking with the physician.
- Avoid alcoholic beverages while taking the drugs (will potentiate CNS action).
- Avoid orthostatic hypotension by rising slowly from a sitting or reclining position.

Antiparkinson Drug Agents

Antiparkinson drug agents are used to relieve the drug-induced extrapyramidal symptoms associated with the antipsychotic drug agents. The two most commonly used are benztropine (Cogentin) and trihexyphenidyl (Artane), synthetic anticholinergic agents that resemble both atropine and diphenhydramine in their chemical structure. They are available only with a prescription, and the dosage is determined by the severity of symptoms.

The main contraindications are hypersensitivity reaction to the drug, narrow-angle glaucoma, myasthenia gravis, urinary retention, peptic ulcer disease, prostatic hypertrophy, and children under 3 years of age. These drugs must be used with caution in older adults because of significant side effects including urinary retention, visual disturbances, palpitations, and increased intraocular pressure.

BOX 11.5

National Institute of Mental Health AIMS Scale Abnormal Involuntary Movement Scale

A. Facial and Oral Movements
1. Muscles of facial expression (frowning, blinking, smiling, grimacing)
2. Lips and periorbital area (puckering, pouting, smacking)
3. Jaw (biting, clenching, chewing, mouth opening, lateral movements)
4. Tongue (thrusting, tremors, athetoid movements)

B. Extremity Movements
5. Upper (include choreic or rapid, objectively purposeless, irregular, spontaneous movements; athetoid or slow, irregular, complex, serpentine movements); Does NOT include tremors (repetitive, regular, and rhythmic)
6. Lower (lateral knee movement, foot tapping, heel dropping, foot squirming, inversion and eversion of foot)

C. Trunk Movements
7. Neck, shoulders, hips (rocking, twisting, squirming, pelvic gyrations)

D. Global Judgment
8. Severity of abnormal movements
9. Incapacitation due to abnormal movements
10. Patient's awareness of abnormal movements

E. Dental Status
11. Current problems with teeth or dentures?
12. Does the patient usually wear dentures?
13. Level of cooperation

Monitoring Scale for Sections A–C
0—Abnormal movements are not observed
1—Minimal or infrequent movements difficult to detect
2—Mild infrequent, but easy to detect
3—Moderate, frequent, easy to detect
4—Severe, almost continuously

Monitoring Scale for Section D
0—No awareness
1—Aware, no distress
3—Aware, moderate distress
4—Aware, severe distress

Monitoring Scale for Section E
0—None
1—Partial
2—Full

AIMS Examination Procedure

Observe the patient unobtrusively at rest. The chair to be used in the examination should be hard, firm, and without arms.
1. Ask patient, whether there is anything in mouth (i.e., gum, candy) and if there is, to remove it.
2. Ask patient about current condition of his/her teeth. Ask if patient wears dentures. Do teeth or dentures bother patient now?
3. Ask whether patient notices any movement in mouth, face, hands, or feet. If yes, ask to describe and to what extent they currently bother patient or interfere with activities.
4. Have patient sit in chair with hands or knees, legs slightly apart, and feet flat on floor. (Look at entire body for movement while in this position.)
5. Ask patient to sit with hand hanging unsupported. If male, between legs, if female and wearing a dress, hanging over knees. (Observe hands and other body areas.)
6. Ask patient to open mouth. (Observe tongue at rest within mouth.) Do this twice.
7. Ask patient to protrude tongue. (Observe abnormalities of tongue movement.) Do this twice.
8. Ask patient to tap thumb, with each finger, as rapidly as possible for 10 to15 seconds, separately with right hand, then with left hand. (Observe facial and leg movements.)
9. Flex and extend patient's left and right arms (one at a time). Note any rigidity separately.
10. Ask patient to stand up. (Observe in profile. Observe all body areas again, hips included.) Ask patient to extend both arms outstretched in front with palms down. (Observe trunk, legs, and mouth.)
11. Have patient walk a few paces, turn, and walk back to chair. (Observe hands and gait.) Do this twice.

TABLE 11.3   Age-Related Physiological Changes and Drugs in Older Clients

PHYSIOLOGICAL CHANGE	DRUG RISK
Higher body fat-to-lean ratio	Increased risk of cumulative effects
Less serum albumin and protein-bound drug	More free drug in bloodstream
Less total body water	Dehydration increases the concentration of drug in body
Decreased liver metabolism	Clearance of drug is delayed or slowed
Decreased renal elimination	Slowed elimination of drug from system

Psychotropic Drugs and the Older Client

For the older clients who have dementia-related aggression, distressing repetitive behaviors, catastrophic reactions, delusions, hallucinations, or agitation, the use of antipsychotic drugs has become a common approach to reducing and managing the incidence of these symptoms. The Omnibus Budget Reconciliation Act (OBRA) of 1987 limited the use of psychotropic medications for residents in long-term care facilities. These guidelines have been modified but with specific diagnostic and monitoring specifications. Antipsychotic medications can cause serious side effects such as tardive dyskinesia and other extrapyramidal side effects. The newer generation of psychotropic drugs is associated with fewer side effects, and they have thus become drugs of choice for older clients. Guidelines set by OBRA specify that these drugs can only be used for specific diagnoses and when behavioral and environmental measures are unsuccessful in managing symptoms. Research data on the safety and response of the older client to psychotropic medications are limited further suggesting a cautious approach to the use of these drugs.

Senior Focus

In the older adult, the half-life of a drug tends to increase by as much as five to six times, increasing the risk of toxicity. The effects accumulate slowly and may not be apparent for days or weeks after the initiation of the drug (Merck, 2014).

The impact of age-related physiological changes on antipsychotic drug therapy accounts for many of the serious side effects that occur in older adults. Many antipsychotic drugs, either by themselves or in interaction with other drugs, can cause the very symptoms they are prescribed to treat, such as agitation or delusions. Because older adults have a higher body fat-to-lean ratio, less serum albumin, less total body water, fewer brain cells, and slower liver metabolism and renal clearance than young adults, they need far less of these drugs to produce a therapeutic effect. The higher fat composition of tissue increases retention of the drug, resulting in effects that persist longer, sometimes even after the drug is discontinued. Because older clients have less protein to bind with the drug, more of the drug is free to circulate. A slowed metabolic rate and renal excretion time allow the drug to remain in the body longer. Table 11.3 shows these physiological changes and their imposed risks to older clients when administering an antipsychotic or other psychotropic agent.

All of these factors highlight the importance of monitoring the response to and recognizing the adverse effects of antipsychotic agents in the older client. It is considered extremely important that all alternative approaches be considered before the use of the drugs and that, if used, treatment is discontinued if the person is adversely affected by the drug.

Senior Focus

In the older client, always consider whether a new symptom or behavior may be related to drug therapy.

Application of the Nursing Process

Assessment

A nursing assessment will include information regarding any previous incidence of mental illness or psychotic episodes. Because the person with schizophrenia may not always be a reliable source of information, be sure to consult family members or other people familiar with the client. Data are most often compiled according to the nature of the symptoms, including perceptual alterations such as hallucinations or illusions.

- Identify the type of disturbance the client is experiencing.
- Ask the client about feelings while thought alterations are evident.
- Determine theme and content of delusional thinking. If the delusion is persecution oriented, assess the nature of the threat and whether there is a risk for violence as a result.
- Assess speech patterns associated with the delusions. Delusional thinking is characterized by speech in which the person jumps from one unrelated subject to another.

> ### Just the Facts
> The manner in which speech is manifested along with the accompanying behavior will usually provide more information about the delusion than the content.

- Note the affect and emotional tone of the client and whether they are appropriate in relation to the present situation. Apathy or a lack of interest in the environment and flatness of affect are characteristic signs of schizophrenia.
- Observe behavior patterns, activity, sleep habits, and interactions with other clients.
- Observe for posturing or other psychomotor disturbances.
- Assess for extrapyramidal side effects of antipsychotic drug agents.
- Assess the person's appearance, hygiene, and ability to perform self-care activities.
- Determine any suicidal intent or recent attempts that may have been made.

Selected Nursing Diagnoses

After careful review of the data, nursing diagnoses can be formulated. Approaches to treatment are usually selected on their ability to reduce and control the symptoms. Nursing care should be planned to focus on symptomatic relief as well, with careful attention to the physical, emotional, and social needs imposed by impaired mental functioning. Nursing diagnoses for the client with schizophrenia may include the following:

- Impaired Verbal Communication, related to fragmented delusional thinking

- Risk for Self-Directed or Other-Directed Violence, related to suspiciousness or command hallucinations
- Dysfunctional Family Processes, related to chronic illness
- Ineffective Coping, related to chronic illness, substance use
- Self-Care Deficit, related to withdrawal and apathy
- Disturbed Thought Processes, related to delusional thinking
- Impaired Social Interaction/Social Isolation, related to lack of trust
- Ineffective Relationship, related to decreased functional ability
- Disturbed Sensory Perception (Audio/Visual), related to hallucinations
- Chronic Low Self-Esteem, related to chronic illness
- Hopelessness, related to chronic low self-worth
- Noncompliance, related to denial of illness

> ### Mind Jogger
> How might the altered cognitive processes of psychosis contribute to noncompliance with drug therapy?

Expected Outcomes

The anticipated outcomes for the client with schizophrenia will depend on the level of functioning demonstrated by the client. This will depend on the severity of symptoms and the effectiveness of antipsychotic drug therapy or other therapeutic approaches. It is important that the goals and time frame for improvement be realistic. Expected outcomes for the schizophrenic person may include the following:

- Develops reality-based ways to communicate and meet self-needs
- Remains oriented to self and the environment
- Interacts appropriately with others
- Has not injured self or others
- Family members express realistic expectations of individual member
- Performs self-care and hygiene with minimal prompting
- Demonstrates increased trust of others
- Exhibits increased ability to associate behavior with misperceived environmental stimuli

- Participates in unit activities with appropriate behavior
- Identifies realistic self-expectations and perceptions
- Has reduced incidence of hallucinations
- Cooperates with staff in taking medications
- Family members express realistic expectations of individual member

Interventions

Selecting appropriate interventions that the client can tolerate requires careful planning. It is important to avoid expecting too much, but at the same time it is important to encourage clients to maximize their ability to function. Understanding the client's ability to focus, process, and follow instructions provides direction for the selection of nursing interventions. It is important to consider the holistic picture of the client, including physiological, emotional, cultural, and spiritual needs.

It is also important to assess the client for escalating behavior and intervene before an "out-of-control" situation occurs. In some instances, when other interventions do not work and he or she is at risk of harming himself or herself or others, a temporary restraint with a time-out in seclusion may be imposed to allow the client to regain self-control. When this situation occurs, nurses must use every measure to show respect for the client. Limits for behavior are reinforced and explained, reassuring the client of the temporary nature of these restrictions. Nutritional, hygiene, and toileting needs should be met in accordance with unit policies.

Interventions for the client with schizophrenia may include the following:

- Show acceptance of the client, separating the person from the behavior.
- Provide a safe environment by removing unsafe objects and diffusing potentially violent situations before they escalate.
- Maintain a reality-based approach to communication with the client. Clients experiencing delusions are mistrusting and suspicious making them resistant to taking medications and accepting information. Avoiding a confrontation or argumentative approach while also not reinforcing the delusional belief will reinforce reality. Make direct statements that shed doubt on the illogical thinking of the client.
- Provide a nonstimulating environment that reduces external stimuli.

Case Application 11.3

"Distortions of the Mind"

Richard is a 25-year-old client with a diagnosis of paranoid schizophrenia who has been coming to the clinic for the past 6 years. He has a history of noncompliance with his medications. Today, he is brought in by the police who state they found him starting fires in trash dumpsters. He told the police there are "devil spirits in the dumpsters that are making his mother ill." He stated, "I must create a fire so the smoke will dissipate them into the universal hierarchy of the sun, moon, and stars." The police tell you that Richard's mother is disabled and unable to continue caring for him. She says that he will not take his medication which makes him quite belligerent at times and then he does very bizarre things.

As you approach Richard, he is sitting with his arms stretched upward, eyes closed, and chanting "who is now in the light, cast a sign to the night, where the blue sky reigns, beware of the sane..."

What is the best way to approach Richard at this time?

What nursing diagnoses will help you develop an initial care plan for Richard?

What outcomes would you anticipate as treatment is implemented?

- Monitor for behavioral clues that indicate hallucinations or delusions (e.g., staring at an inanimate object, whispering, inappropriate giggling, facial or hand gestures).
- Acknowledge the perceptual or thinking alteration as being real to the client while reinforcing reality (e.g., "I understand that the voices must be frightening to you, but I do not hear them.") which helps the client to recognize symptoms as part of the illness.
- Set and maintain limits with expectations on unsafe or inappropriate behavior.
- Provide positive feedback for appropriate behaviors.
- Encourage client to ventilate feelings of anxiety, frustration, or those associated with altered thoughts and behaviors.
- Avoid abrupt touching of the client, which can be perceived as threatening.
- Provide prepackaged foods for clients who are paranoid. Clients are more likely to eat foods they can open themselves than food already prepared. Foods such as casseroles, mashed potatoes, meats, and gravy should be avoided during time of increased paranoia. Instead, items such as cheese slices, potato chips, crackers, milk, and complete nutritional prepackaged drinks can be offered as supplemental foods. Some units keep snacks, fruit, and nutritional drinks in an area that is accessible to clients.
- Monitor number of hours the client sleeps each 24-hour period.
- Encourage participation in social interaction with others while recognizing that a group activity may be threatening to the client with paranoia.
- Promote independence in self-responsibility for hygiene and self-care needs.
- The person with schizophrenia tends to neglect grooming and hygiene. Hair may be dirty or unmanaged and body odor evident. Clothing is usually disheveled and dirty. The client is not aware of the social inappropriateness of this appearance. Nursing interventions should encourage and offer assistance in improved daily bathing, dressing, and grooming behaviors.
- Monitor client's fluid intake, especially when in a hyperactive or agitated state.
- Promote client and family understanding of the illness and treatment regimen.
- Provide sources of information about their illness (Client Teaching Note 11.1).

CLIENT TEACHING NOTE 11.1

 Information Sources for Schizophrenia

- The **Information Helpline** is an information and referral service which can be reached by calling **1-800-950-NAMI (6264),** Monday through Friday, 10 AM to 6 PM, Eastern time.
- You may also e-mail us at **info@nami.org.**
- To sign up for Latino, African American, or Asian American and Pacific Islander E-News e-mail us at MACenter@nami.org or call 703–524–7600.
- National Institute of Mental Health Hotline: (888)826–9438
- National Mental Health Association: (800)969–6642
- http://www.nlm.nih.gov/medlineplus/schizophrenia. html
- http://www.nimh.nih.gov/index.shtml
- http://www.schizophrenia.com
- National Schizophrenia Foundation: http://www. nsfoundation.org

Evaluation

When evaluating the effectiveness of planned interventions, the nurse should look for signs that indicate improved functioning of the client. It is anticipated that compliance with drug therapy will diminish the positive symptoms of psychosis the client experiences. Hopefully, this is accompanied by an increase in the client's understanding of actual and real events that precipitate the perceptual and delusional alterations. This is demonstrated as the client is able to identify these factors and practice diversional techniques to avoid the anxiety that encourages the psychotic behavior.

Communication with staff and other clients in an appropriate and reality-based conversation is evidence of improved thinking processes. A decrease in bizarre and inappropriate behavior will occur as thoughts and perceptions decrease the need for their use. Reduced suspiciousness is evidenced by increased willingness to trust staff and other clients. This is a slow process for a client who has lived with a world of perceived threats and injustice. Any small gain should be viewed as progress. Compliance with taking medications and increased food intake are also evidence that the client has decreased fear of poisoning by ingested substances.

Case @ Application 11.4

"Carmen's Dilemma"

Carmen has been living in an apartment since her discharge from acute care. Since she is also a diabetic taking daily insulin injections, Carmen has been assigned home health visits three times a week to make sure she is taking her medications and appropriately managing living in an independent setting.

On this day, the LVN arrived to visit Carmen and was met with no answer to the doorbell. Voices were heard from inside the apartment indicating Carmen was at home. The nurse gently tried to open the door and found it unlocked. As she opened the door, she noticed Carmen standing on top of the couch talking to the ceiling fan. Carmen did not acknowledge that anyone had entered the room. The nurse spoke Carmen's name softly and told her who she was and the reason she was there. Carmen suddenly spun around facing the nurse and said, "They are telling me the insulin will poison me and I am slowly being destroyed by maggots from my food. They tell me to destroy all the food. Don't come near me."

If you were the nurse, what data would you collect?

_____

_____

How would the nurse best approach Carmen to get her attention?

_____

_____

What steps should the nurse take as a nurse advocate at this point?

_____

_____

Living with a life of losses in personal and social acceptance is difficult for clients with schizophrenia. Their feelings of hopelessness and worthlessness are ongoing. Expression of these feelings is a positive step as they move toward identification of peer and social support systems. Involvement in unit activities is a demonstration of their willingness to engage in the company of others. This also may be seen in the client who follows a task to completion such as in occupational therapy, clearing tables in the dining area, or taking a shower and dressing without assistance.

Outcome evaluations for the client taking antipsychotic medication therapy include the following:

- Experiences reduced incidence of psychotic symptoms and behaviors
- Seeks help when beginning to feel behavior is out of control
- Experiences minimal drug side effects
- Complies with therapeutic drug regimen
- Participates in planning care and long-term drug compliance
- Expresses understanding of relationship between psychotic symptoms, medication compliance, and behavior
- Client and family verbalize an understanding of prescribed medication regimen and potential side effects

Summary

- Psychosis is severe disarray in the mental processes of thinking, perceiving, and behaving. Behavior is directly linked to perceptions and thoughts about environmental stimuli and changes when these processes are distorted and disorganized.
- The characteristic symptoms reveal a loss of touch with reality and those things that give life meaning.

Loss of the ability to communicate meaningfully with others leads to a deterioration of relationships and contact with society.
- Hallucinations are false sensory perceptions that have no relevance to reality and are not supported by actual environmental stimuli. The person has the perception of seeing, hearing, smelling, feeling,

or tasting although there is no stimulus present. Auditory or hearing hallucinations are the most common. "Voices" may originate inside or outside the person's head and may talk to the person about his or her behavior. Some voices are commanding, telling the person to harm himself or others and are very frightening to the individual.

- Illusions are experienced when sensory stimuli actually exist but are misinterpreted by the person.
- Delusions are thought processes that are confused and disrupted, leaving the person inept at carrying on a conversation. The content or theme of the delusions can include depressive, somatic, grandiose, and persecution.
- Individuals who believe that others are sending messages to them or that they can send these messages through inanimate objects or other media are said to be having delusions of reference.
- Behavior alterations are inappropriate, silly, agitated, and unpredictable. The disorganized action most often leads to an inability to perform activities of daily living or to carry out goal-directed activity.
- Schizophrenia is the most common form of psychotic disorder. A prodromal period often precedes the actual first psychotic event during which the person may begin experiencing inability to concentrate and finish things. Thoughts may become distorted and speech patterns reflect a jumble of misplaced words.
- Positive symptoms of schizophrenia are evidenced early in the progress of the disorder and include alterations in thinking, perception, and behavior. The delusional patterns are distorted and often bizarre with no logical connection. The fragmented and disorganized thought processes are demonstrated in speech patterns of word salad and derailed loose associations.
- Negative symptoms of schizophrenia develop slowly over time and are reflected in the person's inability to deal with the way their illness affects their life. These include a blunted or flat affect that is expressionless and blank. Responses are often inappropriate responses to the mood of the real world around them. Behavior may be described as autistic referring to a focus on an inner fantasy world which excludes the external environment.
- The person with schizophrenia struggles with feelings of inadequacy and resists any type of competition with others which leads to withdrawal from personal, work, and social relationships. The losses result in an overwhelming feeling of loneliness, worthlessness, and apathy. Disorganization becomes the central theme of each day as the disease progresses.

- Subtypes of schizophrenia include paranoid, disorganized, catatonic, undifferentiated, and residual types.
- Psychotic disorders related to schizophrenia include schizoaffective disorder, schizophreniform disorder, brief psychotic disorder, delusional disorder, shared psychotic disorder, psychotic disorder due to a general medical condition, and substance-induced psychotic disorder.
- Schizoaffective disorder is characterized by a combined presence of schizophrenic symptoms and those of a mood disorder. The variance from a mood disorder lies in the presence of the primary symptoms of schizophrenia for at least 2 weeks without any mood symptoms.
- Treatment of the client with schizophrenia centers on reduction and control of the debilitating symptoms. A combined approach of antipsychotic drug therapy and psychotherapy is the most common approach. Management of positive symptoms by drug therapy may be limited by side effects and noncompliance.
- Antipsychotic drug agents aid in reducing or reversing the discomfort of the delusions, hallucinations, and disorganized behaviors common to the disorders.
- The incidence of adverse side effects and lack of insight into the need for continued treatment contribute to the noncompliance seen in many clients with psychosis who require antipsychotic medications to stabilize their illness.
- The potency of an antipsychotic drug will influence the level and frequency of side effects experienced by the client.
- The AIMS assessment tool can be used to monitor the extrapyramidal side effects of antipsychotic agents. Antiparkinson or anticholinergic agents are used to decrease the extrapyramidal side effects exhibited in those taking antipsychotic agents.
- Antipsychotic medications and other psychotropic agents are used with caution in the older client because of age-related physiological changes. The drug effects persist longer and remain in the body longer. Careful monitoring is mandated to avoid the adverse consequences of their use.
- Nursing assessment includes the nature of perceptual alterations, disorganized thought processes, and behavior patterns. In addition, the affect and emotional tone of the client and their relationship to the present environment are observed and monitored.
- Nursing care is planned to focus on the symptomatic relief and careful attention to the physical, emotional, and social needs imposed by the impaired mental functioning of the disorder.

Bibliography

American Psychiatric Association. (2013). *Diagnostic and statistical manual of mental disorders* (5th ed.). Washington, DC: Author.

Gold, K. J., Kilbourne, A. M., & Valenstein, M. (2008). Primary care of patients with serious mental illness: Your chance to make a difference. *The Journal of Family Practice, 57*(8), 515–525. Retrieved February 22, 2014.

Herdman, T. H. (Ed.). (2012). *NANDA International - Nursing diagnoses 2012–2014.* Oxford, UK: Wiley-Blackwell Publishers.

Hill, A. L., Sun, B., & McDonnell, D. P. (2014). Incidences of extrapyramidal symptoms in patients with schizophrenia after treatment with long-acting injection (depot) or oral formulations of olanzapine. *Clinical Schizophrenia & Related Psychoses, 7*(4), 216–222. Retrieved March 2, 2014.

Howard, R., Rabins, P. V., Seeman, M. V., & Jeste, D. V. (2000). Late onset schizophrenia and late-onset schizophrenia-like psychosis: an international consensus. *American Journal of Psychiatry, 152*(2), 172–178. Retrieved February 22, 2014, from http//ajp.psychiatryonline.org/cgi/content/fulltext/157/2/172.

Karch, A. M. (2013). *Nursing 2014 drug handbook.* Philadelphia, PA: Wolters Kluwer/Lippincott Williams & Wilkins.

Linden, N., Onwuanibe, A., & Sandson, N. (2014). Rapid resolution of psychotic symptoms in a patient with schizophrenia using allopurinol as an adjuvant, *Clinical Schizophrenia & Related Psychoses, 7*(4), 231–234. Retrieved March 2, 2014.

National Institute of Mental Health. (2009). Schizophrenia. Retrieved March 2, 2014, from http://www.nih.gov/ healthieryou.com/schizo.html.

Pallanti, S., Quercioli, L., & Hollander, E. (2004). Social anxiety in outpatients with schizophrenia: a relevant cause of disability. *American Journal of Psychiatry, 161*, 53–58.

Pawar, A. V., & Spence, S. A. (2003). Defining thought broadcast: semi-structured literature review. *British Journal of Psychiatry, 183*, 287–291. Retrieved February 22, 2014.

Raiji, T. K., Miranda, D., & Mulsant, B. H. (2014). Cognition, function, and disability in patients with schizophrenia: A review of longitudinal studies. *Canadian Journal of Psychiatry, 59*(1), 13–17. Retrieved March 2, 2014.

Rajagopal, S. (2007). Catatonia., *Advances in Psychiatric Treatment, 13*, 51–59. Retrieved February 23, 2014, from http://apt.rcpsych.org/content/13/1/51.full.

Ruscin, J. M., & Linneburm, S. A. (2014). *Pharmacokinetics in the Elderly,* Merck Manual. Whitehouse, NJ: Merck & Co, Inc. Accessed 2 November 2014 from http://www.merckmanuals.com/professional/geriatrics/drug_therapy_in_the_elderly/pharmacokinetics_in_the_elderly.html

Savilla, K., Kettler, L., & Galletly, C. (2008). Relationship between cognitive deficits, symptoms and quality of life in schizophrenia. *Australian & New Zealand Journal of Psychiatry, 42*(6), 496–504. Retrieved February 22, 2014.

Schutz, S. C. (2013). Schizophrenia, *Merck Manual for Health Care Professionals.* Retrieved February 22, 2014.

Townsend, M. C. (2011). *Nursing diagnoses in psychiatric nursing* (8th ed.). Philadelphia, PA: F.A. Davis Co.

Varcarolis, E. M. (2011). *Manual of psychiatric nursing care planning* (4th ed.). St. Louis, MO: Saunders Elsevier.

Weitzel, C. A. (2000). Could you spot this psychiatric emergency? *RN, 9*(63), 35–38.

Wilson, B. A., Shannon, M. T., & Shields, K. M. (2009). Retrieved February 22, 2014, from http://www.merckmanuals.com/professional/psychiatric_disorders/schizophrenia_and_related_disorders/schizophrenia.html.

Wilson, B. A., Shannon, M. T., & Shields, K. M. (2013). *Prentice hall Nurse's drug guide 2014.* Upper Saddle River, NJ: Pearson Prentice Hall.

Wilson, B. A., Shannon, M. T., & Shields, K. M. (2014). *Prentice hall nurse's drug guide.* Upper Saddle River, NJ: Pearson Prentice Hall.

Student Worksheet

Fill in the Blank

Fill in the blank with the correct answer.

1. Low-potency antipsychotic drugs cause more _____ side effects, whereas high-potency antipsychotic drugs cause more _____ side effects.

2. Extrapyramidal reactions are monitored by the _____.

3. _____ are perceptual disturbances in which the person misinterprets sensory stimuli that actually exist.

4. A psychosis-induced metabolic state of overhydration in the schizophrenic client is referred to as _____ _____.

5. Delusions of _____ centralize on false beliefs that the person is very powerful and important.

6. The person with schizophrenia typically has a _____ affect that is expressionless and blank.

Matching

Match the following terms to the most appropriate phrase.

1. _____ Avolition
2. _____ Derailment
3. _____ Clang associations
4. _____ Thought broadcasting
5. _____ Word salad
6. _____ Waxy flexibility
7. _____ Delusion of reference

   a. Person remains in one position until changed by another person.
   b. "I know all the judges can hear what I am thinking."
   c. Lack of motivation to make decisions or do self-care.
   d. "Our bowl is loud star to a wet red noodle carried by the military in excess of the earth."
   e. "Take the pill up the hill winter kill…"
   f. "Tom Brokaw is telling me I hold the key to security in outer space."
   g. Loose associations that are off track or not connected to each other.

Multiple Choice

Select the best answer from the multiple-choice items.

1. The nurse is assessing a client who states, "The radio is sending signals to my intellectual processes to inflict damage on myself." Which of the following would the nurse include in documenting the delusional pattern of this client?
   a. Experiencing auditory hallucinations
   b. Having delusions of persecution
   c. Demonstrating thought insertion
   d. Speaking in loose associations

2. Which of the following statements best describes poverty of speech?
   a. A jumble of unconnected and disorgaized thoughts
   b. Insignificant rhyming of words
   c. Thoughts of others can be inserted in one's mind
   d. Decrease in amount or speed with which a person talks

3. A client approaches the nurse and states, "This little elf keeps following me with a leash, and it really is getting on my nerves." Which of the following would be the most appropriate response for the nurse to make at this time?
   a. "I know seeing the elf is frustrating to you, but no one else sees it."
   b. "Why don't you just tell the elf to sit down and leave you alone."
   c. "You are only making that up in your mind."
   d. "That is silly. There is no one following you."

4. The nurse who observes protruding tongue movements and finger-rolling motions in a client taking the drug haloperidol (Haldol) would recognize this as:
   a. Signs of extrapyramidal side effects to the drug
   b. Normal response to long-term use of the medication
   c. Part of the illness and unrelated to the medication
   d. Indications an increased dosage may be needed

5. The nurse is providing patient teaching to a client for whom the antipsychotic agent risperidone (Risperdal) has been prescribed. Which statement by the client would indicate a need for further teaching?
   a. "I need to take the medication when I eat so it doesn't upset my stomach."
   b. "It may be a week or two before I feel really good."
   c. "I can still go riding on my bike in the afternoon like I usually do."
   d. "I better sit on the edge of the bed awhile before I get up in the morning."

6. The physician has ordered the drug benzetropine (Cogentin) for a client who has been taking the antipsychotic medication haloperidol (Haldol). Which of the following would the nurse expect to assess in this client?
   a. Increased delusional thinking
   b. Intractable hiccups
   c. Diminished drive and apathy
   d. Protruding tongue movements

7. The nurse is documenting observations made during an initial contact with a client who has recently been diagnosed with acute schizophrenia, undifferentiated type. Which of the following behavior assessments would be considered a positive symptom of schizophrenia?
   a. Presents with a blunted affect
   b. Expresses indications of avolition
   c. Having auditory hallucinations
   d. Disheveled and unkempt appearance

8. The nurse administering the antipsychotic agent haloperidol (Haldol) to a client would recognize the importance of which additional intervention to combat the adverse effects of this drug?
   a. Adding extra salt to prepared foods or beverages
   b. Offering sugar-free hard candy or frequent liquids
   c. Rinsing the mouth after taking the drug
   d. Observing for grayish discoloration of tongue

9. The nurse is planning care for a client who has been newly diagnosed with paranoid schizophrenia. Which of the following perceptual changes should the nurse anticipate?
   a. Client does not notice nor respond to changes in the environment
   b. Client recognizes that he is not responding normally to stimuli
   c. Client accepts and understands the irrational nature of his ideations
   d. Client frequently misinterprets social and environmental stimuli

10. A client with paranoid schizophrenia believes her medications are tainted with poisonous substances and refuses to take them. Which action should the nurse take?
    a. Matter-of-fact reinforcement of the need to take the medication
    b. Ask the client what the medication is tainted with
    c. Ask the client why he thinks the medication is tainted
    d. Withhold the medication and try again later

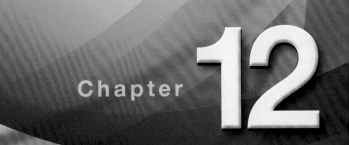

Chapter 12

Personality Disorders

⊙ Learning Objectives

After learning the content in this chapter, the student will be able to:

1. Define what is meant by a maladaptive pattern of personality traits.
2. Describe characteristic behaviors of each personality disorder.
3. Discuss treatment options for the client with a personality disorder.
4. Perform a nursing assessment of the client with a personality disorder.
5. Formulate appropriate nursing diagnoses for a person with a personality disorder.
6. Identify realistic outcomes for the client with a personality disorder.
7. Identify nursing interventions for the client with a personality disorder.
8. Evaluate the effectiveness of planned nursing care.

⊙ Key Terms

entitlement
ideas of reference
magical thinking
narcissism
passive-aggressive

personality disorders
personality traits
self-mutilation
splitting

Each of us is born with a set of traits, temperament, and patterns of behavior that are a unique blend of characteristics that make us who we are. Our thoughts, feelings, and attitudes toward ourselves and the world around us are the distinguishing aspects of our personality. **Personality traits** are persistent ways in which we view and relate to other people and to society as a whole. Those with healthy personalities are able to adapt to life stressors and form interpersonal relationships with reasonable expectations. Some personality traits are seen as negative and may be demonstrated in the difficult people we sometimes encounter in social or work settings. These same negative traits, however, are more severe and more extreme for individuals with personality disorders, creating difficulty for the individuals in adapting to the world around them.

Types of Personality Disorders

Personality disorders are deeply ingrained, persistent, inflexible, and maladaptive patterns of behavior that are in conflict with a cultural norm. Because the behavior does not usually conform to the expectations of society, it leads to distress and impairment in all aspects of a person's life. Behavior characteristics are demonstrated in the person's thinking processes, emotional reactivity, interpersonal relationships, and self-control. Unless they become frustrated with their life pattern or peer relationships, most individuals with personality disorders are oblivious to their problem. They are usually annoying and aggravating to those around them because of their egocentric and demanding behaviors. Most people with these disorders have established the deviant patterns of behavior by adolescence or early adult life. Unlike many other mental disorders where symptoms may alternate in levels, the symptoms seen in personality disorders tend to be consistent and constant. Treatment is rarely sought because of the person's denial or inability to identify the problem. Recent studies show that many individuals with personality disorders have lifelong problems related to their disorder, but respond with limited acceptance of available treatment options. When treatment is obtained, compliance with the treatment plan is inconsistent, doubtful, and less successful.

People with personality disorders tend to share some common characteristics that define them as having inflexible and maladaptive behaviors. Because behavior is the result of the way we perceive and think about the world around us, these characteristic differences tend to permeate their personal and social lives. Individuals with personality disorders tend to view their life in terms of all good or all bad with little understanding that something or someone can have both qualities. They tend to be arrogant and self-indulgent, unable to delay satisfaction of their needs to allow for the wishes of another. Many have unmet needs for dependency that relate back to inconsistent nurturing during the early developmental years.

In addition, there is a **passive-aggressive** tendency in which the person indirectly and subtly acts on hostile feelings. This may be seen as an ambivalent mindset in which the person displays a passive and pleasant effect whereas actions are based on underlying pessimism and bitterness. The person is torn between feelings of dependence and independence, love and hate, and action and inaction, with resulting moodiness, frustration, and stubborn self-will. This ambivalence is demonstrated in acting-out behaviors that allow the person to avoid thinking about the underlying psychological conflict. These behaviors may take the form of self-destructive acts meant to manipulate others into conforming to their wishes. Faults are projected to others to avoid feelings of inadequacy and incompetence. Deadlines are avoided with procrastination and other delay strategies to sabotage the efforts of others. If the passive manipulation fails, the resulting anxiety can precipitate angry emotional outbursts.

There are a number of personality disorders that have been identified, each having a particular set of behaviors and symptoms. The *DSM-5* groups the disorders into three categories or clusters according to the range of characteristics exhibited as shown in Fig. 12.1 (Box 12.1).

Cluster A Personality Disorders

Cluster A personality disorders include paranoid, schizoid, and schizotypal variations. Persons with these disorders tend to demonstrate odd or eccentric behaviors.

Paranoid Personality Disorder

Paranoid personality disorder is defined as a persistent pattern of suspicion and mistrust in which the

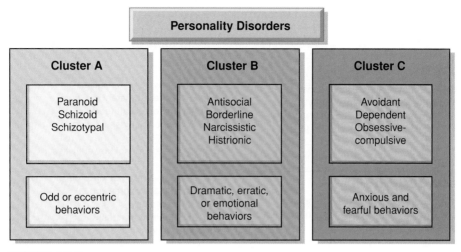

FIGURE 12.1

Categories or clusters of personality disorders grouped according to the range of particular characteristics or behaviors and symptoms exhibited.

actions or motives of others are seen as intentionally threatening or humiliating. Although there is no obvious reason for the suspicion, the person may become hostile and attack without warning. Often people with this disorder think it is necessary to "attack first" before others have the opportunity to harm them.

Signs and Symptoms

People with paranoid personality disorders are often viewed as being cold and aloof. Their suspicious nature leads them to be watchful, resentful, and guarded in their interactions with others. Individuals with paranoia are unable to believe

---

BOX 12.1

Symptoms of Paranoid Personality Disorder

- Cold and aloof manner
- Rigid and inflexible
- Doubts about loyalty and honesty of others
- Watchful and guarded
- Resentful, accusing, and argumentative
- Inability to tolerate criticism
- Mistrustful and unable to confide in others
- Feelings that others are out to deceive them
- Angry or hostile outbursts
- Maintenance of grudges against others
- Controlling relationships
- Extreme jealousy
- Projection of faults to others
- Inability to perceive self as a problem
- Self-sufficiency

---

that others can be good to them. A compliment might be perceived as a ploy to secure something in return, or a well-intended act of kindness may be viewed as a scheme to trick the person. There is a reluctance to share personal information with others for fear that it will be used against them later. Angry or hostile outbursts are perceived as necessary to defend against the disloyalty and deceit of others. The person with this disorder is unable to accept constructive criticism, but at the same time, is being critical of others. Grudges are maintained with no hint of forgiveness for a perceived insult or injustice.

Individuals with paranoid personality disorder usually have a long history of inability to achieve closeness in interpersonal relationships. Many jealous accusations of infidelity and indiscretion are made toward partners or spouses. They attempt to maintain control of the relationship by confronting the partner with demanding questions concerning places they have gone or their intent for going (e.g., vehicle mileage may be monitored to support the perceived disloyalty). This suspicion is further seen in their projection of blame for their own faults onto others. Their need to counterattack for a perceived injustice often leads to lawsuits against those blamed for the action. Their rigid, inflexible nature prevents any type of mutual agreement to resolve a problem. Although they tend to work better independently, people with paranoid personality disorder are often quite efficient and dedicated to their employment situation. Their interests are often in areas such as electronics, physics, and inventive ideas.

Just the Facts

People with physical defects or sensory impairments such as deafness may develop paranoia related to a reduced ability to interpret the reality of the world around them.

Mind Jogger

How would the person with a paranoid personality disorder respond to being given a compliment by a coworker?

Incidence and Etiology

Paranoid personality disorder is more prevalent in men. Typical behaviors are often seen by early adulthood. A possible genetic link to schizophrenia is seen in the tendency for those with this disorder to develop delusional thinking or actual schizophrenia. Some theorists relate this to parental modeling of negative thought processes and paranoid behaviors.

Schizoid Personality Disorder

People with a *schizoid personality disorder* are withdrawn and secluded and demonstrate an emotional indifference toward social relationships.

Signs and Symptoms

Because they are usually self-absorbed in their own feelings and thoughts, people with this disorder tend to avoid close relationships and intimacy. They are viewed as being "loners," usually choosing to pursue activities and interests alone. The person with this disorder derives less pleasure from things that are soothing and sensuous such as music, romance, or beauty. Sexual experiences are usually not desired. Facial expression or affect is usually bland and unresponsive to positive emotions in others. Emotions such as elation or anger are seldom felt or displayed. Delusional thinking can be precipitated by stressful events (Box 12.2).

People with schizoid personality disorder are often described as daydreaming, fantasizing, and without purposeful goals. They are usually oblivious as to how their behavior is being perceived by others. Working situations that require social interaction are usually avoided. However, they may do well in an employment setting where

---

BOX 12.2

Symptoms of Schizoid Personality Disorder

- Withdrawal and seclusion
- Emotional indifference
- Self-absorbed attitude
- Avoidance of close relationships and intimacy
- Loners
- Preference for solitary activities
- Decreased pleasure experience
- Decreased interest in sexual experiences
- Bland facial expression
- Daydreaming
- Emotional barrenness
- Social avoidance

interaction is not necessary and they can work alone. Their interests are often in the areas of mechanics or art.

Just the Facts

The person with schizoid personality disorder is usually not concerned with how his or her behavior is perceived by others.

Incidence and Etiology

This disorder is somewhat more common in men than women. There is an increased incidence in those who have a family history of schizophrenia or other personality disorders. The behavior characteristics are seen in most aspects of the person's life by adolescence or early adult years.

Schizotypal Personality Disorder

In addition to being secluded and withdrawn from social situations, persons with *schizotypal personality disorder* exhibit strange and unusual patterns of thinking and communicating.

Signs and Symptoms

The thinking patterns and opinions of people with this disorder are unusual and bizarre, often with paranoid undertones. They often display a sort of **magical thinking**, or the belief that thoughts, words, and actions can cause or prevent an occurrence by extraordinary means, in which they propose to forecast the future or read the minds of others, for example. **Ideas of reference** are seen in which the person believes that everyday occurrences have a special and significant personal

BOX 12.3

Symptoms of Schizotypal Personality Disorder

- Weird and bizarre thinking and beliefs
- Paranoia and suspiciousness
- Magical thinking
- Ideas of reference
- Perceptual distortions, illusions
- Inflexible emotions
- Eccentric dress habits
- Social isolation
- Remorse over lack of social relationships

meaning. Perceptual distortions and illusions are common. Emotions are rigid and inflexible, and these individuals have little ability to respond to feelings and expressions of others. Dress habits and mannerisms may be eccentric or unusual (Box 12.3).

Increased fear and anxiety are experienced in social situations. This results in a diminished ability to form interpersonal relationships. The person is often unhappy about not having social friends and relationships but is unable to overcome the social ineptness and suspiciousness of others. Psychotic behavior may occur in brief episodes of minutes to hours. It is believed that this disorder is a mild form of schizophrenia but without the continuous thought alterations.

Incidence and Etiology

Schizotypal personality disorder typically is apparent during childhood and adolescence. The odd behavior is often the target of ridicule by other children, leading to early social isolation. It is more common in men than in women. Prevalence is also seen in first-degree biologic relatives of people with schizophrenia. Treatment is usually sought for symptoms of anxiety or depression rather than for the symptoms of the personality disorder itself.

Cluster B Personality Disorders

Dramatic, emotional, or erratic behavior is characteristic of individuals with a cluster B personality disorder. The category includes the antisocial, borderline, narcissistic, and histrionic personality disorders.

"Uneasy Predictions"

Margie is a 25-year-old client who was admitted to the psychiatric unit after employees of a clothing store called the police about a lady who was "acting weird" and saying "all this crazy stuff." She has always worn clothes that were unusual and don't match.

She expresses little emotion as she walks around the unit. Margie seems superstitious, because she avoids mirrors and steps over cracks in the tile floor. It is not unusual to see her gazing out of the window with nodding and hand gestures, seeming to indicate she is communicating with someone. Today the nurse walks into the day room and finds Margie looking into a flower vase and telling the other clients, "I can see the future…there is danger in the air and tomorrow something bad is going to happen!" One of the clients becomes very disturbed and shouts "Shut her up! Shut her up!"

How should the nurse approach this situation?

_____

_____

What characteristics of schizotypal personality does Margie demonstrate?

_____

_____

How could the nurse help Margie continue a therapeutic type of interaction with other clients on the unit?

_____

_____

Case Application 12.1

Antisocial Personality Disorder

Those with an *antisocial personality disorder* exhibit a persistent pattern of disregard and infringement on the rights of others in a society. A false sense of privileged revenge against others is demonstrated by their basic cold indifference to the laws of society and humanity. Also referred to as a sociopath, the person with antisocial personality disorder is selfish and seemingly has no conscience. Lying and stealing are common, along with a failure to accept or follow through with responsibilities of everyday living, parenting, or work-related tasks. A childhood and early adolescence marred with abuse and neglect add to the risk of adults with antisocial behaviors. The disorder tends to be chronic and perhaps one of the most difficult to treat.

Signs and Symptoms

The person with this disorder is suspicious and feels betrayed by the world. Thinking that humans are basically evil and out to undermine, the person performs actions impulsively and recklessly to avoid being sabotaged. Vandalism, fighting, explosive anger, and verbal assault are common. School expulsion, truancy, and delinquency are among the problems in the person's history. Their interactions with others are full of deceit and dishonesty. People with antisocial personality disorder victimize others for materialistic self-gain and are often described as "con-artists." Their way of thinking is cold, calloused, insensitive, arrogant, and ruthless, with insensitivity to the feelings of others. Their behavior results in continued and frequent encounters with law enforcement officials. Despite the continued conflict with the law, these people do not feel remorse or responsibility for the consequences of their behavior. In the mind of a criminal, getting caught is seen as a failure to achieve success. Rarely do they benefit from incarceration or treatment programs. Projection of blame to others is typical as they try to rationalize and minimize their vengeful actions (Box 12.4).

Individuals with antisocial personality disorder may use alias names, relocate, or change jobs in an attempt to avoid recognition by law enforcement or other regulatory agencies. Little regard is given to dependent or financial responsibilities. They often display superficial charm, smooth conversation skills, and excessive self-assurance as they manipulate others for their personal gain and pleasure. There is a reckless disregard for

---

BOX 12.4

Symptoms of Antisocial Personality Disorder

- Suspiciousness of others
- Impulsive and reckless behavior
- Vandalism, fighting
- Explosive anger
- Deceitfulness and dishonesty
- Lying
- Coldness and insensitivity
- Arrogance
- Violation of rights of others
- Lack of remorse or guilt
- Manipulation
- Projection of blame
- Irresponsibility
- Alias names
- Charm and scheming
- Recklessness
- Sexual promiscuity and exploit
- Dysphoria

---

the safety of others as seen in careless driving, actions that put others in danger, or destruction of property. Sexual promiscuity and exploitive relationships with a lack of concern for partners are common. Unable to tolerate boredom, the person with antisocial personality disorder may become dysphoric and may look for something stimulating such as sex, alcohol, gambling, or other compulsive self-indulgence activities to compensate for this feeling.

Mind Jogger

How is the antisocial personality reflected in the mind of the criminal who thinks that getting caught is failure to achieve success?

Incidence and Etiology

Most people with antisocial personality disorder have a history of conduct disorder with an onset before the age of 15. Situations of child abuse, unstable parenting, and inconsistent parental discipline may increase the chances of a person developing antisocial personality disorder by the age of 18. The disorder tends to be more prevalent in men than in women and is most often associated with those in low socioeconomic class and crowded living situations. There is a higher incidence among the prison population and those who have a history of substance abuse. There tends to be a familial pattern with it occurring more often in those who have first-degree biologic relatives

"Smooth Character"

You are assigned to the psychiatric unit where Ed, a 28-year-old, was admitted yesterday under a court order. He was diagnosed with conduct disorder at the age of 10 and has been in conflict with law officials many times during his adolescent years. He has been in custody for driving under the influence of drugs and assault of a peace officer. Because this is not his first substance-related offense, he is court-ordered to receive treatment for substance abuse and anger management.

Ed is very charming and good looking. His manner is very convincing as he freely gives polite compliments and makes friendly gestures. Today Ed tells you that he is really attracted to you and has never felt this way before. He asks for your phone number so he can call you when he is discharged. Although you inform him you cannot give him this information, he is persistent. When confronted with his manipulative behavior, Ed becomes enraged and says, "You wouldn't recognize a good thing if you saw it. You're nothing but a slut anyway."

How should you respond to this situation?

_____

_____

Why is limit-setting so important in dealing with Ed's behavior?

_____

_____

What are the chances that Ed will benefit from the treatment process?

_____

_____

with antisocial personality disorder. The disorder tends to be chronic but may become less evident as the person ages.

Borderline Personality Disorder

Persons diagnosed with *borderline personality disorder* have a persistent pattern of unstable interpersonal relationships, insecure self-image, and mood swings. They are impulsive and intense in their outbursts of anger. Anger is often preceded by anxiety with a recurrent emotional swing between anxiety, sadness, and anger.

Signs and Symptoms

People with this disorder often feel a chronic sense of emptiness and abandonment accompanied by continued anxiety and efforts to avoid the perceived rejection. The fear often leads to clingy, dependent, and needy behavior with rapid attachment to a nurturing partner. Individuals with borderline personality disorder quickly become overinvolved and attached in the relationship, but soon feel threatened that the partner will leave. Without warning, the person may suddenly view the caring partner as evil and cruel, pushing them away to avoid future

rejection. While rallying between the labile emotional states of self-admiration and self-dislike, the person with this disorder becomes confused about self-identity. There are intense episodes of dysphoria and irritable moods that may last hours or days. The quick change from clingy and dependent extremes to angry outbursts in a short period of time is typically referred to as a "Jekyll and Hyde" characteristic. This is very frustrating to those who try to befriend them and dampens most of the person's relationships.

Along with the mood change, the person usually demonstrates an extreme view, or **splitting**, of their relationship to the world. Things are seen as all or none, black or white, love or hate, with no neutral ground (e.g., loss of a partner means I am a bad person). When a relationship ends, the person believes it proves his or her feelings of worthlessness. Dissociation may occur to escape the feeling of being alone. At times, there may be brief episodes of paranoia and hallucinations because the person's ability to maintain a reality state is unstable. This is often the time when repeated threats of suicide or self-mutilation are exhibited. **Self-mutilation** is an intentional act of

---

BOX 12.5

Cutting: What to Look For

- Small, straight cuts
- Frequent injuries with doubtful explanations
- Low self-esteem
- History of relationship problems
- Isolated and loner tendency
- Razor or knife in bag or purse
- Blood stains on clothing
- Clothing with long sleeves in warm weather

---

inflicting bodily injury to oneself without intent to die as a result. It demonstrates an outward focus of control over inner pain and serves to restore the person's sense of realism and value. Self-injury stimulates a release of endorphins that leads to the release of inner tension. This reinforces and feeds the repetitive pattern of the self-injurious behaviors. There is some speculation that the response to endorphin elevation may be related to repeated childhood abuse and pain that has resulted in a type of self-hate and redirected anger toward the person. The physical pain of the self-injury serves as a coping mechanism that distracts from and allows the individual to avoid dealing with the emotional pain. Some of the acts are stereotypic and self-stimulating such as head-banging or cheek-chewing. Other actions may be more intermittent but habitual such as burning and cutting various body sites (Box 12.5), or skin picking the body using fingernails, tweezers, pins, teeth, or other instruments. These behaviors bring a distorted sense of emotional relief to the individual. Although ashamed of their actions, they feel a compelling need to continue the behavior. The person also may engage in impulsive behaviors that have the potential for self-destruction such as substance abuse, gambling, sexual promiscuity, reckless activity, or excessive eating patterns.

People with this disorder may demonstrate caring for others, but with expectation for self-gain. Rarely do they experience any positive emotions of happiness or well-being. If their wishes are ignored, the display of acting-out behaviors demonstrates their inability to delay satisfaction of their needs. These behaviors are usually in the form of temper tantrums, impulsive anger, and sarcasm directed at others. They are easily enraged if authority figures do not provide instant response to their wishes. This behavior often tends to undermine their successes because they often quit before a goal is achieved. Multiple employment

---

BOX 12.6

Symptoms of Borderline Personality Disorder

- Unstable relationships
- Insecure self-image
- Mood swings
- Dissociation
- Impulsive outbursts of anger
- Chronic sense of abandonment
- Clingy, dependent, manipulative behavior
- Splitting
- "Jekyll and Hyde" characteristic
- Self-mutilating behaviors
- Suicidal threats and gestures
- Inability to delay gratification of needs

---

losses, broken relationships, and unfinished education are common (Box 12.6).

Just the Facts

People with borderline personality disorder tend to engage in additional self-destruction by repeatedly becoming involved in no-win relationships with others who are emotionally unstable or abusive.

Mind Jogger

In what way could self-mutilation be described as a manipulative behavior?

Incidence and Etiology

Borderline personality disorder tends to occur more in women than in men. It is more common in those with a family history of the disorder. There seems to be more instability during the early adult years, with some stabilization of moods seen by the 30- to 40-year-old age-group. The incidence of suicide in this group is the highest during young adulthood.

The exact cause of this condition is not known. It is believed that perhaps instances of parental neglect, separation from the primary caregiver, and child abuse may contribute to development of the disorder. An infant who is suddenly removed from the emotional attachment figure learns that a comfortable trusting relationship is followed by anxiety when that person is no longer available. Trust is lost and the separation is viewed as abandonment. Once the security and comfort of the good relationship changes to anxiety in a bad situation, the child learns to see "all good" and

"Hidden Ambivalence"

Sherry is a 24-year-old woman who is admitted to the emergency room for self-mutilation: she cut her forearms 28 times with a kitchen knife. She had just discovered that her live-in boyfriend of 2 years had moved out. Her history reveals many broken relationships and four previous suicide attempts, including two overdoses, walking in front of a fast-moving vehicle, and a gunshot wound to her left leg. Before the present incident, she had telephoned her boyfriend, who abruptly hung up on her. Her mother tells the nurse that she doesn't understand why this is so upsetting to Sherry. She says that 2 months ago Sherry told her boyfriend to "get lost." In between episodes of crying, Sherry tells the nurse, "I must have done something bad for him to do this. If I were a good person he would still be there."

How does Sherry's behavior demonstrate her underlying sense of insecurity?

_____

_____

How is "splitting" evident in her behavior?

_____

_____

How should the nurse respond to Sherry's last statement?

_____

_____

"all bad." There is continued difficulty in being able to integrate these two conditions as coexistent in the same person. This leads to splitting, in which the person reacts to people in either a very positive or very negative way.

Narcissistic Personality Disorder

The term **narcissism** is a Greek word, meaning "excessive love and attention given to one's own self-image." The person with a *narcissistic personality disorder* has a continued need for lavish attention and admiration with little regard for the feelings of others. Other people may be used unfairly to satisfy this person's desires.

Signs and Symptoms

People with narcissistic personality disorder have an exaggerated and grandiose sense of importance. This is exhibited as arrogance and claims of **entitlement** that others owe them because of their superiority. When shopping for services or merchandise, for example, the person will ask to see the manager or owner of the establishment, indicating their sense of importance. Any personal achievement is overexaggerated with demands for praise and approval. Fantasies of power, beauty, and success are believed to be superior and only understood by others who are on this level. They may talk at length about themselves not realizing that others are not showing an interest in the conversation (Box 12.7).

Although people with this disorder perceive an awesome superior self, there is an underlying

> **BOX 12.7**
>
> ### Symptoms of Narcissistic Personality Disorder
>
> - Grandiose sense of self-importance
> - Intense need for admiration and approval
> - Lack of empathy for others
> - Exploitation of others for own needs
> - Sense of entitlement
> - Demand for the best of everything
> - Fantasies of power, beauty, success
> - Underlying feelings of inferiority
> - Hypersensitivity to criticism
> - Anxiety
> - Social withdrawal
> - Poor insight into behavior
> - Arrogance

feeling of inferiority and envy of others. They may inwardly resent and dislike those who are awarded more respect or attention and are usually overly sensitive to failure, which results in feelings of insecurity. The grandiose overinflation of the self is seen as overcompensation for their low self-esteem. Because of their extreme sensitivity to criticism, people with narcissistic personality disorder may experience humiliation, intense anxiety, and shame if reprimanded or disappointed. The need for admiration increases to overcome these feelings of being "bad" if they are not receiving attention. They do not have insight into their behavior and unrealistic thinking. Social withdrawal and mood alterations are common during periods of frustration and anxiety.

Mind Jogger

How are narcissistic attitudes fed by a culture that places excessive value on physical appearance?

Incidence and Etiology

Although there is a tendency for adolescents to have a narcissistic view of themselves as they search for their identity, this does not mean that a personality disorder exists. It is only when the narcissistic traits become inflexible and maladaptive enough to cause dysfunction in the person's life that a disorder may be diagnosed. People who develop the disorder rarely seek treatment and often blame the negative results of their behavior on society. Narcissistic personality disorder is more common in men than women and usually has an onset during early adulthood.

Histrionic Personality Disorder

Typically, the person with *histrionic personality disorder* displays a pattern of egocentric and excessive emotion in a demanding manner to gain personal attention. Individuals with this disorder are uncomfortable in situations where center stage is not afforded to them.

Signs and Symptoms

People with this disorder are overly dramatic and may seem fake or exaggerated in their behavior. By creating a scene that gets the attention of others, they usually receive sympathy or affectionate gestures in return. As a result, they may develop attachments easily but tend to be superficial and

---

BOX 12.8

Symptoms of Histrionic Personality Disorder

- Attention-seeking behavior
- Extreme egocentricity
- Overly dramatic and exaggerated behavior
- Shallow, superficial relationships
- Provocative sexual behavior
- Melodramatic but vague speech
- Manipulation
- Unmet dependency needs

---

easily dissatisfied with the relationship. They may also demonstrate unexpected sexual advances in their interactions with others. Relationships are often described in detail as involving more intimacy than is actually present. Casual acquaintances may be introduced as a best friend or a wonderful, dear person. Provocative dress and mannerisms are often used to draw attention. Speech tends to be melodramatic with numerous hand gestures but is vague and lacking in content. The behavior is described as a manipulative ploy to satisfy underlying needs of dependency and protection. Individuals with this personality disorder may be easily influenced by others and overly trusting of those perceived as able to solve all their problems (Box 12.8).

Incidence and Etiology

Histrionic personality disorder tends to occur more often in women but is seen also in men and is usually evident by early adulthood. The available statistics are limited. There is a strong association between the disorder and dissociative symptoms. It is also common for these clients to demonstrate several personality features of other disorders, such as somatization, manipulative behavior, sexual promiscuity, and self-indulgence. There is speculation that symptoms may stem from the childhood experiences in which recognition was only received if parental expectations were met. Only when the histrionic traits of the person become maladaptive and impair functioning, it is considered a disorder.

Cluster C Personality Disorders

Persons with cluster C personality disorders exhibit anxious and fearful types of behavior such as the avoidant, dependent, and obsessive-compulsive personality disorders.

Avoidant Personality Disorder

The person with an *avoidant personality disorder* is typically shy and very sensitive to negative comments from others. Feelings of inadequacy and intense discomfort are felt in social situations that involve people other than family.

Signs and Symptoms

Because of their extreme fear of ridicule or disapproval, people with this disorder tend to avoid events or situations that involve interaction with others. Educational and work-related opportunities may be rejected out of fear that criticism may follow. The person is afraid that others might become aware of his or her self-doubt and tends to withdraw from relationships if there is a chance these feelings might be exposed. Intense anxiety is experienced when in a group of people. This feeling is linked to those of inferiority and incompetence. Any indication of disapproval will prevent the individual from becoming involved, though he or she may be encouraged and offered support by others in the group. There is a perception of rejection even when it does not exist. Unless individuals with avoidant personality disorder are certain of being liked, there is usually an unwillingness to trust the environment. Although they desire to have intimate interpersonal relationships, this guardedness often prevents them from doing so (Box 12.9).

> **Just the Facts**
>
> Dwelling on perceived inadequacies and previous mistakes, the individual with avoidant personality disorder tends to view himself or herself as inferior in all aspects of life.

BOX 12.9

Symptoms of Avoidant Personality Disorder

- Extreme shyness
- Hypersensitivity to rejection or negative comments
- Feelings of social inadequacy
- Social withdrawal/isolation
- Self-doubt
- Fear of criticism or embarrassment
- Intense anxiety in social setting
- Feelings of inferiority
- Low self-esteem
- Lack of trust in others
- Lack of close friends
- Fear of intimate relationship
- Reluctance to take risks or try new things

Incidence and Etiology

Avoidant personality disorder is equally frequent in men and women. Shyness and fear of new situations exhibited in childhood tend to increase by adolescence in individuals with this disorder. There is some evidence that it decreases with age. People who demonstrate avoidant behaviors often have associated social phobia.

Dependent Personality Disorder

People with *dependent personality disorder* demonstrate a consistent and extreme need to be cared for that leads to a reliance on others. At the same time, they perceive themselves as helpless and incompetent. If one relationship ends, there is immediately a pressing need to begin a new one.

Signs and Symptoms

People with dependent personality disorder have difficulty making decisions that affect everyday life unless prompted and reassured by others. They relinquish control and priority for their own needs to someone else. Feelings of insecurity and doubt prevent them from making self-care decisions. They may not be able to select items to wear, requiring another to choose their daily attire. Although they may disagree with those caring for them, they do not express these feelings for fear of upsetting the other person. It is not uncommon for these people to demonstrate acting-out behaviors to show their inability to make a decision or know what to do in a given situation. For example, a woman who shoves a shopping cart into the wall of a grocery store when her husband asks her to select a package of bacon from the shelf. She states she does not know what brand he wants. Afraid of making her husband upset and being left alone, she relinquishes the selection of groceries to him.

People with dependent personality disorder will search at length to find relationships where the hovering support will continue. Because of the extreme anxiety experienced when someone is not present to make decisions for them, a replacement figure is needed if a relationship ends. Independent or self-initiated involvement in activities is not an option for individuals with this disorder (e.g., a man needs shampoo to wash his hair, but will not buy it until someone tells him what brand to buy). There is an increased incidence of abuse and surrender that is tolerated in these relationships. Because the abused person is so afraid of being alone, the abuse is endured even when help is offered to leave the situation. Their passive

BOX 12.10

Symptoms of Dependent Personality Disorder

- Inability in making decisions without approval from others
- Extreme reliance on others
- Insecurity and self-doubt
- Extreme fear of being alone
- Excessive anxiety
- Feelings of helplessness and incompetence
- Constant need for reassurance
- Self-sacrificing behavior
- Relinquishment of control to others
- Submissive behavior

nature and fear of abandonment overrides any expression of unmet personal needs. For example, a 28-year-old woman who is in an abusive relationship wants to take college classes, but is afraid her husband will leave her if she has skills for making her own living. She does not pursue her dreams and remains dependent on his support. This person is so afraid of being unable to make decisions for living by herself, she remains in the clutch of a controlling and cruel relationship (Box 12.10).

Mind Jogger

How is the dependent personality reflected in the "empty-nest" syndrome experienced by a parent when all his or her children leave home?

Incidence and Etiology

Dependent personality disorder is diagnosed more often in women than in men. The disorder usually occurs by early adulthood and follows a chronic pattern. It is one of the most frequently reported personality disorders. Age and cultural factors can contribute to the behavior. In some cultures, women are expected to be subservient to men. The distinction between what is considered respectful and what is excessive must be made. Children and adolescents who experience chronic physical illnesses or separation anxiety disorder have an increased risk of developing this disorder.

Obsessive-Compulsive Personality Disorder

People with *obsessive-compulsive personality disorder* are conscientious, highly organized, and preoccupied with order and perfection. They are usually dependable but want rigid control and lack the flexibility to allow for compromise.

Signs and Symptoms

Individuals with obsessive-compulsive personality disorder pay excessive attention to details and rules to the point that tasks are left unfinished. For example, a businessman is so concerned that specific rules of order be maintained during a meeting that nothing is accomplished. Compulsive people tend to insist that their way is the only right way to do things and have a desire to be in charge of situations. As a result, they have difficulty delegating to others, preferring to do the task their way so it is done right. If tasks are assigned, lengthy detailed instructions are given. They are highly critical of others and of themselves if mistakes are made or deviations made from the instructions. It is difficult for people with this disorder to feel satisfaction for their accomplishments. They experience high anxiety levels if deadlines or prioritizing are expected of them.

Miserly spending and hoarding are part of their stubborn refusal to waste or throw away items that "might be needed" at some future time. It is common for items such as magazines or paper sacks to be saved and arranged precisely in piles with all corners exactly in line to perfection. There is an inability to discard items that are worthless or no longer functional. Their need to keep things is often an annoyance to those around them. People with obsessive-compulsive disorder rarely take time off from work for leisure activities or vacation, believing that to do so is a waste of time. Relationships are often more serious and shallow. The person believes that public display of emotion or affection is foolish and typically exhibits a limited ability to express feelings or intimacy toward another (Box 12.11).

BOX 12.11

Symptoms of Obsessive-Compulsive Personality Disorder

- Preoccupation with orderliness
- Rigidness and controlling behavior
- Focus on details
- Unrealistic expectations, inflexible
- Missed deadlines
- Inability to relax
- Rigid moral and ethical standards
- Hoarding of items
- Inability to delegate
- Stubbornness
- Miserly with material things
- Shallow display of emotions

Just the Facts

The person who has an unconscious feeling of powerlessness may attempt to achieve self-control by controlling others.

Incidence and Etiology

Obsessive-compulsive personality disorder is seen twice as often in men than in women. The disorder tends to appear in the late teen years in males, and early twenties in females. People with this disorder are often employed in situations such as research where precision and detail are required. They rarely seek treatment because to do so would require change. Any diversion from their rigid nature is highly threatening to them. There is usually little insight into the psychological origin of their discomfort.

Treatment of Personality Disorders

Members of the health care community join together in providing an environment in which the client with a personality disorder can affect behavior change. In order to accomplish this, the client must gain perspective into the problem underlying his or her maladaptive response to the world. This is often difficult because most people with these disorders lack insight and resist attempts to impose change. If the person is admitted for an associated mental disorder such as anxiety, depression, substance abuse, or other mood disorders, he or she may comply with treatment for that problem while avoiding the personality symptoms completely. Many individuals with personality issues also have trouble trusting others which leads to difficulty in their social relationships. This factor often prevents them from forming a therapeutic relationship with a therapist. Their ineptness in social interactions also leads to a poor self-image and feeling of personal despair.

Just the Facts

No-harm contracts, journals, and behavior logs can help the client who self-mutilates or engages in cutting to track their thoughts and behavior patterns. This can prove beneficial by encouraging them to explore ways of regaining self-control.

Various types of psychotherapy are used including individual, group, and family approaches. The type used for any given client will depend on the underlying mental problem.

Cognitive-behavioral therapy deals with one's thinking in relation to subsequent actions, while interpersonal therapy focuses on human relationships. In the case of personality disorders, the benefit of individual therapy is limited by the lack of trust and personal comfort boundaries. If accepted however, it can help clients gain insight into their thinking and how his or her thoughts and perceptions are distorted. Ways can be explored for them to modify their behavior to a more functional level. Some behavior therapy involves weekly individual therapy along with group sessions to help the clients understand their actions while working toward improved adaptive behaviors. Other disorders that involve dependency, mistrust, manipulation, and arrogance may involve a longer course of treatment. Since many of these individuals have deeply ingrained beliefs and attitudes, the resistance to change is greater and outcomes are less favorable.

Group therapy and behavior modification help clients improve interaction skills in addition to gaining an understanding of how they are perceived by others. Clients can learn how to ventilate anxiety and trust others in a safe environment. Problem-solving methods can be practiced within the group to resolve community issues.

Occupational therapy allows clients to increase their level of functioning so they can become more independent. Task completion skills can also be evaluated and enhanced by these activities. Recreation therapy can assist clients to ventilate feelings and increase socialization skills. Interaction and guidance by the therapist can provide clients with constructive ways to deal with anger and other self-destructive behaviors.

A combination of psychotherapy and medication is the preferred approach to treatment of personality disorders, although the symptoms of these disorders are less responsive to drugs. Thinking errors can be somewhat improved with antipsychotic medications such as risperidone (Risperdal) and olanzapine (Zyprexa). Anxiety and depression can be treated with antianxiety and antidepressant agents. Reducing environmental stress is often the first step in treatment goals.

Typically, treatment also involves family members and friends of the client. Often, the actions of those most closely associated with the person may affect the behavior issues and are useful in the treatment process. Treating personality disorders is a prolonged process and requires diligent patience and understanding on the part of the therapist and/ or family members and friends.

Senior Focus

Medications are used with caution in the older client because of potential side effects and drug interactions. In addition, other medical problems may be affected by these drugs. Focus should be on identifying recent stressors that may intensify current behavior problems.

Application of the Nursing Process

Assessment

It is not often that a client is admitted with a personality disorder as a primary cause for treatment. Treatment may be sought by the person or family members as the maladaptive traits become problematic and disrupt the person's life. Other disorders such as depression, substance abuse, or suicidal acts may be the trigger that leads to admission. It is important to first develop a trusting relationship by using an empathetic and nonjudgmental approach.

Some assessment techniques that could be used with individuals with personality disorders may include the following:

- Use direct questions to find out what events or behaviors led to the admission.
- Observe nonverbal behaviors and symptoms that indicate appropriate affect.
- Assess thought processes for content and clarity, all or none thinking, magical thinking, or narcissism.
- Look for inconsistencies between what is said and mannerisms or behavior.
- Determine social habits and present or past relationships in which the person is involved.
- Assess the level of anxiety and emotional state during the initial history intake.
- Note any resistance to questioning or indication of impulsive reaction to requested information.
- Ask about usual coping methods used to deal with life stressors.

- Note any scars or cuts that may indicate self-mutilating behaviors.
- Ask if suicidal thoughts have occurred and verify whether a plan has been made.
- Establish what type of situations may have led to the self-destructive behavior.

Because clients with personality disorders tend to be irritating and demanding, it is important for you to recognize and deal with your own feelings toward such clients. Your feelings are often the same feelings being demonstrated in the client and caregivers. The client with a personality disorder can be manipulative and conniving with nurses and other clients. It is important to view the situation objectively. Therapeutic intervention can only occur if self-awareness allows you to project an appropriate attitude of caring and concern for the well-being of the client.

Selected Nursing Diagnoses

A nursing diagnosis is made after a thorough analysis of the data collected through the nursing assessment process. Any data that can provide new or useful information should be considered when developing the diagnosis statement. Nursing diagnoses may be applicable for more than one personality disorder because many share similar symptoms and problems. These may include the following:

- Social Isolation, related to suspicious view of others
- Anxiety, related to unconscious conflicts
- Impaired Verbal Communication, related to social withdrawal
- Ineffective Coping, related to suspiciousness, ambivalence, or projection
- Impaired Social Interaction, related to indifference toward others
- Disturbed Personal Identity, related to social withdrawal
- Risk for Self-Directed Violence, related to self-mutilating behaviors
- Risk for Other-Directed Violence, related to rage and inability to tolerate frustration
- Chronic Low Self-esteem, related to unmet dependency needs
- Powerlessness, related to extreme feelings of dependency
- Disturbed Personal Identity, related to splitting and unmet dependency needs
- Decisional Conflict, related to ineffective problem-solving ability

- Compromised Family Coping, related to maladaptive relationships
- Hopelessness, related to feelings of inadequacy and incompetence

Expected Outcomes

Expected outcomes provide criteria by which the effectiveness of nursing interventions can be measured. Nurses and clients work together to facilitate change within a reasonable time. If the expected changes have not occurred within the given time frame, the plan of care is revised at the time of evaluation. Anticipated outcomes for a client with a personality disorder may include the following:

- Expresses thoughts and feelings appropriately
- Increases interaction with others
- Exhibits decreased hostility and anger
- Exhibits relaxed posture
- Participates in unit activities
- Conforms to unit rules
- Gains control over impulses
- Decreases manipulative behaviors
- Manages anxiety without acting-out behaviors
- Refrains from harming self or others
- Associates anxiety with precipitating factors
- Refrain from using splitting or clinging behaviors
- Claims ownership of own feelings and thoughts
- Verbalizes positive qualities about self
- Makes independent decisions about self-care

Interventions

Providing nursing care for people with personality disorders is very challenging. Identify personal feelings about the client's behaviors and maintain a continuous awareness to provide appropriate interventions. Nursing interventions for the client with a personality disorder may include the following:

- Show acceptance of the person at all times by separating the person from the behaviors.
- Provide a safe environment, especially important for clients who exhibit self-mutilating behavior.
- Set and maintain limits with consequences.
- Explain all unit rules and enforce them fairly and consistently.
- Require the client to take responsibility for his or her own behavior.

- Identify inappropriate behavior and discuss possible alternative behavior with the client.
- Do not make exceptions or show favoritism.
- Encourage the client to openly express feelings and thoughts.
- Identify triggers of acting-out behaviors.
- Maintain alertness to manipulative behaviors of clients.
- Communicate problems with manipulative clients to other team members.
- Provide positive feedback to clients who are making efforts to change behavior.
- Approach clients from the front and speak clearly. This is especially true for the client with paranoia.
- Monitor for cheeking of medication.
- Encourage the client to participate in unit activities.
- Assess for suicidal ideation.
- Develop a no-harm contract with the client with self-destructive tendencies.
- Assist and educate the client in the problem-solving process.
- Demonstrate a matter-of-fact attitude when clients act out or exaggerate events.
- Point out "all or none" behavior to the client when it occurs.
- Encourage the client to keep a private journal of thoughts and feelings.
- Discuss with the client how his or her behavior affects others and assist to explore alternative actions.
- Observe and intervene before escalation of behavior occurs.
- Use time-out for curbing acting-out behavior if client is resistant to redirection.
- Educate client and family on information resources about their disorder (Client Teaching Note 12.1).

Evaluation

The effectiveness of implemented interventions for clients with personality disorders is difficult to measure. Changes do not occur quickly and are often not recognizable during the brief treatment period. Your ability to set boundaries and maintain a therapeutic approach to the behaviors is often one indicator of progress. Short-term outcomes that involve interaction with other clients and impulse control can be evaluated within the confined milieu. The client's behavior following discharge will demonstrate whether

CLIENT TEACHING 12.1

Information Resources for Personality Disorders

Contact your local Mental Health Association, community mental health center, or:

National Mental Health Association
2000 N. Beauregard Street, 6th Floor
Alexandria, VA 22311
Phone: 703-684-7722
Fax: 703-684-5968
Mental Health Resource Center 800-969-NMHA
TTY Line: 800-433-5959

National Mental Health Consumer Self-Help Clearinghouse
Phone: 800-553-4539

Center for Mental Health Services
National Mental Health Information Center
PO Box 42490
Washington, DC 20015
Phone: 800-789-2647

Personality Disorders Awareness Network (PDAN)
www.BPDCentral.com

National Educational Alliance for Borderline Personality Disorder (NEA-BPD)
Phone: 914-835-9011
www.borderlinepersonalitydisorder.com

National Institute of Mental Health (NIMH)
6001 Executive Boulevard
Bethesda, MD 20892
Phone: 301-443-4513
Toll-free: 1-866-615-6464
http://www.nimh.nih.gov/health/publications/

actual improvement has occurred. Regardless of efforts expended by the mental health team, the potential for improvement is limited by the deeply ingrained patterns of pervasive behaviors that have developed over time. Unlike an acute medical problem, the maladaptive personality traits are usually hidden to those who exhibit them. They cannot solve the problem because they are unable to identify the reason for the problem.

Summary

- Personality traits and characteristics that are deeply embedded, inflexible, and maladaptive are the defining picture of the personality disorder. The paradox is that although the feelings that accompany the disorder cause misery, the person usually does not recognize the problem and sees the behavior as normal.
- Failure to identify the problem is what contradicts the benefit of treatment programs and interventions. Most people with personality disorders endure a lifetime of unsuccessful attempts to secure stability in their personal and social situations.
- According to the DSM-5, three cluster groups of personality disorders have been identified. Regardless of the disorder, commonalities exist between the groups. All tend to view the world from an ambivalent perspective, conforming to rigid thinking that objects, people, and events are either all good or all bad. This tunnel vision rejects the possibility of these two extremes coexisting in one situation. With this mindset, the individual often passively and indirectly projects hostility to others in subtle,

deceitful ways to avoid feelings of inadequacy and incompetence.
- Cluster A disorders include paranoid, schizoid, and schizotypal variations. Persons with these disorders tend to demonstrate odd or eccentric behaviors.
- Paranoid personality disorder is defined as a persistent pattern of suspicion and mistrust in which the actions or motives of others are seen as intentionally threatening or humiliating. Although the suspicious is unfounded, the person may become hostile and attack without warning.
- Those with schizoid personality disorder are withdrawn and secluded, demonstrating an emotional indifference toward social relationships.
- In addition to being secluded and withdrawn from social situations, persons with schizotypal personality disorder exhibit strange and unusual patterns of thinking and communicating.
- Dynamic, emotional, or erratic behavior is characteristic of individuals with a cluster B disorder. These include the antisocial, borderline, histrionic, and narcissistic personality disorders.

- Those with antisocial personality disorder exhibit a persistent pattern of disregard and infringement on the rights of others in a society. A false sense of privileged revenge against others is demonstrated by their basic indifference to the laws of society and humanity.
- Persons with borderline personality disorder have a persistent pattern of unstable interpersonal relationships, insecure self-image, and mood swings. An extreme view called *splitting* describes their relationship to the world in which things are seen in terms of black and white, all or none, love or hate with no neutral ground. They are impulsive and intense in their outbursts of anger. A pattern of self-mutilation or self-injury tends to restore the person's sense of realism and value, demonstrating an outward focus of control over inner pain.
- Narcissistic personality disorder indicates a continued need for lavish attention and admiration with little regard for the feelings of others. Other people may be used unfairly to satisfy this person's desires.
- The person with histrionic personality disorder displays a pattern of egocentric and excessive emotion in a demanding manner to gain personal attention.
- People with cluster C disorders exhibit anxious and fearful types of behavior and are categorized as avoidant, dependent, and obsessive-compulsive personality disorders.
- The person with an avoidant personality disorder is typically shy and very sensitive to negative comments from others with feelings of inadequacy and intense discomfort in social situations that involve people other than family. They exhibit an intense fear of criticism or embarrassment adding to feelings of inferiority and low self-esteem.
- People with dependent personality disorder demonstrate a consistent and extreme need to be cared for that leads to a reliance on others. Viewing themselves as helpless, incompetent, and unable to make decisions, they have a profound insecurity and sense of self-doubt with an extreme fear of being alone.
- Those with an obsessive-compulsive personality disorder are conscientious, highly organized, and preoccupied with order and perfection. They are usually dependable, but insist on rigid control and are inflexible without room for compromise.
- Most clients with personality disorders receive treatment in connection with care received for another disorder. In many cases, the person may have engaged in self-destructive behaviors that bring them to the attention of the health care system.
- The ability of nurses to participate in the treatment plan is diverted by the manipulative, annoying, and disruptive nature of the behaviors which lead to frustration and irritation. Although the maladaptive behaviors are obvious to nurses and others, the individuals with these disorders are oblivious to the impact their actions have on those around them.
- It is important that boundaries and limits be set and strictly enforced for behavior. Nurses must have an awareness of their own feelings and be alert for the manipulative efforts of the client.
- A therapeutic climate mandates the nurse be accepting and nonjudgmental as attempts are made to evoke change in the client who is so resistant to the treatment strategies.
- Efforts to invoke therapeutic intervention are limited by the deeply ingrained patterns of pervasive behaviors that have developed over time. Improvement can only occur if self-awareness allows the client to identify the reason for the problem.

Bibliography

American Psychiatric Association. (2013). *Diagnostic and statistical manual of mental disorders text revision* (5th ed.). Washington, DC: American Psychiatric Association.

Goethals, K., Willigenburg, L., Buitelaar, J., & Van Marie, H. (2008). Behavior problems in childhood and adolescence in psychotic offenders: An explanatory study. *Criminal Behaviour and Mental Health, 18*(3), 153–165. Retrieved March 04, 2014.

Gunderson, J. G. (2013). Personality disorders. *The Merck Manual Online Medical Library* (Reviewed/revised May 2012). Retrieved March 04, 2014, from www.merck.com/mmpe/sec15/ch201a.

Herdman, T. H. (2012). *NANDA International nursing diagnoses: Definitions & classification 2012–2014.* Oxford, UK: Wiley-Blackwell Publishers.

Jacobson, C. M., Muehlenkamp, J. J., Miller, A. L., & Turner, J. B. (2008). Psychiatric impairment among adolescents engaging in different types of deliberate self-harm. *Journal of Clinical Child and Adolescent Psychology, 37*(2), 363–375. Retrieved March 04, 2014.

Jansson, I., Hesse, M., & Fridell, M. (2008). Personality disorder features as predictors of symptoms five years post-treatment. *American Journal on Addictions, 17*(3), 172–175. Retrieved March 04, 2014.

King, G. (2014). Staff attitudes towards people with borderline personality disorder. *Mental Health Practice, 17*(5), 30–34. Retrieved March 04, 2014.

Linehan, M. M., McDavid, J. D., Brown, M. Z., Sayrs, J. H., & Gallop, R. J. (2008). Olanzapine plus dialectical behavior therapy for women with high irritability who meet criteria for borderline personality disorder. *Journal of Clinical Psychiatry, 69*(6), 999–1005. Retrieved March 04, 2014.

National Institute of Mental Health. Borderline personality disorder. Retrieved March 04, 2014, from www.nimh.nih.gov

National Mental Health Association. Personality disorders. Statistics. Retrieved March 04, 2014, from http://www.nimh.nih.gov/statistics/1ANYPERS.shtml

O'Connell, B., & Dowling, M. (2013). Community psychiatric nurses' experiences of caring for clients with borderline personality disorder. *Mental Health Practice, 17*(4), 27–33. Retrieved March 01, 2014.

Perry, J. C., Presniak, M. D., & Olson, T. R. (2013). Defense mechanisms in schizotypal, borderline, antisocial, and narcissistic personality disorders. *Psychiatry: Interpersonal and Biological Processes, 76*(1), 32–52. Retrieved March 04, 2014.

Schmeck, K., Sehluter-Muller, S., Foelsch, P. A., & Doering, S. (2013). The role of identity in the DSM-5 classification of personality disorders. *Child and Adolescent Psychiatry and Mental Health, 7*(1), 1–11. Retrieved March 04, 2014.

Sternberg, R. J. (2000). *In search of the human mind* (3rd ed.). Philadelphia, PA: Harcourt Brace.

Student Worksheet

Fill in the Blank

Fill in the blank with the correct answer.

1. The symptoms in personality disorders tend to be _____ and _____.
2. People with personality disorders tend to have a(n) _____ mindset in which underlying hostility is indirectly exhibited in subtle behaviors.
3. A type of self-destruction is involvement in _____ relationships with people who are emotionally unstable and abusive.
4. Those who exhibit a sense of _____ feel that others owe them because of their superior and powerful status.
5. _____ is an intentional act of inflicting bodily injury to oneself that demonstrates an outward focus of control over inner pain.
6. A persistent pattern of disregard and infringement on the rights of others in a society is characteristic of the _____ personality.

Matching

Match the following terms to the most appropriate phrase.

1. _____ Personality traits
2. _____ Splitting
3. _____ Narcissism
4. _____ Dependency
5. _____ Projection
6. _____ Acting-out behavior
7. _____ "Jekyll and Hyde" characteristic
8. _____ Sociopath
9. _____ Avoidance

a. Defense mechanism in which faults are attributed to others
b. Person who disregards the rights of others without remorse
c. Withdrawal related to extreme self-doubt and fear of disapproval
d. Aggressive response to underlying negative feelings
e. Extreme view of all good or all bad
f. Persistent ways of viewing and relating to the world
g. Perceived state of helplessness leading to extreme reliance on others
h. Extreme mood shift from clingy dependent behavior to angry outbursts
i. Grandiose sense of self-importance

Multiple Choice

Select the best answer from the multiple-choice items.

1. The nurse is caring for a client admitted with self-inflicted burns to her abdomen. While the nurse is doing an assessment of the wounds, the client says, "I deserve to be in pain." Which of the following best describes the underlying feelings in this statement?
   a. Arrogance
   b. Worthlessness
   c. Suspicion
   d. Egocentricity

2. The nurse notes that a client is monopolizing most of the conversation during breakfast. He is loud and criticizing other clients. Which of the following is the most appropriate intervention for the nurse to make at this time?
   a. Reprimand him for his inappropriate behavior
   b. Provide him with medication to calm him down
   c. Put him in seclusion until he can control his actions
   d. Redirect and reinforce limits on his behavior

3. Which of the following statements is true regarding clients with personality disorders?
   a. They are aware that they have a behavior problem
   b. Manipulative patterns often render treatment ineffective
   c. Most have a sincere motivation to change behaviors
   d. Most recognize how their behavior affects others

4. Which of the following types of behavior could be interpreted as a form of self-destruction?
   a. Avoiding close relationships and intimacy
   b. Involvement in no-win relationships
   c. Eccentric dress habits and mannerisms
   d. Exaggerated sense of importance

5. A young man who loudly demands to see the manager of a restaurant when he and his date are not seated immediately upon their arrival is displaying the narcissistic behavior referred to as:
   a. Projection
   b. Splitting
   c. Entitlement
   d. Ambivalence

6. Which of the following indicators is most demonstrative that improvement has occurred related to treatment strategies?
   a. Is able to define what is meant by a personality disorder
   b. Ability to recognize personality traits in others
   c. Relates the requirements for compliance with treatment plan
   d. Demonstrates behavior changes following discharge

7. The individual with an antisocial personality demonstrates a false sense of privileged revenge against others. Which of the following best describes the result of this thinking?
   a. An outward focus of control over inner pain
   b. Repeated unsuccessful attempts to secure stability in relationships
   c. Persistent disregard and indifference to laws of society and humanity
   d. Unrealistic expectations and standards of perfection

8. Creating an overly dramatic scene of emotional behavior to attract the attention of others is typical in which of the following personalities?
   a. Schizotypal
   b. Histrionic
   c. Dependent
   d. Obsessive-compulsive

9. Which of the following correctly describes the person with a narcissistic personality disorder?
   a. Has a profound insecurity, sense of self-doubt, and a fear of being alone
   b. Rigid and controlling with unrealistic expectations and standards
   c. Exhibit strange and unusual patterns of thinking and communicating
   d. May use other people unfairly to satisfy a selfish need for lavish attention

10. Which of the following terms would be characteristics common to all personality disorders?
   a. Inflexible and maladaptive behaviors
   b. Odd or eccentric behaviors
   c. Cold, aloof, and suspicious tendencies
   d. Display ideas of reference in everyday occurrences

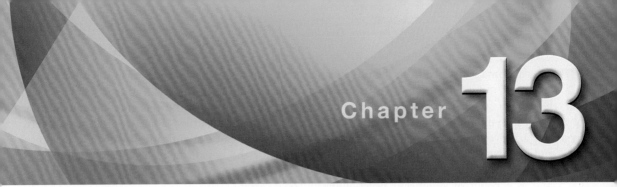

Chapter 13

Somatic Symptom and Related Disorders

⊙ Learning Objectives

After learning the content in this chapter, the student will be able to:

1. Define the psychophysiological syndrome of a somatic disorder.
2. Identify the signs and symptoms of the somatic disorders.
3. Identify etiological factors in the development of a psychophysiological disorder.
4. Discuss treatment options for the client experiencing somatic symptoms.
5. Perform a skilled data collection in assessing the client with a somatic disorder.
6. Identify nursing diagnoses and outcomes to address problems common to clients with somatic disorders.
7. Identify appropriate nursing interventions for psychophysiological behaviors.
8. Describe evaluation methods for determining the effectiveness of planned interventions.

⊙ Key Terms

conversion disorder
factitious disorder
hysteria
illness anxiety disorder
la belle indifference
Munchausen syndrome
primary gain

pseudoneurological
psychophysiological
psychogenic
secondary gain
soma
somatization
somatic symptom disorder

The term **soma** is derived from the Greek language and refers to the body. Historically, the connection between stress, anxiety, and physiological symptoms has been delegated to **hysteria**, a nervous disorder marked by ineffective emotional control. The predictable syndrome of physical complaints and symptoms that are expressed as a result of significant psychological stress are defined as **somatization**. These physical symptoms suggest that a medical condition exists, but often the diagnostic findings do not support a medical diagnosis for the symptoms. Because the persistent symptoms are accompanied by psychological distress, they may be described as **psychophysiological** or somatic.

Somatization is considered a defense mechanism. Unlike an individual who intentionally creates symptoms to remain in the role of client, the person with somatization is not consciously aware of the psychological factors underlying the disorder and does not intentionally continue the complaints. The person is not in control of the symptoms, which are an involuntary expression of psychological conflicts. The somatic symptoms provide a psychological or **primary gain** as the anxiety is relieved and focus is diverted to the physical problem. **Secondary gain** comes from the subsequent attention the person receives from a physician or family member. Other mechanisms that are used by people with this disorder include repression of trauma or conflict, denial that psychological factors exist, and displacement of anxiety and conflict to body symptoms.

> ### Just the Facts
> Somatic disorders are characterized by disturbances in sensory or motor functioning, while dissociative disorders (see Chapter 14) affect the sense of identity or memory.

Types of Somatic Disorders

The DSM-5 has realigned the somatic disorders with prominent somatic symptoms (previously somatoform disorders) into a new category of Somatic Symptom and Related Disorders that includes somatic symptom disorder (includes previous pain disorder), illness anxiety disorder (previously hypochondriasis), conversion disorder, factitious disorder, and unspecified somatic symptom–related disorder. These disorders share the common feature of physical symptoms that

seem to suggest that a medical problem or condition is their cause, but typically, the clinical findings do not support the existence of a medical or other mental disorder. The symptoms are severe enough to cause significant distress and dysfunction for the person in his or her daily life. The autonomic nervous system response to stress may be associated with an increased awareness of physiological symptoms such as acceleration of the heart rate, muscle tension, and increased gastrointestinal motility. These symptoms may initially seem to indicate a medical problem for which the person seeks treatment. Individuals with these disorders are more commonly seen in primary care and medical settings rather than in mental health settings. The new classification in the DSM-5 defines somatic symptom disorders on the basis of these medically unexplained somatic symptoms, but places more emphasis on the disproportionate abnormal ideas, feelings, and behaviors experienced by the individual in response to the symptoms.

Clients with a somatic disorder often have long histories of medical and unnecessary surgical treatments by several different doctors. This fact, in addition to the automatic nature of the symptoms over which the person has no control, tends to complicate the process of distinguishing the symptoms from actual medical problems. The client tends to perceive the presence of an illness or injury despite reassurance to the contrary by the physician. The impact of the perceived problem stretches to the number of sick leave days taken from employment situations, and imposed early retirement for the disabling nature of the symptoms.

> ### Just the Facts
> Somatic disorders are a significant issue for the health care system due to the fact clients with these symptoms tend to overuse physician services and resources.

Somatic Symptom Disorder

Somatic symptom disorder is typically characterized by one or more somatic symptoms that are disturbing to the individual and cause disruption in his or her daily functioning. Individuals with this disorder typically have multiple somatic symptoms although one—most commonly pain—may be more severe than others. Symptoms may be described specifically (e.g., localized pain as abdominal or back pain), or nonspecifically, such as "hurting all over" or fatigue. Typically, these symptoms are not explained or supported by medical testing but continue to cause significant distress for the client. With the new diagnostic standard, more emphasis is placed on the disproportionate distress and behaviors related to the symptoms than the lack of a diagnosed medical condition.

The client often goes from one physician to another seeking a medical diagnosis for their symptoms. Any reassurance from the physician that the symptoms are not serious is disregarded by the client. Feeling their medical attention has been inadequate, the client will seek out another physician. This in turn leads to a series of repeated diagnostic tests and x-ray studies in an attempt to support a medical problem. The potential hazard of concurrent medical treatments (e.g., drug interactions or potentiation), when seeing several different physicians is also a definite consideration.

Signs and Symptoms

A somatic complaint is considered to be valid if it requires medical treatment such as medication. In this disorder, there are one or more somatic complaints that cannot be completely explained by medical findings. The individual's description of the somatic symptoms and recurrent thoughts and feelings related to the somatic symptoms are often exaggerated with little supportive factual information. Symptoms of persistent moderate to severe levels of anxiety and depression are commonly seen in addition to the somatic complaints. The intensity and persistence of the symptoms, and the time and energy the person devotes to the perceived health problem indicate the person's desperate need to be cared for in all aspects of living. While the previous emphasis in DSM-IV was on the lack of a medical explanation for the symptoms, the current DSM-5 places the emphasis for this disorder on the degree to which excessive thoughts, feelings, and behaviors about their illness are disproportionate to the illness itself. The individual may or may not have an underlying medical condition, but if the client's concern and behavior indicate excessive mental distress over the symptoms, a diagnosis of somatic symptom disorder may be made.

The somatic subjective symptoms cannot be controlled by the person and are perceived as real by the person experiencing them. The common thread of the complaints is the accompanying

---

BOX 13.1

Signs and Symptoms of Somatic Symptom Disorder

- Somatic symptoms that suggest physical illness or injury, but are unexplained by medical findings
- Recurring somatic complaints usually continue for several years (may include pain)
- Excessive worry or anxiety over physical health symptoms that is disruptive to the person's life
- Exaggerated belief in the severity of their symptoms and health
- Excessive time is devoted to investigating his or her health symptoms
- Anxiety and depression

---

behaviors and feelings of primary gain obtained as the anxiety is relieved and the secondary gain, or attention the person receives in response to the symptoms. These factors are usually not apparent to the client demonstrating the behavioral pattern. The person becomes extremely dependent both in doctor–patient and personal relationships with an increasing demand for attention and emotional support, often getting enraged when they feel their needs are not being met. In an attempt to manipulate others, the demand for attention may in some instances result in threats or attempts to commit suicide. Signs and symptoms for somatic symptom disorder are found in Box 13.1.

Incidence and Etiology

The percentage of the US population affected by DSM-IV criteria for somatoform disorder is around 5% to 7%, and it is seen much more prominently in women than men. The coexistence of excessive anxiety, PTSD, or depression is common and may increase the symptoms and imposed disability. Somatic symptom disorder tends to run in families, with a likely occurrence of other mental disturbances (e.g., anxiety, depression, or substance use) as well. Familial patterns of behavior are often replicated by children and adolescents, especially when those behaviors receive the attention of others. This imitation as well as differences in the perception of pain may be factors in the generational tendency.

With the major changes to the diagnostic criterion for somatic symptom disorder in the DSM-5, the actual statistics of occurrence are yet to be determined. A 2012 study by Voight, Wollburg, Weinmann, Herzog, Meyer, Langs, and Lowe in the Journal of Psychosomatic Research, concluded that the current diagnostic criterion in DSM-5 might increase the disorder's prevalence.

Mind Jogger

How might the secondary gain received by the parent with somatic symptom disorder encourage a child to copy the behavior?

Illness Anxiety Disorder (Formerly Hypochondriasis)

Individuals with **illness anxiety disorder** may or may not have a medical condition, but do have increased body sensations and are extremely anxious about the possibility of an existing serious undiagnosed illness. The individual devotes a great deal of time and energy to researching the health concerns. Persons with illness anxiety disorder experience considerable distress over their presumed and undiagnosed health issues, and are not readily reassured if no medical problem is found.

Signs and Symptoms

The person with illness anxiety disorder is preoccupied with the possibility of having or acquiring a serious illness despite reassurance to the contrary. Somatic symptoms are usually absent or of mild intensity. A thorough medical examination usually fails to support the medical condition for which the person has sought medical attention, or if a diagnosable condition exists, the person's concern and anxiety are disproportionate to the disorder itself. The person's distress related to fears and worry about the suspected medical diagnosis is evident. If a physical symptom is present, it usually is a normal physiological sensation (e.g., positional dizziness or food-related indigestion).

Individuals with this disorder tend to become alarmed and overconcerned when reading or hearing about someone having a health-related problem (e.g., case of West Nile virus or HIV). Attempts by medical personnel to reassure the individual or suggested home remedies for insignificant complaints do not alleviate the person's anxiety and concern. The overconcern and worry about health issues consumes the individual's everyday life and becomes a central theme for their identity and conversation with others. They fervently research their suspected illness (e.g., on the Internet) and seek continued support and reassurance from family and friends. Family gatherings and community

---

BOX 13.2

Signs and Symptoms of Illness Anxiety Disorder

- Unwarranted fear or preoccupation with body functioning misperceived as a major illness
- Repeated health care visits seeking verification of fears
- Excessive anxiety about having a serious medical condition or acquiring a serious disease or illness
- Disproportionate level of anxiety and worry if symptoms are minor
- Symptoms reported in specific detail, but do not follow those typical of pathological condition
- Perceived illness focal point of existence
- Client is unconvinced by repeated examinations and reassurance that disease does not exist
- Physician shopping
- Perception of incompetent medical care
- Impaired social and family relationships

---

activities may be avoided as the fear of becoming ill intensifies. The individuals often consult multiple physicians for the same problem and feel they are not taken seriously if negative test results indicate a lack of support for their suspected condition. Signs and symptoms for illness anxiety disorder are found in Box 13.2.

Incidence and Etiology

The actual etiology of illness anxiety disorder is not known. It is suggested that, like other somatic disorders, it is related to an overindulgence in self-concern with a need to satisfy strong dependency needs. The prevalence of this disorder tends to be similar in males and females, with the peak incidence in the late 30s for men, and late 40s for women. The disorder tends to be chronic in nature, with a pattern that reflects a heightened awareness of body functions with an obsessive preoccupation that a problem exists. Because of the underlying psychological need for dependency, only a few people are able to associate the somatic symptoms with their mental state. Depression is common as they continue to believe their fears and refuse to accept reassurance to the contrary.

Conversion Disorder (Functional Neurological Symptom Disorder)

The person with a **conversion disorder** exhibits symptoms that indicate a sensory or neurological impairment that is not supported by results of diagnostic testing. Usually there are related stress

"Jerry's Displaced Fear"

Jerry is a 47-year-old heavy equipment operator. His wife, Angela, has been a homemaker and mother to their three children for the past 12 years. Now that the children are all in school, Angela has decided to fulfill a lifelong dream and enroll in college classes to become a nurse. She has asked Jerry to help her with the children so she can have more time to study. She reminds him that once she is a nurse, she can supplement the family income. Three months after Angela begins her classes, Jerry develops severe back pain that requires him to take a leave of absence from work. He undergoes extensive imaging studies, but no medical reason is found for the pain. He states that the analgesics and muscle relaxants just don't seem to help. He tells you that he wants a referral to a large medical clinic 400 miles from his present location because the local doctors don't seem to want to help him. He states that he cannot help with the children or household chores because of the pain. Two months later, Jerry quits his job and Angela must become the family support. She drops her classes and finds a job as a receptionist for a local insurance agency.

What underlying psychological conflict may be causing Jerry's symptoms?

_____

_____

What are his primary and secondary gains?

_____

_____

Case Application 13.1

or trauma factors that have occurred concurrent with the onset of the symptoms. Because the symptoms essentially involve voluntary motor or sensory functioning, they are considered **pseudo-neurological**, or false neurological, disturbances. The actual conversion aspect of this disorder refers to the transfer of psychological conflict or stressors into a perceived paralysis of body parts or sensory functioning. For example, a person loses functional use of her dominant arm and hand before a piano recital she does not want to perform.

Just the Facts

Family stress and physical or sexual abuse are thought to be the most common causes of conversion disorders in children and adolescents.

Signs and Symptoms

The conversion symptoms contain the factor of anxiety, which serves to divert attention away from the underlying stress situation. The transfer of this anxiety to a loss of physical functioning serves as a primary gain for the client. The changes in social, work-related, or family circumstances that result from the temporary disability may provide the secondary gain of avoiding unpleasant tasks or responsibilities along with the accompanying attention the person receives. People with conversion disorder may exhibit an attitude of **la belle indifference**; that is, they demonstrate little anxiety or concern over the implications of the symptoms.

Motor symptoms may include impaired coordination or balance, paralysis of a limb, the inability to speak, difficulty swallowing, or urinary retention. Sensory deficits may relate to a loss of pain sensation, visual or hearing malfunction, and hallucinations. Occasionally episodes of abnormal generalized shaking with apparent loss of consciousness that resemble a seizure may occur, or episodes of unconsciousness that are similar to syncope. The symptoms tend to differ from actual neurological deficits in that the person's description of the problem does not exhibit a dysfunction of the typical nerve pathway. Typically, the symptoms do not lead to any physical changes or disabilities, as are seen in neurological disorders. There may be an inability to perform a particular movement, but other functions of the body part

BOX 13.3

Signs and Symptoms of Conversion Disorder

- Sensory or neurological impairment that is not supported by diagnostic testing
- Lack of conscious control over the symptoms
- Loss of balance or paralysis of limb
- Loss of swallowing, speaking, seeing, or hearing
- Loss of pain or touch sensation
- Impaired functioning in social or work-related areas caused by symptoms
- A la belle indifference
- Seizures or convulsion-type behavior inconsistent with usual symptom pattern
- Lack of physical change or disability
- Functional ability and symptoms inconsistent with usual neurological disorders

may be intact. Sometimes the extremity described as dysfunctional will inadvertently be moved when attention is temporarily directed away. Although a limb is described as nonfunctional, the neurological reflexes are intact. Unlike a pathological seizure, a conversion or **psychogenic** (nonepileptic) seizure will vary from one incident to the other without a distinct pattern of activity and may resemble a seizure that has been described to the individual. Signs and symptoms for conversion disorder are found in Box 13.3.

Mind Jogger

What symptoms usually seen in a pathological or epileptic seizure might be missing in a conversion or psychogenic seizure?

Incidence and Etiology

Conversion disorder may begin at any age but tends to develop during adolescence or early adulthood, and is more common in women. This disorder does not seem to run in families. Cross-cultural studies show a variation in prevalence of this disorder. The prevalence of prior exposure to traumatizing life events tends to be higher in persons with conversion symptoms (Brown and Lewis, 2011).

Adolescents with this disorder often have overprotective parents with a subdued need to see their child as "ill." The symptoms then become the focus of the family's attention and lifestyle. Conversion disorder tends to be of short-term duration, with most clients recovering in 2 to 4 weeks without reoccurrence. Those with symptoms of

paralysis or loss of speech or vision tend to have a better outcome than those experiencing tremors or seizures.

Factitious Disorder

In the DSM-5, **factitious disorder** is divided into two types, the disorder is imposed on oneself, or the disorder is imposed on another (previously termed factitious disorder by proxy). The primary characteristic of both types of *factitious disorder* is the falsification of medical or psychological signs and symptoms without obvious external benefits. It is estimated that the unnecessary medical tests and wasted medical resources caused by this disorder costs the United States millions of dollars each year. The term **factitious** stems from a Latin word that means artificial or false. The individuals are often referred to as "frequent" or "problem patients" by health care clinics and hospitals.

Signs and Symptoms

Individuals with factitious disorder deliberately falsify signs and symptoms of illness for the primary purpose of assuming the sick role. They may describe a false history of illness or surgeries, and may present falsified lab reports or other assessment findings. The description of symptoms is vague and stereotyped. Absence of typical symptoms that would usually be seen in persons presenting with the same complaint is common (e.g., absence of bacteria in urine with complaints typical of bladder infection). The symptoms may be intentionally induced in oneself or another (e.g., intentional infliction of an infectious agent or excessive medication ingestion) that guarantees a hospital admission or explorative surgery. The inconsistencies between history and objective findings raise doubts about the legitimacy of the subjective symptoms and atypical presentation. Knowledge of a textbook description of the illness or unusual use of medical terminology also raises the possibility of a factitioius disorder. The individual usually has a long history of frequent medical clinic and emergency room visits, along with numerous hospital admissions.

It must be noted that **Munchausen syndrome** or faking illness for attention, is not specified as a factitious disorder. However, many clinicians associate this syndrome with the factitious disorders related to the abuse or manipulation of another person, often a child, in order to seek attention or secondary gain for the perpetrator

Signs and Symptoms of Factitious Disorder

- Deliberate falsification of physical or mental symptoms primarily to assume the sick role
- Inconsistencies between history and findings on objective examination
- Falsification of objective symptoms or self-inflicted conditions
- Extensive knowledge of medical terminology and medical testing procedures
- Evidence of self-induced physical signs
- Evidence of multiple surgical scars

from the health care the child receives. Their knowledge of the fake illness is quite deliberate and their ability to mimic the disorder is planned. The deception results in a deep-seated emotional manipulation of the health care system leading to treatment and hospital stays based on a pathological need for attention. Although well aware of their actions, the person may be unaware of the underlying motivation for the behavior. Referrals to mental health professionals are resented and rejected. Because the repeated false symptoms tend to build strained doctor–patient relationships, the presence of a real medical condition may be overlooked. Social and family relationships also become disturbed as the focus is constantly drawn to the person's physical well-being. Signs and symptoms for factitious disorder are found in Box 13.4.

Incidence and Etiology

Studies show the incidence of factitious disorder among hospital patients is probably from 0.2% to 1%. The most prevalence of the disorder is seen in individuals who present to medical clinics and hospitals with persistent skin rashes or wounds that do not heal, unexplained blood disorders such as anemia, hematuria, or neurological problems such as numbness of a body part or reported seizures that have only been witnessed by the person reporting them. The disorders are most common among women ages 20 to 40 years who are working in the medical field with a knowledge of how diseases might be acquired or have access to the means with which to accomplish the intended falsification of symptoms. Onset is usually in early adulthood and often occurs after a hospitalization for the individual, the individual's child, or other dependent. The disorder tends to be chronic and lifelong.

Application of the Nursing Process

Because the somatic disorders are associated with physical symptoms, the person is often first seen by a medical physician for the subjective complaints. The reorganization of the DSM-5 has allowed a better view of the interlacing of the mind and body in which the client may or may not have a diagnosed medical condition in addition to a somatic-related disorder.

Before a somatic determination is made, physical examination and diagnostic testing are necessary to determine any underlying pathology or medical condition for which the individual may need to be treated. It is of major importance that nursing observations and data collection contain information that will be of help in this process. Considering the client with somatic symptom disorder or illness anxiety disorder is unaware of possible underlying psychological issues and is unable to consciously control the symptoms, health care professionals are challenged by clients with these disorders. In factitious disorder, the false illness behavior is conscious and intentional, but is considered to have an unconscious psychogenic origin.

Mind Jogger

Clients who repeatedly access the health care system searching for answers often undergo many diagnostic tests and exploratory surgeries. What risks could this pose for the client?

Nursing Assessment

It is first important for the nurse to create an accepting, safe, and supportive atmosphere that allows open communication with the client and his or her family. This nurturing environment encourages the client to express feelings and needs more honestly. The nurse should focus on the whole person, including psychological, social, and family factors in addition to the physical symptoms.

A careful assessment of physical complaints and the accompanying behavior should be made, taking into consideration any statements made by the client, thoughts and feelings about the symptoms, and the manner in which they are expressed. Note any preoccupation with the symptoms and any inconsistency between what is being described and what is observed in the client. Elicit any pattern of repeated complaints by taking a history of current and past health status. Because most clients with somatic complaints are frequent users of both outpatient and inpatient health care services, it is important to include a history of previous symptoms, hospital admissions, surgeries, and current medications along with a medication history. It is important to note the client's attitude toward the symptoms and how he or she may view any limitations caused by them. It should also be noted whether the client is aware of events surrounding the onset of symptoms. In addition, the client's level of stress or anxiety and previous coping skills should be assessed. Evaluate the type and amount of medications the client is taking. Questions should be asked to determine whether the symptoms have imposed any limitations related to the person's lifestyle and whether the client's role has changed within the family system. Any behavior that indicates an increased dependency need, such as repeatedly turning on a call light for assistance, should also be noted and documented.

Just the Facts

Secondary gains may be assessed by asking questions concerning any previous work or activity the client is now unable to perform as a result of the symptoms. The nurse can also ask in what way the client's life has been altered by the symptoms.

Just the Facts

Clients with somatic disorders who are overconcerned about their symptoms may become dependent on analgesic or antianxiety medication. A pattern of repeat physician office and emergency room visits for medication, or seeking prescriptions from a number of physicians and having them filled at alternating pharmacies assures the availability of a constant supply.

Selected Nursing Diagnosis

Planning care for the client with a somatic disorder must consider that the client is often frustrated and angered by the implication that the symptoms are psychological. Nursing diagnoses to address the problems related to these disorders may include the following:

- Anxiety, severe, related to repressed trauma or unmet dependency needs
- Ineffective Denial, related to avoidance of possible psychological causes for symptoms

- Chronic Pain, related to severe anxiety or unmet dependency needs
- Ineffective Coping, related to anxiety, repression, or unrealistic perceptions
- Disturbed Body Image, related to severe anxiety or low self-esteem
- Self-Care Deficit, related to perceived loss of function or paralysis of body part
- Sensory Perception Disturbed, related to psychological stress or chronic pain
- Disturbed Sleep Pattern, related to anxiety, depression, or chronic pain
- Social Isolation, related to preoccupation with self and chronic state of perceived illness
- Deficient Knowledge, related to psychophysiological nature of illness
- Sexual Dysfunction, related to perceived loss of body function or fear of contracting major disease
- Situational Low Self-Esteem, related to repressed unmet dependency needs and unsatisfactory interpersonal relationships

Expected Outcomes

Once problems have been identified for the individual client situation, planning will include realistic outcomes in the course of treatment. Expected outcomes for an individual with a somatic disorder may include the following:

- Expresses feelings of anxiety and effective means of dealing with the illness
- Acknowledges understanding and perception of present health problem
- Discusses present health problem with health care provider and family
- Acknowledges that physical pain may be associated with psychological stress
- Participates in development of a plan for effective pain control
- Demonstrates reduced use of manipulative behavior to secure attention
- Expresses positive feelings about self
- Verbalizes realistic perception of minor body defect and related positive feelings
- Performs self-care needs independently and willingly
- Verbalizes understanding of psychological factors associated with alteration in physical functioning
- Reports a decrease in sleep-related problems
- Participates in social activities and interaction without discomfort

"Nathan's Search for a Cure"

Nathan is a 36-year-old who has been to four different physicians attempting to find an answer to his repeated bouts of chest pain that radiates to his arms and back. Despite an extensive diagnostic work-up by a cardiologist that reveals no cardiovascular abnormalities or problems, Nathan is convinced that he has angina. He believes it is only a matter of time before he has a major heart attack. Last week, his employer told him his sick time had run out. Rather than face having to work everyday, Nathan quits his job. He tells his wife that he is afraid to overwork his heart by going to work every day. He refuses to go with her to family gatherings or outings with their friends, stating he will get too tired and start having chest pain.

Today, Nathan comes into the emergency room stating, "I know I am having a heart attack. The pain is in my chest, then goes down my arms and back. What do I have to do to get someone to listen to me?"

_____

_____

What assessment data should the nurse gather related to the symptoms Nathan is experiencing?

_____

_____

Nathan tells the nurse there have recently been a lot of layoffs where he worked and that his department was in the process of reorganization before he quit because of his illness. What underlying feelings may be contributing to Nathan's anxiety and somatic symptoms?

_____

_____

What secondary gain does Nathan receive from the physical symptoms?

_____

_____

Case Application 13.2

- Reduces statements that demand a focus on self and physical symptoms
- Identifies realistic illness-related goals and self-perceptions

Interventions

Establishing a trusting relationship with clients experiencing a somatic disorder is the first step in helping them overcome a low self-concept. A safe and supportive environment will also help lower their anxiety to a level that allows expression of underlying feelings. It is important to identify and come to terms with any anger or negative feelings that you may have related to clients with this disorder. Remember that they are not consciously trying to be sick or avoid responsibilities. Other interventions may include the following:

- Recognize that the physical complaints are real to the client even though supportive medical evidence is lacking.
- Avoid any confrontation concerning the psychological defense nature of the symptoms.
- Respond to client with understanding and patience.
- Encourage discussion of person's life history, recent emotional events, and fears.
- Document observations and behaviors related to physical complaints.
- Continue to monitor physical complaints to assist in determining any actual cause for the symptoms.
- Identify unfulfilled dependency needs of the client.
- Identify types of primary and secondary gain achieved by symptoms.
- Minimize time and attention given to physical symptoms.
- Help the client to use words rather than physical means to express feelings.
- Encourage client to keep a diary of daily happenings and feelings, along with physical symptoms.

- Listen actively to determine what the client may be omitting when describing the symptoms or for discrepancies between occurrences.
- Observe for incongruence between the described symptoms and client's behavior.
- Encourage the client to make decisions and take responsibility for situations related to them.
- Help the client to identify more effective coping mechanisms rather than the somatic symptoms.

Evaluation

Evaluation of implemented nursing actions focuses on the client's ability to recognize the underlying psychological stress and anxiety that are contributing to the physical symptoms. Determine whether the client has developed an awareness of increased anxiety and initiated more effective coping mechanisms to deal with the stress level. Once the client can look realistically at the connection between repressed emotional turmoil and the somatic symptoms, a decrease in complaints or full recovery from the previous level of altered physical functioning or pain is anticipated. As the need to use somatic symptoms to fill unmet dependency needs is reduced, the client should return to a functional state in self-care activities, social interaction, and family responsibilities. Because these disorders tend to reoccur, it is important to recognize that the symptoms can reappear if psychological defenses and coping strategies fail.

Summary

- Somatic disorders are characterized by the transfer of anxiety and psychological conflict into somatic or physical symptoms with varying degrees of abnormal thoughts, feelings, and behaviors. Typically seen in medical nonpsychiatric settings, clients with these disorders may or may not have a diagnosed medical condition.
- The person with a somatic disorder is not consciously aware of the psychological implications of his or her disorder. The symptoms are involuntary and cannot be controlled by the person experiencing them. Once it has been determined that no disease state exists, the person is not content with the outcome. Despite reassurance that a disease does not exist, the person remains unconvinced and continues to seek health care and may dwell on the symptoms to the point of dysfunctional living.
- Two common psychological factors in somatic disorders are the history of emotional conflict or trauma about the time the symptoms originated and the unmet dependency needs that are objectively evident in the person's behavior.
- Somatic symptoms provide a psychological or *primary gain* as the anxiety is relieved and focus is diverted to the physical problem. *Secondary gain* comes from the subsequent attention the person receives from a physician or family members.
- Somatic symptom disorder typically is characterized by one or more somatic symptoms that are disturbing to the individual and cause disruption in his or her daily functioning. Unexplained by medical testing, the symptoms continue to cause significant distress for the person. The disproportionate distress caused by the abnormal thoughts, feelings, or behaviors related to the symptoms is the primary factor in diagnosis of this condition.
- Illness anxiety disorder is characterized by an excessive fear or preoccupation with having a serious illness that is based on a misinterpretation of somatic signs and symptoms. Excessive time and energy is used by the individual in researching the suspected health concern. Despite medical testing and reassurance that a disease does not exist, the person continues to experience fear and distress over the symptoms. Access to health care for verification of their fears results in a pattern of "physician-shopping" to find a practitioner who will substantiate their illness.
- Conversion disorder consists of a sensory or neurological impairment that is not supported by diagnostic testing. There is a lack of conscious control over the symptoms. People with this disorder may exhibit an attitude of *la belle indifférence*, demonstrating little anxiety or concern over the implications of their symptoms.
- In factitious disorder, the key feature is the deliberate falsification of medical or psychological signs and symptoms, or the induction of an injury or disease to oneself or another without obvious external benefits. The deceitful behavior is done with the primary purpose of assuming the sick role. The individuals with this disorder squander much time and resources through unnecessary medical visits, laboratory testing, and hospital stays.

- The goal of treatment is to develop a trusting relationship with the client and family that will foster an understanding of the psychophysiological symptoms. Interventions are planned to help the person acknowledge the anxiety issues and their connection to the somatic complaints. Once this occurs, the resolution of the symptoms will hopefully follow as more effective coping strategies are employed.
- Somatic disorders tend to reoccur. If the underlying emotional conflict is confronted and resolved, the need for the somatic retreat will be unnecessary.

Bibliography

American Psychiatric Association. (2013a). *Diagnostic and statistical manual of mental disorders* (5th ed.). Washington, DC: American Psychiatric Association.

American Psychiatric Association. (2013b). Somatic symptom disorder. Accessed March 7, 2014, from http://www.dsm5.org/Documents/Somatic%20Symptom%20Disorder%20Fact%20Sheet.pdf

American Psychiatric Association. (2013c). DSM-5 self exam: Somatic symptom and related disorders. *Clinical and Research News*. Retrieved September 20, 2013, from http://dsm.psychiatryonline.org/news Article.aspx?articleid=1741905&RelatedWidget Articles=true. DOI: 10.1176/appi.pn.2013.9b22

Bhalchandra, D. A., Hatti, S., Thippeswamy, H., & Kumar, C. S. (2014). Factitious disorder-experience at a neuropsychiatric center in southern India. *Indian Journal of Psychological Medicine, 36*(1), 62–65. Retrieved March 8, 2014.

Dimsdale, J. E., Creed, F., Escobar, J., Sharpe, M., Wulsin, L., Barsky, A., Lee, S., Irwin, M. R., Levenson, J. (2013). Somatic symptom disorder: An important change in DSM. *Journal of Psychosomatic Research, 75*(3), 223–228. Retrieved March 8, 2014.

Frye, E., & Feldman, M. (2012). Factitious disorder by proxy in educational settings: A review. *Educational Psychology Review, 24*(1), 47–61. Retrieved March 8, 2014.

Hassan, I., & Ali, R. (2011). The association between somatic symptoms, anxiety disorders and substance use. A literature review. *Psychiatric Quarterly, 82*(4), 315–328. Retrieved March 8, 2014.

Herdman, T. H. (2012). *NANDA International nursing diagnoses: Definitions & classification 2012–2014.* Oxford, UK: Wiley-Blackwell Publishers.

Kinns, H., Housley, D., & Freedman, D. B. (2013). Munchausen syndrome and factitious disorder: The role of the laboratory in its detection and diagnosis. *Annals of Clinical Biochemistry, 50*(3), 194–203. Retrieved March 8, 2014.

Mayo Clinic. DSM-5 redefines hypochondriasis – For medical professionals. Retrieved March 7, 2014, from http://www.mayoclinic.org/medical-professionals/clinical-updates/psychiatry-psychology/diagnostic-statistical-manual-mental-disorders-redefines-hypochondriasis

Todd, S. E. (2014). Factitious disorder imposed on self, medscape reference, drugs, diseases & procedures. Accessed March 8, 2014, from http://emedicine.medscape.com/article/291304-overview

Voigt, K., Wollburg, E., Weinmann, N., Herzog, A., Meyer, B., Langs, G., & Lowe, B. (2012). Predictive validity and clinical utility of DSM-5 somatic symptom disorder – comparison with DSM-IV somatoform disorders and additional criteria for consideration. *Journal of Psychosomatic Research, 73*(5), 345–350. Retrieved March 8, 2014.

Student Worksheet

Fill in the Blank

Fill in the blank with the correct answer.

1. A predictable syndrome of physical complaints and symptoms that are expressed as a result of psychological stress are defined as _____.

2. The attention the person with a somatic disorder receives from physicians and family in response to the symptoms is referred to as _____.

3. In a conversion disorder, the transfer of anxiety into a loss of physical functioning serves as a _____ as the emotional conflict is avoided and relieved.

4. The lack of concern or anxiety over the implications of functional loss in the person with a conversion disorder is known as _____ indifference.

5. _____ is the term given to the search by the person with illness anxiety disorder for a physician to substantiate their feared illness.

Matching

Match the following terms to the most appropriate phrase.

1. _____ Factitious disorder
2. _____ Conversion disorder
3. _____ Munchausen syndrome
4. _____ Illness anxiety disorder
5. _____ Psychogenic seizure

a. Abuse or manipulation of another person, often a child, in order to seek attention
b. Fear of having a serious illness based on a misinterpretation of somatic symptoms
c. Nonepileptic or nonpathological seizure
d. Sensory or neurological impairment not supported by medical testing
e. Deliberate falsification of symptoms or medical testing for sole purpose of assuming sick role

Multiple Choice

Select the best answer from the multiple-choice items.

1. The nurse is doing an assessment of a client with a known diagnosis of illness anxiety disorder. Which of the following statements made by the client would the nurse recognize as most typical of a client with this disorder?
   a. "I don't eat much because I will have diarrhea if I do."
   b. "I can't understand why no one can find out what is wrong with me."
   c. "I know I have colon cancer just like my dad."
   d. "I just don't have the energy I used to."

2. The nurse is caring for a client who was functioning without difficulty until today when she suddenly developed numbness in her right arm. No apparent reason is found for the paralysis. Which of the following is most important for the nurse to remember concerning the client's symptoms?
   a. Cause is related to actual neurological dysfunction
   b. Symptoms represent a primary gain for the client
   c. Client is probably aware that emotions may be the cause
   d. Inability to use her arm will be of major concern to the client

3. When interacting with the client with a somatic symptom disorder, it is most important for the nurse to use which of the following interventions?
   a. Diversion from the sick role to other more productive activities
   b. Supportive interventions that focus on dependency needs
   c. Confrontation with the client over the underlying feelings of anxiety
   d. Avoidance of conversation related to fears and recent traumatic events

4. A client has been repeatedly seen in the clinic for evaluation of severe lower back pain radiating into the left leg that prescribed medication has not relieved. Diagnostic testing does not indicate a medical cause for the level of pain described by the client. In reference to the client's symptoms, which of the following is likely to remain unchanged?
   a. Amount of time lapse between repeat office visit related to the pain
   b. Impairment in functioning as a result of the pain
   c. Amount of analgesia being taken for relief of the pain
   d. Location and description of the symptomatic pain

5. When addressing the self-care needs of a client with a known somatic symptom disorder, the nurse should utilize an approach that focuses on what outcome?
   a. Dependency needs of the client are met
   b. Attention is placed on the physical symptoms
   c. Independent involvement in activities of daily living
   d. Increased descriptive statements of neediness are encouraged

6. Which of the following best describes the result of a client using somatization as a defense mechanism?
   a. An awareness of the psychological factors underlying the symptoms
   b. Underlying anxiety and feelings are effectively resolved
   c. Anxiety is relieved as focus is diverted to physical problem
   d. The person acknowledges that a disease may not exist

7. In addition to substance dependence, which of the following poses the most significant mental health risk to the client experiencing chronic pain?
   a. Sleep disturbances
   b. Depressed mood
   c. La belle indifference
   d. Lack of attention

8. During a routine clinic visit a client tells the nurse she suddenly experienced an inability to use her left arm. She is unable to initiate movement upon command. Which of the following observations would alert the nurse to a possible conversion disorder?
   a. Rotates left wrist for assessment of radial pulse
   b. Husband demonstrates serious concern over her symptoms
   c. Extends right arm for blood pressure assessment
   d. Client has received prior treatment for unrelated problem

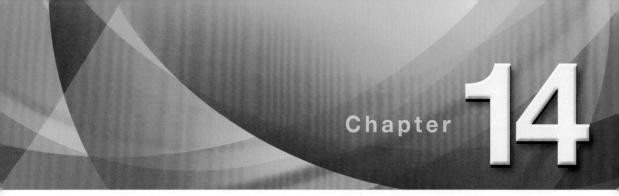

Chapter **14**

Dissociative Disorders

⊙ Learning Objectives

After learning the content in this chapter, the student will be able to:

1. Identify the essential feature of the dissociative disorders.
2. Describe characteristics of the four main categories of dissociative disorders.
3. Assess the primary signs and symptoms of mental disorders of dissociation.
4. Describe treatment available for the client with a dissociative disorder.
5. Identify appropriate nursing diagnoses for the client with a dissociative disorder.
6. Develop expected outcomes for persons with dissociative states.
7. Plan appropriate nursing interventions for the dissociative mental disorders.
8. Evaluate the effectiveness of planned nursing care and make needed revisions.

⊙ Key Terms

continuous amnesia
depersonalization
derealization
dissociation
dissociative amnesia
dissociative fugue

dissociative identity
generalized amnesia
localized amnesia
malingered fugue
selective amnesia
switching process

Dissociation is the mechanism that allows our mind to separate certain memories, most often of unpleasant situations or traumatic events from conscious awareness. These separated parts are kept in the unconscious, or are repressed, and may re-emerge at any time. Repression, the most basic and widely used defense mechanism, may keep painful thoughts and memories buried until we encounter a situation similar to the original trauma. We cannot prevent or control the reoccurrence of these thoughts. However, because the unconscious mind also contains learned behaviors, we can go on "automatic pilot" to carry on with routine activities of daily living such as driving the car, parenting, reading, writing, and cooking.

Just the Facts

Dissociation, or the "not me," is a systematic process used unconsciously to minimize or avoid certain events or experiences to decrease the anxiety that accompanies them.

Mind Jogger

In reality, don't we all have periods of dissociation? For example, while driving a car, you suddenly realize that you don't remember what has happened during the trip. Or, while listening to someone talk, you did not hear part or all of what the person said. Why do you think this happens? Can this be a situation of divided consciousness in which the action and the person's thought go in two different directions at the same time?

The dissociative disorders are described as a disturbance in the ordinarily organized functions of the conscious awareness, memory, identity, and view of oneself in relation to the environment. These disorders tend to occur in response to severe trauma or abuse as the brain is believed to process and store traumatic events in a different, more distant way than it handles and maintains normal or pleasant memories. The mental disturbance may be sudden or gradual, intermittent or chronic. This disorganization causes significant interference of the person's general functioning, social relationships, and work environment. The disruption of functioning is characterized by a dissociation or interruption in the ability to recognize personal information such as identity, background, and family history. These mental disorders tend to occur in response to severe trauma or abuse. The brain is believed to process and store traumatic events in a different, more distant way than it handles and maintains normal or pleasant memories.

Types of Dissociative Disorders

In the DSM-5, the disorders include three main categories that include dissociative amnesia (includes dissociative fugue), dissociative identity disorder, and depersonalization/derealization disorder.

Dissociative Amnesia

Dissociative amnesia is characterized by an inability to remember important personal information, usually of a traumatic or stressful nature. This lack of recall includes a loss of information beyond ordinary forgetfulness. The void may cover the entire scope of the person's life or may be confined to certain details related to the traumatic event itself. The types of dissociative amnesia are listed in Box 14.1.

Signs and Symptoms

Localized amnesia usually occurs within a few hours following the event or traumatic incident. This acute form is more common in response to war combat, natural disasters, or severe trauma. For example, a mother who experiences the activity of a tornado may not remember the hours immediately following the storm that has destroyed her home and taken the life of her child. The mother retains an overall understanding of who she is but forgets fragments of her identity. In **selective amnesia**, a person retains memory of some portions of the event, but not all details are remembered. The woman whose home was destroyed by the tornado may remember the storm but not that her child was killed by flying debris. A person with **generalized amnesia** is

---

BOX 14.1

Types of Dissociative Amnesia

- Localized amnesia: Usually occurs within hours after incident
- Selective amnesia: Retention of overall identity, but fragments are forgotten
- Generalized amnesia: Inability to recall any aspect of one's life
- Continuous amnesia: Inability to recall any aspect of identity, both past and present

BOX 14.2

Common Signs and Symptoms of Dissociative Amnesia

- Inability to recall portions or all of memory or identity inconsistent with normal forgetting
- Depression
- Anxiety
- Depersonalization
- Trance state
- Loss of sensation
- Impaired social and occupational relationships
- Suicidal gestures or acts

With dissociative fugue:

- Inability to recall some or all of one's past or identity
- Sudden travel away from home
- Assumption of new identity
- Mood swings
- Anxiety
- Grief
- Shame or guilt
- Suicidal behaviors

Just the Facts

The person with amnesia usually appears alert and may give no indication to observers that anything is wrong.

Incidence and Etiology

Dissociative amnesia can occur in any age group from children to adults. The main manifestation is a gap in memory for past events that may cover minutes or years. There is a recent increase in incidence, perhaps because of more awareness and newer therapeutic approaches that address traumatic childhood memories. The diagnosis is made with caution in those who may claim symptoms to avoid accountability for personal actions.

Just the Facts

Using the mental mechanism of dissociation can change our ability to look at ourselves and our actions objectively and prevent us from making positive changes in our behavior. Providing a safe and nondemanding environment encourages the client to reconnect with the feelings and perhaps painful events that underly the mental escape of dissociation.

unable to recall any aspect of his or her life. **Continuous amnesia** encompasses a period up to and including the present that is lost from conscious recollection. Common signs and symptoms of dissociative amnesia are found in Box 14.2.

Case Application 14.1

"Displaced Guilt"

Elizabeth is a 23-year-old married mother of 2-year-old twin boys who moves in the apartment adjacent to yours. Despite her ability to state her first name, she is unable to recall her last name or that she has a husband and family. Her husband, Seth, tells you that 3 weeks prior to the onset of the symptoms Elizabeth was in a car accident in which the other vehicle involved was thrown into the path of a semi-truck. The mother and two children who were passengers in the vehicle were killed on impact. Seth states that after the accident she was treated for minor cuts and released from the local hospital. Now, several weeks later, Elizabeth is unable to recall any details of the accident or recognize him or the twins as familiar. She has been spending most of her days sitting in the porch swing. She has not attempted to care for the boys or to interact with them since the accident. Seth is crying and afraid she will never mentally come back to them.

How are Elizabeth's symptoms characteristic of localized dissociative amnesia?

_____

_____

What is the best way to approach Elizabeth?

_____

_____

How can the nurse help Seth to cope with his present situation?

_____

_____

Mind Jogger

What approach would the nurse use to initiate a therapeutic relationship with the client who is experiencing amnesia?

Dissociative Amnesia with Dissociative Fugue

Dissociative amnesia with **dissociative fugue** is demonstrated by the inability to recall some or all of a person's past or identity, accompanied by the sudden and unexpected travel of the person away from home or place of employment. The person often assumes a new identity in the new geographic location. Travel may include simple short trips for a few hours or days, or more extensive travel across many miles over a period of weeks or months. The person usually does not demonstrate outward indications of a psychological problem and adapts to a new social setting without being noticed.

Signs and Symptoms

Although people with dissociative fugue forget their name, family, and where they live, they seem to remember things unrelated to their identity, such as how to drive a car or how to read. When they suddenly return to their former self, they are unable to remember the time of the altered identity or fugue itself. This escape from their identity is usually caused by a traumatic event that has resulted in severe psychological stress, none of which they are able to remember. Most cases of fugue are seen in adults and occur during times of disaster or periods of environmental or personal chaos when there is an actual threat of death, injury, or loss. It is important to recognize that this type of dissociation may also occur in people who are trying to avoid a legal, financial, or unwanted personal situation. This is referred to as **malingered fugue** and is especially relevant in forensic or criminal activity.

Most cases of the disorder are brief—hours or days—with most people experiencing full recovery. A person typically recovers abruptly from dissociative fugue in a state of disorientation and dismay with no recollection of what happened during the time they were in the fugue state or how they got to the unfamiliar place. They may be picked up and questioned by law enforcement authorities. Some resistant amnesia can persist for an extended period of time. The extent and length of the fugue may result in a loss of employment or severely disrupt marriage and family relationships.

Mind Jogger

How might dissociative fugue be compared with manipulative behavior?

Incidence and Etiology

Few people have actually been diagnosed with dissociative fugue. However, its prevalence may increase during times of extremely stressful events. These can include the impact of war and combat, events such as the terrorist attacks of September 11, 2001, or natural disasters as seen in the devastation of hurricanes, earthquakes, or tornadoes.

Dissociative Identity Disorder

In **dissociative identity disorder** (formerly known as multiple personality disorder), two or more distinct identities or personalities are present in the same person. These identities alternate in assuming control of the person's behavior. In addition, there is an inability to recall important personal information that cannot be explained as simple forgetfulness. People with this disorder are unable to connect various aspects of their identity with the past and the present, resulting in fragmentation of the original personality. It is believed that people with severe sexual, physical, or psychological abuse during childhood are predisposed to the development of this disorder. The child who endures severe stress may be unable to integrate all of their experiences into one cohesive identity. An intolerable traumatic event at a time when the psychological defenses are inadequate to deal with the anxiety may result in dissociation of the event and feelings associated with the memory, resulting in the split of the personal identity.

Signs and Symptoms

The dissociated part of the personality takes on characteristics of its own. This subpersonality learns to deal with feelings and emotions that could overwhelm the primary personality. Each

BOX 14.3

Fragmented Personality States of Awareness

- Original personality is usually unaware of the alternate personalities.
- Alternate states are aware of the original one and have varying awareness of each other.
- Alternate personality states often display traits that are foreign to the original personality, such as a giddy, extroverted personality in a person who is naturally very shy.

BOX 14.4

Signs and Symptoms of Dissociative Identity Disorder

- Inability to recall relevant personal information
- Inability to associate the identity with the past and present in organized way
- Multiple personality states, switching from one identity to another
- Migraine headaches
- Nightmares
- Flashbacks
- Hyperactive startle reflex
- Self-injurious behaviors
- Suicidal gestures or acts
- Aggression
- Repetitive abusive relationships

personality character may appear as if it has a distinct personal history, self-concept, identity, and name with its own memories, behavior patterns, and social relationships that are evident when that personality is in control (Box 14.3). These behavior patterns may include aggression, sexual promiscuity, pleasure seeking, or childlike fearfulness. Only one personality is manifested at a time, with one of them usually being dominant during the course of the illness. Psychiatrists refer to this main personality as the "host" person. This primary or host personality usually assumes the person's given name and is passive, dependent, self-blaming, and depressed; it is often the personality that seeks treatment. The host is unaware of the other states during their dominance, but the others may be aware of each other to some extent. The alternate identities usually emerge in a pattern and are often in conflict and critical of the others. The changing of one personality to the other usually occurs very abruptly and is referred to as the **switching process**. This switch is most often triggered by psychosocial stress and may be preceded by behaviors such as rapid eye blinking, facial changes, changes in voice and persona, or a sudden break in the continuity of thought processes. The number of identities can range from as few as 2 to as many as 100 (Box 14.4).

Persons with this disorder have memory gaps for both recent and remote memory. The passive aspects of the personality tend to have less recall, whereas the more hostile and controlling states retain a more complete memory. Sometimes an identity that is not in control will introduce auditory or visual hallucinations to gain control of the conscious state, such as a voice that criticizes the present identity for something he or she is doing.

Mind Jogger

How would a person with dissociative identity disorder differ from one who has a personality disorder?

Incidence and Etiology

Adult dissociative identity disorder is diagnosed more frequently in adult women, and they also tend to have more identities than adult men. The disorder tends to run a lengthy and chronic course from symptom recognition to diagnosis, with the average onset during the early school years. The disorder is less pronounced after age 40. People with this disorder often report a history of severe physical and sexual abuse, particularly during childhood. There is some question that these memories may be distorted, especially if the trauma occurred during periods when imaginary and fantasy play is considered normal. Many times, however, the abuse is validated by actual evidence such as scars from the trauma.

Depersonalization/ Derealization Disorder

Depersonalization is marked by a persistent and repetitious feeling of being detached from one's mental thoughts or body without the presence of disorientation. The person with this disorder has a feeling of not recognizing himself or is unsure about his personal information and identity. The person may sense that his body is imaginary, in an altered state, or disappearing.

Signs and Symptoms

People who actually have this disorder are socially dysfunctional because of the intensity imposed by the feelings of detachment. In **derealization**, the person perceives the external environment as unreal or changing. He or she may see other people as mechanical but be able to recognize the illogical nature of these feelings. There may also be accompanying anxiety, panic, depression, or obsessive and somatic complaints. The person may perceive an unusual change in the size or shape of objects or people may seem unfamiliar and mechanical. People with this disorder may not seek treatment until adolescence or early adulthood, although symptoms may have been present since childhood. The condition tends to be chronic with recurrent brief episodes related to traumatic or stressful events in the person's life. The episodes or feelings of detachment may occur periodically or continuously. Signs and symptoms for depersonalization/derealization disorder are listed in Box 14.5.

Incidence and Etiology

The prevalence of this as a chronic disorder is unknown. It is estimated that perhaps half of all adults may have experienced a single brief episode of depersonalization, usually precipitated by severe stress or life-threatening situational experience. This feeling can also occur with sleep deprivation or after taking certain mind-altering drugs such as marijuana, hallucinogens, Ectasy, or PCP.

BOX 14.5

Common Sign and Symptoms of Depersonalization Disorder

- Feelings of detachment from one's body or thoughts
- Inability to recognize oneself or personal information
- Anxiety or panic
- Depression
- Somatic complaints
- Obsessions
- Perceptual changes of size or shape
- People seem unfamiliar and mechanical

Treatment of Dissociative Disorders

Many people with dissociative disorders achieve complete recovery without treatment. Treatment is sought only if the disorder continues to persist or causes the person considerable anguish. Diagnostic testing must be done to determine if there are any coexisting mental health conditions or substance abuse involved. Antianxiety drugs and antidepressants may be useful for symptoms of anxiety or depression associated with these disorders.

Various types of psychotherapy are the usual approach to the dissociative states. Cognitive techniques can allow the person to talk and identify the underlying negative thoughts associated with the traumatic events. Understanding that these thoughts determine resulting behavior can aid the individual in realizing that changing the way one thinks about a situation can also lead to a more positive behavior outcome. Some therapists use hypnosis to aid in recollection of events and feelings associated with repressed trauma. Other forms of therapy include creative art processes to facilitate expression of feelings and thoughts. All types of psychotherapy are intended to help the person work through the trauma that triggered and resulted in the dissociative symptoms.

Application of the Nursing Process

Nursing Assessment

During the diagnostic process, any physical condition that could produce the symptoms of amnesia and dissociation must be ruled out. These conditions include head injury, epilepsy, brain disease, pharmacological side effects, or substance abuse. Psychotic disorders such as schizophrenia must also be ruled out. Psychological tests are used to further evaluate the authenticity of the symptoms.

Case Application 14.2

"Art's Disappearance"

Art is a 47-year-old division dean of a university extended campus location. He is married and the father of two teenage children. He has been active in campus and community affairs, including assisting with productions of the local amateur theater. Art is scheduled to board an 8:15 AM flight to meet a professional colleague in a city 300 miles from his hometown. At 7:00 AM the day of his intended arrival, the colleague notifies the university and Art's wife that Art did not arrive on his scheduled flight. When his wife checks with the airport, she is told that her husband never boarded the flight. Art's car is found at the airport with the keys locked inside.

Six months later, investigators have uncovered no clues as to Art's whereabouts or what may have occurred in his disappearance. Several months later, Art walks into his office at the university accompanied by an unfamiliar woman whom he introduces as his wife. It is apparent to the office personnel that he does not recognize them or his previous position in the division office. He states that a young man saw him at a restaurant in a neighboring state and told him about his real identity. Art states he has no recollection of the institution or his family. He is admitted for treatment in a state of severe anxiety with suicidal ideation.

What symptoms indicate that Art is experiencing a dissociative state?

_____

_____

What type of dissociative disorder do Art's symptoms suggest?

_____

_____

How should the nurse approach Art when discussing past traumatic events?

_____

_____

A clinical interview is included to ascertain any significant childhood or adult trauma.

Along with a physical assessment, a baseline psychosocial assessment is done to determine behavioral alterations such as disorientation, level of anxiety, amnesia, any depression, and the extent to which functioning in the social and work environment is affected. It is important for the nurse to describe the client's behavior and verbalized statements because clients with dissociative disorders can present ambiguous pictures or personalities to various staff members as a manipulative means of causing conflict.

Nursing Diagnoses

Once assessment data are obtained, nursing problems are identified. Common nursing diagnoses used to address problems seen in clients with dissociative disorders include the following:

- Altered Thought Processes, related to memory loss and repressed trauma
- Sensory Perceptual Alteration, related to depersonalization and view of self
- Personality Identity Disturbance, related to childhood trauma or more than one personality state
- Self-Care Deficit, related to mechanical trancelike state or aimless wandering
- Ineffective Individual Coping, related to repressed memories and issues, loss of identity, or travel away from home
- Anxiety, related to repressed traumatic events or loss of identity
- Risk for Violence, related to self-destructive behaviors
- Family Coping Ineffective, related to loss of identity

Expected Outcomes

The ultimate goal of the therapeutic process is to help the person integrate the fragmented personalities into one identity. Extensive psychotherapy is used to help clients retrieve repressed ideas and memories. The process includes the planning of nursing outcomes that are anticipated with the implementation of nursing interventions to address the nursing problems. The time frame in which a realistic expectation can be anticipated for symptom resolution differs with the type of dissociative disorder. Expected outcomes for the client may include the following:

- Associate memory deficit with past stressful events
- Recover memory deficits and develop improved coping mechanisms to deal with stressful events
- Verbalize reality-based perception of environmental stimuli in stressful situations
- Verbalize understanding of multipersonality states and the need to consolidate all the personalities into one
- Perform self-care activities independently
- Demonstrate more adaptive coping methods in response to stressful situations
- Verbalize feelings and identify positive effective ways of managing fear and anxiety
- Verbalize understanding of personality conflict in dissociative state
- Demonstrate self-control over behaviors toward self and others

Expected outcomes for the family may include the following:

- Verbalize realistic expectations for client's behavior and treatment process
- Demonstrate support of the client and of the family unit

Nursing Interventions

The nurse must first establish a trusting and supportive therapeutic relationship with the client. It is important to use active listening and communication techniques that encourage verbalization of feelings, conflicts, and information regarding the traumatic events that led to the current dissociative state. This process assists the client to develop personal insight and an awareness and understanding of the self and behaviors that are self-defeating and damaging, along with alternative plans for behavioral changes. Clients need encouragement and support to achieve control over their anxiety and previous dissociative response to those situations that trigger the symptoms. People with these disorders are overwhelmed with fear of not knowing or being out of control.

Other interventions include the following:

- Encourage the client to keep a daily journal of thoughts and feelings.

- Develop a contract between the client and staff for dealing with self-destructive behaviors.
- Promote a safe environment to protect the client from self-injury or injury to others.
- Assist the client in developing effective coping skills.
- Model positive and desired behaviors.
- Identify environmental stressors that trigger the dissociative symptoms.
- Decrease anxiety-producing stimuli.
- Use stimuli that stimulate pleasant memories and pleasurable feelings for the client. This assists the client to remember past experiences without the risk of precipitating increased trauma.
- Avoid flooding the client with details of past traumatic events. This may cause the client to regress further into the dissociative state that is serving to protect the person from the emotional pain.
- Help the client to understand that periods of imbalance are to be expected and will decrease as the personal identity is restored.
- Maintain an awareness of behavioral changes that may indicate self-destructive behavior.
- Assist the client to identify alternatives to self-injury such as physical exercise, written methods of expression, or creative art and task-oriented activities, which provide a means of nonverbal expression of thoughts that the person may not be able to verbalize.
- Assist the client to identify the purpose that each subpersonality (dissociative identity disorder) serves in the total personality of the person.
- Identify contributing factors within the family dynamics and the environment.
- Help the family to provide encouragement and reinforcement of positive client behaviors.

Evaluation

During the evaluation process, it is important to note the progress the client has made toward identifying and demonstrating a more adaptive response to stressful stimuli. This step is helpful in decreasing the dissociative response. The client must also come to an understanding of the relationship between the dissociative state and the increased anxiety that is felt as repressed past trauma is triggered by environmental factors.

"Home But Lost"

Phillip has just arrived in his hometown after recovering from shrapnel wounds received during military action in Iraq. He is brought to the emergency room after he is found wandering on a boat dock incoherent and bleeding from his wrists. When asked his name, it is obvious that he has no recollection of his identity or what he was doing on the pier. However, when he is asked about recent events in his life, he states he attended class at the high school the day before. When Phillip's family is located, they tell the nurse that Phillip is 26 years old and has not attended high school in 8 years. Once his lacerations are treated, Phillip is admitted to the psychiatric unit with a diagnosis of dissociative generalized amnesia.

What feelings may be responsible for Phillip's attempted suicidal acts?

_____

_____

Why is it important to obtain information from the family about Phillip's likes, dislikes, activities, or hobbies?

_____

_____

What is the purpose of reintroducing things and people from his past that represent pleasant experiences for him?

_____

_____

Why is it important not to flood Phillip with information about his recent past in Iraq?

_____

_____

Recalling past traumatic events is crucial to this understanding. In dissociative identity disorder, evaluation centers on the client's acknowledgment of the existence of more than one personality and how these various states function as protection from the anxiety related to traumatic memories. It is also important to note the client's progress toward the ultimate goal of integrating all personalities into a single personality.

Nurses are faced with a challenging and frustrating task of accepting the client's behavior while trying to understand the complex nature of the dissociative states. Providing a safe and trusting environment with acceptance and support allows the client to develop a sense of power and self-control in a consistent, caring milieu with a positive forward progression in the treatment process.

Summary

- The dissociative disorders are characterized by an interruption from the conscious acquaintance with identity, personal background, and family history. These disorders are most often seen in people who have experienced severe trauma or abuse.
- Dissociation is the mechanism that allows the mind to separate these traumatic memories from the conscious awareness. These repressed memories can resurface at any time, usually triggered by environmental factors. The repetition of these thoughts cannot be controlled or prevented by the client when they are occurring.
- Dissociative amnesia takes two forms. It may be a localized amnesia that occurs shortly after an incident where the person retains an overall understanding of who he or she is but forgets pieces of

the identity picture. The second form is a generalized amnesia in which the whole life span is beyond recall.

- When the amnesia is accompanied by sudden travel away from home or place of employment with the establishment of a new identity, it is referred to as a dissociative fugue. The person functions in this new location without drawing any attention to the false identity. When the fugue is terminated, the person may return home with no recollection of the events before or during the fugue.
- Another type of dissociative disorder occurs when two or more distinct identities or personalities are present in the same person and alternately assume control of the person's behavior.
- Depersonalization occurs with a persistent and repetitious feeling of being detached from one's mental thoughts or body. The person retains orientation but is socially dysfunctional because of the intensity created by the feelings of detachment. Treatment of an identity disorder may be extensive and focuses on reintegration of the personalities into the original personality.

- Treatment of dissociative disorders involves psychotherapy to help the individual recapture the feelings and thoughts associated with the trauma toward understanding how these are connected to their current behavior and symptoms.
- The nurse must first establish a trusting and supportive therapeutic relationship with the client. The client is then supported to develop an awareness of the self-defeating behaviors with alternative plans for changing these patterns.
- Interventions are directed at helping the client to develop a sense of power and self-control toward a predictable and positive outcome.

Bibliography

American Psychiatric Association. (2000). *Diagnostic and statistical manual of mental disorders text revision* (4th ed.). Washington, DC: American Psychiatric Association.

Chu, J. A., Frey, L. M., Ganzel, B. L., & Matthews, J. A. (1999). Memories of childhood abuse: Dissociation, amnesia, and corroboration. *American Journal of Psychiatry, 156,* 749–755. Retrieved May 04, 2009, from http://ajp.psychiatryonline.org/cgi/content/full/156/5/749

Foote, B., Smolin, Y., Kaplan, M., Legatt, M. E., & Lipschitz, D. (2006). Prevalence of dissociative disorders in psychiatric outpatients. *American Journal of Psychiatry, 163,* 623–629. Retrieved May 04, 2009, from http://ajp.psychiatryonline.org/cgi/content/full/163/4/623

Herdman, T. H. (2012). *NANDA International nursing diagnoses: definitions & classification 2012–2014.* Oxford, UK: Wiley-Blackwell Publishers.

National Alliance of Mental Illness Factsheet. (2000). Reviewed by Maser, J. D. Retrieved May 04, 2009, from http://www.nami.org/Content/Content Groups/Helpline1/Dissociative_Disorders.htm

Simeon, D. (2008). *Merck manual home edition: dissociative disorders.* Section 07, Chapter 106. New Jersey: Merck & Co., Inc. Full review/revision June 2008. Retrieved May 04, 2009, from http://www.merck.com/mmhe/sec07/ch106.html

Simeon, D., Guralnik, O., Knutelska, M., & Schmeidler, J. (2002). Personality factors associated with dissociation: Temperament, defenses, and cognitive schemata. *American Journal of Psychiatry, 159,* 489–491. Retrieved May 04, 2009, from http://ajp.psychiatryonline.org/cgi/content/full/159/3/489

Varcarolis, E. M., Carson, V. B., & Shoemaker, N. C. (2006). *Foundations of psychiatric mental health nursing* (5th ed.). Philadelphia, PA: W. B. Saunders.

Student Worksheet

Fill in the Blank

Fill in the blank with the correct answer.

1. An interruption from the conscious knowledge of personal identity and background history is termed _____.

2. When certain memories are removed from conscious awareness, the separated parts are _____ in the unconscious and may resurface at any time.

3. In dissociative identity disorder, the main personality is referred to as the _____ person.

4. The changing of one personality or the _____ process in dissociative identity disorder usually occurs very abruptly and is most often triggered by psychosocial stress.

5. A persistent and repetitious feeling of being detached from one's mental thoughts or body without noted disorientation is referred to as _____ disorder.

Matching

Match the following terms to the most appropriate phrase.

1. _____ Fugue
2. _____ Localized amnesia
3. _____ Malingering
4. _____ Depersonalization
5. _____ Derealization

a. Acute inability to recall personal information shortly after a traumatic event
b. Persistent feeling of being detached from one's mind or body
c. Seeing the external environment as unreal or changing
d. Sudden travel from one's home setting accompanied by the inability to recall one's past
e. Inability to recall one's past accompanied by unexpected travel to avoid unwanted situation

Multiple Choice

Select the best answer from the multiple-choice items.

1. A woman who claims to be Ryan's biological sister visits him in his home. She tells him that he has a family in another location. When she asks Ryan why he doesn't come home, he replies, "I'm sorry, but I don't know who you are." Ryan is demonstrating symptoms of:
   a. Derealization
   b. Malingering
   c. Dissociative fugue
   d. Depersonalization

2. Alice has been admitted to the psychiatric unit with a diagnosis of dissociative identity disorder. The nurse observes that during interaction with other clients, Alice is laughing and quite talkative. When the nurse approaches Alice to administer her medications, Alice slumps her shoulders as she looks away with tears in her eyes and says in a child-like voice, "Are you going to hurt me?" The nurse's best response in this situation is:
   a. "You were laughing a minute ago. What happened to Alice?"
   b. "These medications are to help Alice feel better."
   c. "I'll come back later when you feel better."
   d. "Why do you think I am going to hurt you?"

3. Ralph is a client with dissociative amnesia. The nurse has identified a nursing diagnosis of personal identity disturbance. An appropriate expected outcome for this client is:
   a. Client will discuss past experiences that have influenced self-concept
   b. Client will verbalize understanding of need to integrate personality
   c. Client will demonstrate an understanding of the role of each personality
   d. Client will function independently in all self-care activities

4. The nurse is addressing past memory deficits with a client who has a dissociative disorder. To avoid flooding the client, it is important for the nurse to:
   a. Instruct the client to focus on the current stress factors
   b. Reorient the client to time, place, and person at each contact
   c. Observe for cues that the client is ready to revisit the traumatic incident
   d. Include details of the traumatic events surrounding the memory loss in the first session

5. A client tells the nurse a rather confusing story of recent events surrounding her symptoms of amnesia. The nurse's best response is:
   a. "You must be very angry that it is difficult for you to remember this."
   b. "You seem to overreact each time you try to talk about this."
   c. "Let me see if I correctly understand what you are telling me."
   d. "We will try this again when you can tell the story like it happened."

6. A client tells the nurse she knows she is married and has three children but does not remember she recently had a baby who died from sudden infant death syndrome. The nurse would recognize this type of dissociation as:
   a. Localized amnesia
   b. Selective amnesia
   c. Generalized amnesia
   d. Continuous amnesia

7. Which of the following would be true of the primary or host personality in the person with dissociative identity disorder?
   a. Usually dominant and critical of the others
   b. Often in conflict with other personality states
   c. Is aware of all alternate personalities
   d. Is passive, dependent, and self-blaming personality

8. A client who describes recurring feelings that he is "out of his body" and sees himself as fragmented with disconnected body parts. Although feeling detached from his body, which of the following would this client likely demonstrate?
   a. Inability to recall all or most of past identity
   b. A lack of disorientation
   c. Assumption of a new identity
   d. Alternate personality states

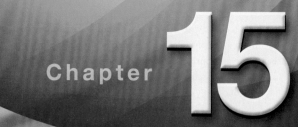

Substance-Related Disorders

⊙ Learning Objectives

After learning the content in this chapter, the student will be able to:

1. Demonstrate an understanding of substance abuse and addiction.
2. Describe etiological factors that contribute to substance abuse.
3. Discuss the term *codependency* and its relationship to substance abuse.
4. Describe treatment goals for the client and family toward long-term sobriety.
5. Assess the client with substance intoxication and withdrawal symptoms.
6. Identify nursing diagnoses common to clients with disorders related to chemical dependency.
7. Determine expected outcome criteria for the client in the acute withdrawal phase and the recovery period of substance-abuse disorders.
8. Plan effective nursing interventions to address the detoxification phase and the recovery period of treatment in chemical dependency.
9. Identify evaluation criteria to determine the effectiveness of the treatment intervention.

⊙ Key Terms

addiction
blackout
codependent
craving
delirium tremens
detoxification
enabling
inhalants

relapse
substance
substance abuse
substance intoxication
tolerance
Wernicke–Korsakoff
 syndrome
withdrawal

230

Substance Use, Abuse, and Addiction

The term **substance** is used in reference to any drug, medication, or toxin that shares the potential for abuse. According to the National Institute on Drug Abuse, 23.6 million persons aged 12 or older required treatment for use of an illegal drug or alcohol use problem. Of these, approximately 11% ever received treatment. The economic impact of illicit drug abuse combined with alcohol and tobacco costs in the United States alone is estimated at over $500 billion annually, or $6,120 per second. These figures include the extended costs of health care, the criminal justice system, unemployment, and social welfare programs.

Substance Abuse

Substance abuse is a maladaptive pattern of substance use that demonstrates physiological, cognitive, and behavioral indications that the person continues to use the drug despite the adverse substance-related problems he or she may be experiencing. In the new diagnostic criteria, the terms substance abuse and substance dependence have been combined into a single category centering around the issue of compulsive drug-seeking behaviors. Substances can decrease the energy use and activity in the brain, alter the shape of brain cells, and change the function of the signals and networks within the CNS. This underlying change triggers the brain's reward system with an intense **craving**, or strong desire to use the substance for the reward of the intense feelings of euphoria or "high" it produces. This extreme desire for the substance often is pursued even if other aspects of the person's life are neglected. It is these mental and behavioral aspects of substance use that comprise the basis for the substance-use disorders.

Substance abuse results in repeated absences from work, school, or home with repeated poor performance in these areas because of hangover effects. The incidence of abuse is more common in episodic substance use, such as when the person becomes inebriated on a weekend or at a particular event. There tends to be an increase in encounters with disciplinary authorities as a result of abuse-related behaviors (e.g., arrests for disorderly conduct, public intoxication, driving while intoxicated, suspension or expulsion from school, involvement of child protective services). Despite the persistent negative personal and interpersonal problems that result from repetitious abuse of the substance, the person does not abstain from continued use.

Mind Jogger

What are the extended personal costs of substance abuse and dependency?

Addiction

Addiction is a physiological and psychological dependence on alcohol or other drugs that affect the central nervous system (CNS) in such a way that withdrawal symptoms (discussed later in the chapter) are experienced when the substance is discontinued. A **tolerance** develops as the brain adapts to repeated doses of the drug with a declining effect as it is taken repetitively over time. This results in the need to use greater amounts of the substance to obtain the same effect. The tolerance may be varied in degree depending on the drug involved and its effect on the CNS. Substantial levels of tolerance may develop with heavy drug use that would be lethal to a person who does not use drugs. In people who smoke cigarettes, a habit of 2 to 3 packs per day indicates a tolerance to nicotine that would produce toxic effects in the nonsmoker. High blood levels of a drug without obvious symptoms of intoxication often signify tolerance.

Substance abuse and addiction can result in serious health problems that in turn invoke enormous cost to the health care system in the way of treatment, detoxification, and rehabilitation programs. With the surging incidence of drug-related HIV/AIDS infection, hepatitis, and other diseases, the expense of prevention, research, and treatment has soared to new levels. Society is additionally burdened by drug-related criminal behaviors that involve both the participation in usage or sale of drugs and the violence associated with the drug industry. The cost of arrest and incarceration in drug-related crimes has risen steadily in the past decade. In addition, there is the cost of lost jobs and families who, as a result of these behaviors, are reduced to dependence on welfare and other subsidiary means of support. Increases in child abuse and neglect are fostered by the violence and degradation that accompanies the use and abuse of substances.

Finally, the number of premature deaths attributed to drug abuse enlarges this picture to include not only financial losses but also human lives shortened as a result of the detrimental extension of its effects. Despite the fact that substance abuse and dependency are among the most preventable of the mental disorders, millions of people continue to abuse drugs each day. Alcohol continues to be the drug most often abused by Americans.

Phases of Substance Dependency

Although there are many proposed theories about the etiology or cause for chemical dependency, research is ongoing to help us understand this condition. An estimated one third of hospital admissions are alcohol related, although the incidence of alcohol as a contributing factor in motor vehicle accidents, falls, trauma, and other disorders may not always be readily apparent.

Substance abuse and dependency is a destructive and progressive process from the first use of a substance to the far end of the harmful decline. Most people who become substance dependent do not intend to become alcoholics and drug abusers. They often start with a need to belong, to escape, or to experiment, unaware of the destructive process ahead. Substance dependency is a progressive and predictable continuum of symptoms that increase in severity and frequency.

There are four phases that occur from the first use of a substance to the eventual dependency with continued use (Fig. 15.1). In *phase one*, or first use, the user experiences a mood of euphoria or "high" and learns that the substance can provide a temporary escape or altered emotional state each time it is used. The user learns to control the effects by regulating the amount of substance and prioritizing the opportunities to use it.

During *phase two*, the user experiences hangover effects and starts to feel guilty for behaviors related to use of the substance. A need for the drug may develop, leading to tolerance and increased use to obtain the same effect. The person's friends and companions may change to a group who approve of and indulge in similar drug-related behaviors.

As the user enters *phase three*, a dependent lifestyle begins, with periods in which control over substance use is lost. The person can no longer predict the outcome and begins to engage in behaviors that compromise his or her values. As the substance assumes control, insight is lost and a revolving cycle begins in which the drug use becomes the priority.

In *phase four*, the user demonstrates dependency or addiction with periods of blackout, paranoia, and helplessness. Engaging in the acquisition of the substance is no longer seen as a social activity, but as survival.

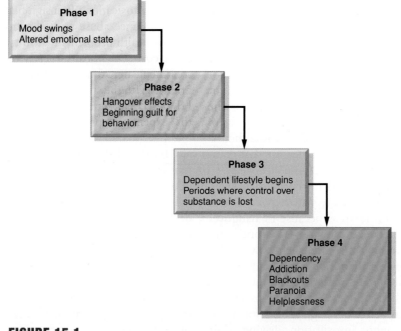

FIGURE 15.1

Phases of chemical dependency and the consuming nature of its hold on the substance user.

Just the Facts

Blackout is a form of amnesia for events that occurred during the drinking period (e.g., client does not remember conversations or activities engaged in during the time of drinking).

The characteristic warning signs that exist in the series of events leading to chemical dependency are described in Table 15.1.

Classes of Substances

Substances are grouped by the *DSM-5* into 10 classes that are listed in Box 15.1. A category for other substance intoxication includes those substances that cause a severe, unfamiliar intoxication response from a street-available unknown sub-

BOX 15.1

Substance Classifications Recognized by DSM-5

- Alcohol
- Caffeine
- Cannabis
- Stimulants (amphetamines, cocaine)
- Hallucinogens (includes PCP)
- Tobacco
- Inhalants
- Opioids
- Sedatives, hypnotics, or anxiolytics
- Other (or unknown) substance intoxication

stance. Prescription drugs and over-the-counter medications, originally intended as harmless treatment, can also become part of the web of addiction. Prescription drug abuse is the nation's fastest-growing drug problem and has been identified as an epidemic by the Centers for Disease Control and Prevention. For most people who use pain relievers, CNS depressants, or stimulants as prescribed, the risk is small. However, when these drugs are used in ways other than that intended by the physician, the risk for addiction exists. Symptoms of substance-related disorders usually appear at higher dosages and usually disappear as the dose is decreased or the drug is discontinued. Medications included in this category are seen in Box 15.2.

Exposure to toxins and other chemical substances can result in a mental disorder as well.

TABLE 15.1	Warning Signs of Substance Dependency
Early	Uses substance to relax in social situation
	Avoids situations where drugs/alcohol will not be available
	Is preoccupied with drugs and their usage
	Has occasional blackouts (periods in which person cannot remember drug use)
	Experiences personality change during substance use
Abuse and Dependency	Shows increase in tolerance
	Denies drug problem—hides drug use from others
	May switch to other chemical use
	Neglects and loses friends
	Blames others for problems—projection
	Has increased craving
	May have aggressive behaviors with drug use
	Has physical withdrawal symptoms when use is interrupted
	Consumes unpredictable amounts of substance
	Neglects nutritional needs
Chronic	Shows irreversible physical damage (liver, brain, and other medical problems)
	Has decreased tolerance
	Has severe withdrawal symptoms
	Feels persistent remorse
	Has drug-related arrests
	Has delirium tremens (DTs)
	Hallucinates
	Has seizures
	Death may occur

BOX 15.2

Classifications of Drugs That May Cause Substance-Related Disorders

These classifications include, but are not limited to:
- Analgesics
- Anesthetics
- Anticholinergics
- Antihistamines
- Antihypertensives
- Antimicrobials
- Antiparkinson agents
- Cardiovascular medications
- Chemotherapeutic agents
- Corticosteroids
- Gastrointestinal medications
- Muscle relaxants
- Nonsteroidal anti-inflammatory drugs
- Over-the-counter medications such as sleep aids, antihistamines, decongestants, weight-loss agents, gastrointestinal aids, and pain-relief drugs

Toxins and Other Chemical Substances

- Heavy metals (lead, aluminum, iron)
- Pesticides (nicotine)
- Nerve gases
- Carbon dioxide
- Ethylene glycol (antifreeze)

Toxic substances that may cause substance-related illness include those listed in Box 15.3.

Volatile substances such as gasoline and paint, if used for the purpose of intoxication, are referred to as **inhalants**. The most common symptom associated with these toxic substances are alterations in cognitive functioning or mood, which usually resolve over a period of weeks or months once exposure is terminated.

Theoretical Approaches to Substance Use and Abuse

Why does a person advance down this path of self-destruction? There are several theoretical approaches to explain causation and motivational factors leading to drug abuse and addiction.

Genetics and Family Influences

Social learning involves the effects of modeling, imitative, and identification behaviors that begin at an early age. Children of substance-abusing parents are at a greater risk for substance abuse and subsequent problems because of both genetic and environmental factors. There is an apparent link between heredity and the development of substance-use disorders. Studies show this tendency to be especially true for alcoholism, where the risk for alcohol abuse is increased by 50% in first-generation relatives of alcoholics. Research also shows that the younger a person is when drug usage begins, the greater the probability that it will progress to abuse and addiction. Chaotic home environments and association with peers who engage in drug-related behaviors also increase the likelihood that this will occur. This scenario is often accompanied by weak parent–child attachment with ineffective parenting and hostile, troubled relationships.

Mind Jogger

In what way does a strong solid family system aid in reducing the risk of adolescent drug use?

Peer Pressure

Adolescence is a time when new things are exciting and the pressures to conform to one's peers are at its highest. Teenagers may get involved with illicit drugs for various reasons, and experimentation is common. They often do not see the connection between their present actions and the consequences these actions may impose. Teenagers with a family history of substance abuse, those who are depressed or have low self-esteem, and those who feel like a misfit among the crowd are at particular risk for developing a drug problem. Adolescents tend to perceive the drug-using behavior on the part of family, peers, and community as an endorsement of drug usage.

Environmental Stress Factors

Stressful situations increase the need for coping strategies to manage the resultant anxiety, which is usually the excuse or reason the person uses to justify the repeated use of the substance. Stress is cited as a major factor in the initiation and continued use of alcohol and other drugs. It is a significant factor when the person relapses and returns to a pattern of self-destructive behaviors.

Mind Jogger

What environmental issues are likely to be contributors to substance use and abuse?

Chronic Physiological Disease

Addiction or dependency is also described as a chronic disease in which there are changes in brain chemistry that bring about the perceived need to continue usage of the drug. It is suggested that herein lies the reasoning that one substance is often replaced with another as the individual travels the path to addiction. The brain cells have become adapted to functioning with the substance or substances and cannot function properly without it for long. The drug must be continued to avoid symptoms of withdrawal.

Personality Characteristics

Dependency cannot be discounted as a component of the personality in people who abuse drugs. The need to depend on an external force to provide a sense of self is reflected in the form of a weak

BOX 15.4

Determinants of Our Sense of Self

External Control

- Primary motivation is acceptance by others
- Will compromise values under peer pressure
- Depends on external source of strength (other people, drugs, activities)

Internal Control

- Acts on clearly defined self-chosen beliefs and convictions
- Accepts responsibility for decisions and consequences of those choices
- Recognizes and is willing to act on the need for change

self-esteem and an inability to define values and boundaries for behavior (Box 15.4). Conformity and blending into the social drug culture result in the substance taking control of the person's existence. The person is painfully aware of the craving for the drug in order to fulfill a need for affection and power. Most people who abuse drugs have difficulty expressing feelings and may release these explosively as the drug diminishes their ability to control them. Feelings of emotional isolation and a low frustration tolerance are further indicators of the need to borrow a feeling of strength and security from an external substance.

Codependence: A Family Disease

Codependency is a multigenerational pattern of coping mechanisms that lead to self-defeating behaviors. This state evolves from a transmission of family dynamics in which the person is discouraged from feeling or expressing needs, leading to suppressed anger and emotional pain. People in this situation often mistake feelings of control within the family as security and learn to tolerate and excuse the maladaptive behavior. This tolerance results in adjustment to the circumstances and the appearance of normalcy to the outsider.

Just the Facts

Codependency is an emotional behavior that is learned by watching and imitating other family members who demonstrate this type of behavior.

A theoretical approach based on the family systems model proposes that substance abuse is a family disease in which members either are drug users or codependent, and that these factors are interrelated in a way that enables or feeds the problem. Families often display defensive actions that in a way normalize and excuse the behavior of the drug user, and thus unintentionally increase the likelihood that the abusive pattern will continue.

People who are **codependent** tend to feel a responsibility for the drug user's problem and internalize a form of guilt for the behavior of that person. As a result, they continue to do everything possible to sustain the relationship and are unable to recognize the detrimental effects of the codependency on their own physical and mental health. This pattern of either consciously or unconsciously helping the maladaptive behavior to continue is referred to as **enabling**. The enabler commonly makes excuses or lies to others about behaviors related to the substance abuse. They may also cover up financial and legal problems out of a false sense of responsibility. Social events may be avoided because of shame or fear of ramifications related to the drug use, such as questioning or abusive language and actions. Codependent people deny their own needs while living and doing for another what they need to do for themselves. The passive nature of enablers is seen as they silently comply with the choices and decisions of the user even though they may not agree with them. This yielding behavior allows the user to maintain a perceived sense of control over the dependency and provides a false permission for the addiction to continue.

Despite attempts to protect the user from the consequences of substance abuse, the enabler often feels powerless and, in all actuality, is controlled by the person with whom he or she is codependent. Enablers are caught in a cycle of thinking they are helpless to change the situation because to stop these actions would bring greater disaster. Rigid, inflexible family rules predispose the codependent person to a feeling of being trapped in this dysfunctional situation.

Mind Jogger

In what other situations might codependency be a factor?

Substance-Induced Disorders

The category of substance-induced disorders is inclusive of substance intoxication, withdrawal, and other substance or medication-induced mental disorders (e.g., substance-induced psychosis, mood, and anxiety disorders).

Substance Intoxication

Substance intoxication is the development of a reversible pattern of behavior caused by recent ingestion of a substance. This syndrome is clinically seen as maladaptive behavioral and psychological changes that are related to the effects of the substance on the CNS.

Signs and Symptoms

The person with substance intoxication may have belligerence, a labile mood, impaired thinking and judgment, and impaired functioning in the social or work setting that are unrelated to any other medical condition. The most common changes that occur with intoxication involve disturbances in the areas of perception, sleep–wake cycle, attention, concentration, thinking, judgment, psychomotor activity, and interpersonal relationships. The person who is intoxicated may have a flushed appearance, eyes may be red or blood-shot, an increased heart rate or elevated blood pressure, and may be nauseated or vomit. Some symptoms are drug specific (listed in the substance-specific section of this chapter) and others may be indicative of the abuse of several drugs.

Substance Withdrawal

A maladaptive change in behavior or **withdrawal** occurs as the blood or tissue concentrations of a substance decline in a person who has engaged in heavy prolonged use of the substance. Once these unpleasant symptoms occur, the person is likely to seek relief by reingesting the substance. This cycle typically begins on awakening and continues throughout the day. The pattern of compulsive use is demonstrated as larger amounts of the substance are taken over a more extensive period than was intended. The person may indicate a desire or attempt to decrease the substance use but is unsuccessful in these efforts. Much time and energy is devoted to planning activities necessary to obtain the substance. What once may have been valued and enjoyable time spent with family, friends, and colleagues in recreational activities is surrendered to substance use. Even though the person may have recurrent physiological and psychological ill effects from drug usage, it continues.

As psychological dependence develops, the person feels they cannot function without continued use of that substance. This failure to refrain from using the substance even when the harmful effects are known is the key symptom found in those diagnosed with substance-use disorders.

> **Just the Facts**
>
> The presence of withdrawal symptoms poses a higher risk for medical problems and relapse rate.

Signs and Symptoms

The signs and symptoms of withdrawal develop within several hours to a few days after drug cessation and vary with the substance involved (see Table 15.2).

> **Just the Facts**
>
> Short-acting substances tend to have a higher potential for withdrawal than do those substances with a longer duration of action. The duration of the withdrawal period tends to parallel the half-life of the substance (e.g., the longer the action of the drug, the longer the withdrawal period).

Incidence and Etiology

There is a strong association between familial predisposition and the substance-induced disorders. Children of a person with a substance-related disorder are also more likely to develop substance-related problems. There is some evidence that genetics may determine the variances in the doses necessary to produce intoxication in different people. Because of their smaller body mass and slower body metabolism, women tend to become intoxicated more easily than men.

It must be noted that tolerance and withdrawal are not unique to substance addiction as these features of physical dependence can be normal responses to prescribed medications that affect the CNS. As is the case with some substances (e.g., marijuana or cannabis), there are no physical symptoms of tolerance and withdrawal although the substance severely impairs the functional ability of the individual. In the diagnostic criteria, the conditions causing the physical response are referred to as substance-induced disorders (e.g., intoxication, withdrawal, psychosis, delirium).

TABLE 15.2   Substance-Related Information

INTOXICATON	WITHDRAWAL	SUBSTANCE-RELATED INFORMATION	SIGNS AND SYMPTOMS OF ASSOCIATED DISORDER
Alcohol			
Drug-related maladaptive behavior, odor on breath or clothes, slurred speech, incoordination and unsteady gait, difficulty focusing with glazed appearance of eyes, very passive or very argumentative manner, memory impairment, poor concentration, stupor	Autonomic response: (diaphoresis, increase in pulse rate), tremors or "shakes" 24–48 hrs after cessation, insomnia, nausea and vomiting, easily startled, irritable, flushed face Hallucinations: auditory (buzzing, ringing, clicking, voices); visual (people, animals, insects); tactile (insects or spiders crawling) Psychomotor: agitation, increased anxiety, grand mal seizures, delirium tremens	Tends to loosen inhibitions Most common cause of preventable birth defects Devastating effects on health Alcohol equivalents (1 oz spirits = 5 oz wine = 12 oz beer) Legal level of intoxication is 0.08%–0.10% in most states Average age for first use is 12 y of age Examples: Beer, wine, bourbon, scotch, gin, vodka, rum, tequila, liqueurs Common substances containing alcohol that may be used by dependent people to satisfy craving (liquid cough or cold preparations, mouthwash, isopropyl rubbing alcohol, nail polish, remover, cologne, aftershave, extracts used in food)	Increased risk of accidents, violence, suicide Criminal behaviors Absenteeism Wernicke–Korsakoff syndrome Delirium tremens
Amphetamines/Methamphetamine			
Dilated pupils, dry mouth and nose, halitosis, lip-licking, hyperventilation tachycardia or bradycardia, hypertension or hypotension, nausea and vomiting, perspiration, chills, weight loss, difficulty staying still, excessive activity, confusion, seizures, dyskinesias **Methamphetamine:** Hyperthermia, violent behavior, anxiety, confusion, insomnia, paranoia, auditory hallucinations, mood disturbances, delusions, out-of-control rages	Fatigue, insomnia or hypersomnia Vivid unpleasant dreams Increase in appetite Increased or decreased psychomotor activity Dysphoric mood, apathy, anhedonia Drug craving, marked symptoms or "crashing" often followed intense use or "speed-run" Chronic user may experience depression, anxiety, fatigue, paranoia, aggression, intense craving for drug Methamphetamine can cause extensive long-term damage to dopamine-producing cells	Can be smoked, snorted, swallowed, or injected Smoking or injecting followed by rush or "flash" lasting a few minutes (described as pleasurable by user) Snorting or smoking produces euphoria, but not intense rush Snorting produces effects within 3–5 min, oral within 15–20 min May take episodic (intense drug use separated by periods of nonuse) or daily Intensive high dose called "speed-runs" or "binges"—usually by injection Tolerance for methamphetamine occurs within minutes, after which user tries to maintain high by binging on drug Ice smoke is odorless, but leaves a residue that can be res-moked—high for 12+ h Longer lasting and more toxic effect on the brain and dopamine cells than amphetamine Street names: Ice, crank, Cristal, Krystal Meth, speed, meth, chalk, glass	Decreased appetite with extreme weight loss, severe dental problems, insomnia, mood disturbances, Hepatitis B and C, HIV and other diseases via contaminated injection use Cognitive impairment with structural and functional changes in areas of brain associated with emotion and memory

(continued)

TABLE 15.2   Substance-Related Information *(Continued)*

INTOXICATON	WITHDRAWAL	SUBSTANCE-RELATED INFORMATION	SIGNS AND SYMPTOMS OF ASSOCIATED DISORDER
Marijuana/Cannabis			
Red and bloodshot eyes, increased appetite, dry mouth, tachycardia, loud rapid talking with bursts of laughter, silly and giggly for no reason, strong odor on breath or clothing Loses train of thought easily distorted sense of time, short-term memory impairment, impaired judgment and perception Negative developmental effects in youth Sleepiness, stupor, dizzy with trouble walking	Physical and mental lethargy, anhedonia, depression, anxiety, hallucinogen-like mental effects, paranoid ideation	Most widespread and frequently used illicit drug Long-term use can lead to loss of ambition and purpose Teens who smoke are eight times more likely to use marijuana Average age for first use is 14 y of age Drug available today can be five times more potent than 20 y ago Street names: Joint, pot, herb, grass, hay, stick, weed, Mary Jane, reefer, Aunt Mary, skunk, boom, gangster, kif, ganja, Texas tea, Maui wowie, chronic, locoweed, hashish, bhang, cha-ras, Sweet Lucy, Yerba, Grifa, Sinsemilla	Euphoria and inappropriate laughter Grandiosity Sedation Lethargy Impaired short-term memory Delayed mental processing Impaired judgment Distorted sensory perception Impaired motor function Anxiety Dysphoria Social withdrawal Conjunctival redness Increased appetite Dry mouth Tachycardia
Cocaine			
Increasing difficulty to abstain from use, with need for frequent dosing for "high" (short half-life) Cardiac arrhythmias, dilated pupils, blood pressure changes Runny nose, chronic sinus problems, nosebleed Nausea/vomiting, weight loss Diaphoresis, chills, muscle weakness, chest pain, respiratory depression Confusion, seizures, dyski-nesias, coma, death	Fatigue, insomnia or hypersomnia Increased appetite Unpleasant dreams, delusions, hallucina-tions (auditory and tactile "coke bugs") Psychomotor increase or decrease Mood changes (depression, suicidal ideation, irritability, anhedonia, attention disturbance) Craving with seeing any white powder	"Crack," the chunk or "rock" form is ready to use or freebase Is generally snorted or dissolved in water and injected (rarely smoked because it is destroyed by high heat temperature) Snorting reaches brain in 3–5 min; injectable produces rush in 15–30 s; smoking produces immediate experience Euphoric effects almost indistin-guishable from methamphet-amine, but do not last as long Gives temporary illusion of enhanced power and energy Depression occurs as elevated mood fades Can lead to permanent vegetative or zombie-like state One million plus chronic users in United States Street names: Coke, flake, snow, dust, happy dust, girl, Cecil, blow, crack, coca, Blanca, perico, nieve, soda	Paranoid ideation Aggression Anxiety Weight loss Rambling speech Headache Ringing in ears "Coke bugs" tactile hal-lucinations Auditory hallucinations Erratic behavior Social isolation Mood changes Suicidal ideation Irritability Anhedonia Emotional swings Inattentiveness Use during pregnancy associated with miscar-riages, stillbirths, or drug-dependent babies
Hallucinogen/Club Drugs			
Extremely dilated pupils, blurred vision, (LSD-low-ered body temperature), (Ecstasy-elevated body temperature), "goose bumps," diaphoresis, body odor, nausea, tachycardia, tremors, incoordination Mood and behavior changes	Flashbacks with per-sisting perception disorder days or even months after an LSD "trip"	Drugs such as LSD (acid) or "designer" drugs such as Ecstasy (MDMA) Used as "raves" or "trances" at clubs and bars Many are tasteless, colorless, and odorless—undetectable in beverages, and may be admin-istered to person without his or her knowledge	Mood swings Fearfulness Anxiety Feelings of going insane Perceptual disturbance Impaired judgment Increase in blood sugar Increase in cortisol hor-mones

TABLE 15.2   Substance-Related Information *(Continued)*

INTOXICATON	WITHDRAWAL	SUBSTANCE-RELATED INFORMATION	SIGNS AND SYMPTOMS OF ASSOCIATED DISORDER

Distorted sensory perception
Unpredictable flashbacks with symptoms similar to those during usage (geometric forms, peripheral field images, flashes of color, intensified colors, images left suspended in path of moving object, afterimages or shadows, halos around objects)
Perceptual disturbance and impaired judgment (may cause accidents or attempts to fly from high places)
		After oral ingestion, effects felt within 30–45 min, peak at 60–90 min, and last 4–6 hr
		Usually sold in form of impregnated paper with colorful graphic designs (blotter acid), tablets (microdots), thin squares of gelatin (window panes), and in sugar cubes
		Street names:
		  LSD—acid, blotter, dots, L, sugar, cubes, big D, angel dust, hog, peace pill, Mesc
		  Ecstasy—XTC, Adam, Georgia Hoe Boy, Businessman's trip, serenity
		  Ketamine-K—Special K, cat, Valium (Veterinary anesthetic used as liquid applied to marijuana or tobacco powder for sniffing)
		  Rophypnol—Roofies, roche, forget-me (illegal but similar to Valium)
			Psychiatric disturbances with long-term cognitive impairment
			Increased body temperature can result in organ failure and death

Inhalants			
Odor of paint or glue on breath or clothes Runny nose, watery eyes, conjunctival irritation, coughing, dyspnea, blurred vision, slurred speech Poor coordination, drowsiness, stupor, lethargy, depressed reflexes and muscle weakness, tremors Euphoria Possession of bags or rags with dried solvents, discarded pressurized aerosol containers, or bags of balloons Glue-sniffer's rash around nose or mouth May be painted on hands, fingernails, or placed on shirt sleeves or wrist bands to allow continuous use such as in a classroom	Clinically meaningful withdrawal syndrome has not been established, but many first-time users have serious respiratory problems and permanent brain damage Among first drugs children use, as many as 6% use by fourth grade	Sniffed directly from open container, huffed from a rag soaked in substance, or filled balloon held to the face Open container or soaked rag can be placed in bag where vapors concentrate before being inhaled Lungs allow rapid absorption with rapidly peaking blood levels that penetrate the brain Known on street as huffing, sniffing, and wanging Solvent: nail polish remover, rubber glue or varnish, pocket lighters are "huffed," felt-tip markers are placed in sandwich bag and stepped on or crushed to breathe the vapors Nitrous oxide gas: propellant in canned whipped cream and in "whippets," hair spray, vegetable oil spray, deodorant spray, computer cleaner, fabric protector spray Amyl nitrate: poppers or snappers—tiny ampoules Butyl nitrite: Sold as tape head cleaner referred to as "rush," "locker room," or "climax" Street names: glue, kick, bang, sniff, huff, poppers, whippets, Texas shoeshine	Confusion Belligerence Aggression Apathy Impaired judgment and social functioning Hallucinations and delusions Perceptual changes Respiratory distress Sinus problems Gastrointestinal disturbances Slowed psychomotor response Cardiac arrhythmias Death (SSDS)

(continued)

TABLE 15.2   Substance-Related Information *(Continued)*

INTOXICATON	WITHDRAWAL	SUBSTANCE-RELATED INFORMATION	SIGNS AND SYMPTOMS OF ASSOCIATED DISORDER
Opiods (Morphine, Codeine, Oxycodone, Hydrocodone)			
Drowsiness, lethargy, slurred speech, constricted pupils that are nonreactive to light, scars on inner arms from injecting, memory and attention impairment	Anxiety, restlessness, irritability Fever, muscle aches in back and legs Increased sensitivity to pain Nausea and vomiting Lacrimation and rhinorrhea, dilated pupils, sweating, diarrhea Insomnia Craving	Oxycodone and hydrocodone are often dissolved and injected—most frequently encountered opiate pharmaceutical in forensic evidence Hydrocodone ranked no. 6 among all controlled substances for abuse by DEA Street names: Harry, horse, Miss Emma, Schoolboy, lords, dollies, perkies, T's, BigO, black stuff	Use during pregnancy causes miscarriages, stillbirths, and drug-dependent babies Initial high followed by dysphoria, apathy Incoordination and impaired judgment Memory lapse Respiratory depression Death Sharing needles are leading cause of HIV, Hepatits B and C
Heroin			
Converts to morphine Particularly addictive because of rapid entry across blood–brain barrier "Rush" is accompanied by warm flushing of skin, dry mouth, and heavy feelings in extremities Nausea/vomiting Severe itching Drowsiness and mental lethargy Slowed cardiac and respiratory function	May occur within a few hours after last use Restlessness and leg movements Muscle and bone pain Diarrhea Vomiting Cold flashes with goose bumps (cold turkey) Insomnia Symptoms usually peak between 24–48 hr after last use	Can be injected, smoked or snorted Regular use can lead to tolerance and dependence Black tar (Mexican) heroin sold in chunks weighing about 1 oz "Cheese" is new face of heroin (Tylenol PM + Black tar heroin)—use coffee grinder to make powder for snorting "Cheese" packaged in small baggies known as "bumps" for snorting through straws or tubes from ball-point pens Can be hid in hoodies, pants, underwear, tennis shoes, backpacks, hair buns Street names: H, junk, skag, smack, "black tar," "bag" (small unit sold on street usually mixed with sugar, starch, acetaminophen, or other cutting agents)	Miscarriages Heart infections Death from overdose HIV/AIDS Hepatitis B and C Collapsed veins Abscesses Arthritis and rheumatological problems Liver or kidney disease
Phencyclidine (PCP)			
Unpredictable behavior, violence Mood swings, disorientation, fear, terror Feeling of detachment, distant, and estranged from surroundings Slurred speech Numbness Poor coordination, ataxia, strange gait, rigid muscles Nystagmus (constant involuntary movement of eyeball) Dilated pupils and blank stare Masklike facial appearance Decreased response to pain and sensory perception Hypertension, tachycardia Hyperacusis (abnormal sensitivity to sound) Seizures and coma	Peak effects 2 hr after oral use with mild effects resolving after 8–20 hr/severe in several days Psychotic disorder may persist for weeks Dependence on other substances complicates withdrawal	White crystalline powder readily dissolvable in water Most PCP on illicit market contains contaminants Also sold in tablets, capsules, and liquid Commonly applied to a leafy material such as parsley, mint, oregano, or marijuana and smoked Street names: angel dust, supergrass, killer weed Also found in embalming fluid, rocket fuel	Inability to control emotions, anxiety, rage, aggression, panic Flashbacks Disorganized thinking Hyperthermia Hypertension Seizures Needle tracks Hepatitis B and C HIV/AIDS Delirium Psychosis Catatonic posturing Coma

TABLE 15.2   Substance-Related Information *(Continued)*

INTOXICATON	WITHDRAWAL	SUBSTANCE-RELATED INFORMATION	SIGNS AND SYMPTOMS OF ASSOCIATED DISORDER
Sedatives, Hypnotics, or Anxiolytics			
Slurred speech Incoordination, seeming intoxicated but without an odor Flat affect Impaired attention and memory Nystagmus Stupor and coma	Sweating Tachycardia Increased hand tremors and psychomotor agitation Insomnia Nausea/vomiting Hallucinations Anxiety Grand mal seizures	Newer drug of abuse GHB, an odorless, colorless liquid or white powder Includes barbiturates, benzodiazepines, flunitrazepam (utilized as party or "date rape" drug), paraldehyde, chloral hydrate, meprobamate, Ambien, and Sonata Street names: liquid ecstasy, scoop, easy lay, Georgia Home Boy, grievous bodily harm, liquid X, goop, "rophies," "roofies," "roach"	Maladaptive behavior change Labile mood Impaired cognitive and CNS functioning Inappropriate sexual behavior Aggression Impaired mobility and coordination Cardiac arrhythmias Hypertension Insomnia
Caffeine			
Recent consumption in excess of 250 mg Restlessness and nervousness Excitement and insomnia Flushed face Diuresis Gastrointestinal complaints More than 1 g/d may cause muscle twitching, rambling thoughts and speech, cardiac arrhythmias, hyperactivity and agitation	Headache Lethargy Decreased alertness, drowsiness, and sleepiness Depressed mood Difficulty concentrating Irritability Onset usually begins 12–24 hr after abstinence with peak at 20–51 hr Duration of symptoms from 2 to 9 d Research continues on whether caffeine is addictive		Tachycardia, cardiac arrhythmias Gastrointestinal disturbances Agitation and restlessness
Anabolic Steroids			
Hypertension Elevated cholesterol levels Severe acne Premature balding Reduced sexual function Testicular atrophy Gynecomastia in males Masculinizing effect in females Premature growth retardation in adolescents Psychotic reactions and manic episodes Anger or hostility Aggression and violence	Drugs used to prevent or treat adverse effects of anabolic steroid use include tamoxifen, diuretics, and human chorionic gonadotropin	Illicit users tend to "stack" the drugs, using multiple drugs concurrently "Cycling" is period of 6–14 wk followed by abstinence to avoid tolerance "Pyramiding" slowly escalates steroid use by increasing number of drugs used at one time or the dose and frequency of one or more drugs, peaking at mid-cycle, and gradually tapering doses toward end of cycle Most are sold at gyms, competitions, and mail-order operations Various preparations are intended for human or veterinary use are smuggled from other countries Many bogus or counterfeit products sold	Not definitely known Increasing concern of cardiovascular damage, cerebrovascular toxicity, and liver damage related to abuse

(continued)

TABLE 15.2   Substance-Related Information (*Continued*)

INTOXICATON	WITHDRAWAL	SUBSTANCE-RELATED INFORMATION	SIGNS AND SYMPTOMS OF ASSOCIATED DISORDER
Nicotine			
Dizziness	Depressed mood		Risk of lung/oral cancer
Nausea	Insomnia		Risk of cardiovascular and
Tobacco odor on breath, clothes, hair	Irritability and frustration		cerebrovascular disease
Cough	Anxiety		
COPD	Difficult concentration		
Excessive skin wrinkling	Bradycardia		
	Increased appetite with weight gain		
Bath Salts (Synthetic Methamphetamine Cocaine or MDVP)			
Euphoria	Hallucinations, paranoia, extreme psychosis (similar to LSD), insomnia, leg cramps, nausea/vomiting, runny nose, sneezing, extreme sweating, hot/cold flashes, severe headaches, tachycardia, hypertension, extreme weakness	Found in many bath products	Permanent psychosis with delusions and flashbacks, paranoia, can cause death
Makes user talkative		May also contain mephedrone	
Sexual arousal		Recently made Schedule I drugs in United States	
Enhanced creativity, and emotional high		Difficult come down period	
Tachycardia and chest tightening		Sold in drug paraphernalia stores under names: Ivory Wave, Purple Wave, Red Dove, Blue Silk, Zoom, Bloom, Cloud Nine, Ocean Snow, Lunar Wave, Vanilla Sky, White Lightning, Scarface, Hurricane Charlie, Super Coke, meow, drone	
Anorexia			
Disturbed sleep pattern			
Involuntary body movements (smacking lips or twitching)			
Hyperactivity		May be ingested, smoked, sniffed, injected	
anxiety, paranoia, hallucinations, psychotic episodes, Agitation			
K2 Spice (Synthetic or Designer Marijuana)			
Elevated mood, relaxation, altered perception, extreme anxiety, paranoia, hallucinations, possible psychotic effects	Loss of control, lack of pain response, pale skin, profuse sweating, uncontrolled spastic body movements, increased heart rate, palpitations, dysphoria, hallucinations, psychotic effects	Wide variety of herbal mixtures marketed as safe legal alternatives to cannabis and produce similar experiences	Rapid heart rate, vomiting, agitation, confusion, hallucinations, hypertension, myocardial ischemia, heart attack
		Sold under names K2, fake weed, Yucatan Fire, Skunkm, Moon Rocks, Bliss, Black Mamba, Bombay Blue, Blaze, Genie, Zohai, Yucatan Fire, JWH-018, 073, 250	Some effects still unknown
		Contains dried, shredded plant material and chemical additives responsible for the psychoactive effects	
		DEA has designated the five active chemicals found in Spice as Schedule I controlled substances	
		Sold in small silvery plastic bags as "incense" and resemble potpourri	
		May be smoked or used as herbal drink	

BOX 15.5

Common Signs of Substance-Induced Disorders

- Substance-specific symptoms that may include the following:
  - Anxiety, depression, and withdrawal
  - Possible manic or psychotic reactions
  - Hyperactivity
  - Elevated blood pressure and heartrate
  - Agitation
  - Shakes
  - Drowsiness
  - Memory problems
  - Inability to concentrate
  - Impaired problem solving

Signs of a substance-induced disorder are found in Box 15.5.

Substance-Specific Use Disorders

Substance-use disorders are patterns of cognitive, behavioral, and physiological symptoms resulting from continued use of a substance regardless of the problems experienced as a result. A 2010 National Household Survey on Drug Abuse estimated the number of users of illicit drugs in the United States at over 22 million. The diagnosis of substance-use disorder can be applied to all 10 classes of drugs listed in Box 15.1, except caffeine. Although the ingestion of caffeine can produce effects on the CNS, the diagnostic criteria for a substance-use disorder are not associated with this substance.

The symptoms can occur from mild to severe depending on the number of the diagnostic indicators that are present. Mild is usually indicated with two or three symptoms, moderate by four to five symptoms, and severe by six or more symptoms. Common signs of substance-use disorders are found in Box 15.7. Each substance is associated with one or both of the substance-induced disorders of intoxication and withdrawal. Alcohol, amphetamines, cocaine, inhalants, cannabis, and hallucinogens all have the potential of causing the psychoactive symptoms. The substances are also associated with some or all of the mental disorders listed in Box 15.6.

BOX 15.6

Other Substance-Related Conditions

- Delirium
- Amnesic disorder
- Psychotic disorder, with delusions
- Psychotic disorder, with hallucinations
- Mood disorder
- Anxiety disorder
- Sexual dysfunction
- Sleep disorder

Alcohol-Use Disorder

Alcohol is the most commonly used brain depressant in most cultures and the cause of considerable associated physiological problems and sometimes death. Ninety percent of adults in the United States have used alcohol to some degree, but most people are able to moderate their drinking and avoid related problems. Statistical data show that nearly 7% of Americans over 12 years of age are binge drinkers of alcohol. According to the National Council on Drug Abuse, alcohol abuse was associated with nearly half of all fatal motor vehicle accidents.

Signs and Symptoms

The use of alcohol is associated with a significant increase in the risk of accidents, violence, and suicide. In people with antisocial personality disorder, there is also an increase in the incidence of related criminal acts. An increase in absenteeism from work, job-related accidents, and decreased employee productivity are commonly linked to alcohol.

BOX 15.7

Common Signs of Substance-Use Disorders

- Denial of the drug problem
- Tolerance and withdrawal from continued use of a substance
- Strong urge or desire to use drug despite negative consequences or craving of the substance
- Substance is taken in larger amounts over longer period than was intended
- Unsuccessful attempts and inability to control substance use
- Much time is spent in pursuit of obtaining the substance
- Important activities are given up because of substance use

In addition, chronic use of alcohol can result in an encephalopathy and psychosis known as **Wernicke–Korsakoff syndrome**. This is a nutritional disease of the nervous system found in alcoholics, caused primarily by thiamine and niacin deficiency. Significant cerebral deterioration and actual brain cell death occur with chronic and permanent impairment. With Wernicke's encephalopathy and Korsakoff's psychosis, there is progressive memory loss and disorientation with emotional lability and apathy, weakness, and fatigue.

Alcohol-induced delirium, or **delirium tremens** (DTs), is a state of profound confusion and delusions along with all of the usual withdrawal symptoms that are seen within a short period following cessation of alcohol use. The episode generally ends after several days of insomnia and rigorous activity when the person falls into a deep sleep. On awakening, the person is coherent but without memory of the events during the delirium. The delirium may last from 72 to 80 hours, during which there is a 20% fatality rate.

Just the Facts

The development of seizure activity during DTs is a life-threatening situation and must be considered a medical emergency.

Withdrawal from alcohol can cause anxiety, tremors, seizures, and hallucinations. Repeated intake of high doses of alcohol can affect nearly every body system and may result in liver failure, heart enlargement, and cancer of the pancreas, stomach, and esophagus.

Incidence and Etiology

Alcoholism is prevalent across all educational and socioeconomic levels. Alcohol abuse and dependence is more common in men. Women are reported to start drinking at a later age than do men, but dependence progresses more rapidly in women. Women also tend to develop a higher blood alcohol concentration because of their lower body water, higher percentage of body fat, and slower metabolic rate and thus may be at greater risk for subsequent liver damage than men.

There is a strong familial pattern of alcohol-related problems, with an estimated 40% to 60% of occurrences thought to be genetically linked. Environmental factors account for the remainder (see previous discussion on theoretical causation).

Mind Jogger

Research shows women tend to use alcohol as a "hidden habit." Why do you think this happens?

Cannabis-Use Disorder

Cannabis or marijuana (bhang) is derived from the cannabis plant and is used widely in the form of rolled cigarettes. Although usually smoked, marijuana may be taken orally mixed in tea or food. The cannabinoid chemicals present in the plant are primarily responsible for the psychoactive effects (Table 15.2).

Signs and Symptoms

The essential features include a high feeling followed by euphoria, inappropriate laughter, grandiosity, sedation, lethargy, impaired short-term memory, delayed mental processing, impaired judgment, distorted sensory perceptions, and impaired motor function. There may be accompanying anxiety, dysphoria, or social withdrawal as the use increases. Within 2 hours after marijuana use, there is conjunctival redness, increased appetite, dry mouth, and increased heart rate.

Just the Facts

Cannabis drug effects usually last 3 to 4 hours. Because the drug is fat soluble, the effects may be detected in the urine for 7 to 10 days and up to 4 weeks in heavy users.

Cannabis is often used with other substances such as alcohol, cocaine, and nicotine. It can also be mixed and smoked with opioids, Phencyclidine (PCP), or hallucinogenic drugs. In people who use high doses, regular use commonly results in depression, anxiety, and irritability, with psychoactive effects similar to those of the hallucinogens. High use can also result in severe anxiety or panic attacks, as well as episodes of paranoid delusional thinking or depersonalization. Chronic cannabis use is associated with weight gain, sinusitis, pharyngitis, bronchitis with persistent cough, and emphysema. Although there is an increase in respiratory illnesses among people who smoke marijuana frequently, the actual carcinogenic effects of cannabis or risk for lung cancer have not yet been determined.

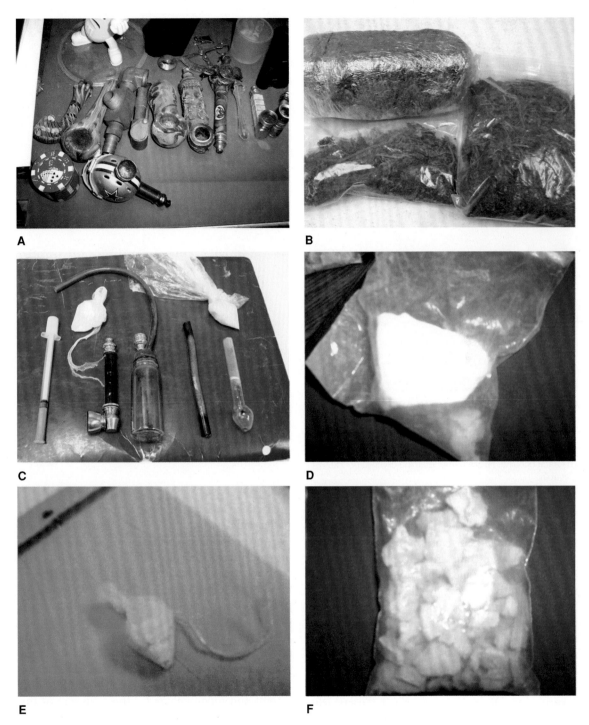

FIGURE 15.2

Common illegal drugs and paraphernalia. **A:** Various pipes used to smoke marijuana. **B:** Bricks of marijuana. **C:** Items used to freebase or inject drugs. **D:** Block cocaine. **E:** "Street buy" of powder cocaine. **F:** Crack cocaine. (*Continued*)

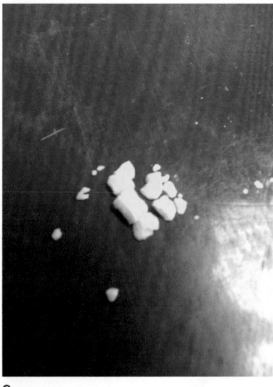

G

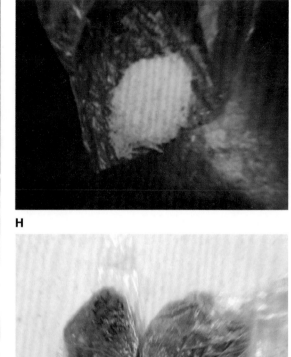

H

I

FIGURE 15.2

G: Crack cocaine. **H:** Methamphetamine crystals or "ice."
I: Heroin.

Incidence and Etiology

The cannabis drugs are the most widely used illicit psychoactive substance in the United States. Statistics demonstrate little gender difference in onset of drug usage, but studies show women tend to enter treatment with fewer years of regular use. The highest prevalence is seen in 18- to 34-year-olds. Surveys show that around 40% of adolescents have used marijuana. It is known that marijuana affects brain development, and with heavy use, its effects on thinking and memory may be permanent. According to the National Institute on Drug Abuse, marijuana users who started using marijuana in adolescence showed a significant decrease in the functioning of the brain areas responsible for learning and memory. It is not known how many reported cases of cannabis-related disorders exist.

Hallucinogen-Use Disorder

Hallucinogens are usually taken orally, although injection does occur. Tolerance to the euphoric and psychedelic effects of these substances develops rather quickly, but there is no clear documented evidence regarding a withdrawal pattern that falls into the criteria for a disorder. However, most users continue to use hallucinogens despite knowledge of the adverse effects, such as memory impairment, panic reactions, or flashback episodes (bad trips) that may occur during drug intoxication.

PCP is not a difficult drug to obtain and is commonly used several times a week by those with dependence on the substance. Users often demonstrate dangerous behaviors because of lack of insight and judgment under the influence of the drug. Aggressive behaviors such as fighting are a particular problem with PCP use. The drug can be taken orally, injected, or smoked. PCP is the most commonly abused substance of the drug compounds in this category.

Signs and Symptoms

Under the influence of a hallucinogenic drug, the person may display mood swings, fearfulness, anxiety, and feelings of going insane or dying.

Many of these drugs have stimulant effects similar to those of amphetamine intoxication. The perceptual disturbances and impaired judgment seen in toxic episodes or flashbacks may result in fatal accidents such as users believing they can fly and subsequently jumping from a building or bridge. Associated physiological changes include increases in blood glucose and cortisol hormones. LSD intoxication is usually confirmed through urine sampling.

Psychological effects of PCP may include inability to control emotions, anxiety, rage, aggression, panic, flashbacks, and disorganized thinking. Medical problems such as hyperthermia, hypertension, and seizures can compound the picture with recurrent PCP use. Other indicators of use may be nystagmus, hypertension, evidence of needle tracks, hepatitis, or HIV disease. Those with substance intoxication may exhibit delirium, psychotic symptoms, catatonic posturing, or coma.

Incidence and Etiology

Use of and intoxication with hallucinogens usually begins during adolescence. Younger users may experience more intense emotional states as a result of the drug effects. Use is shown to be three times more common in men than women. There was an increased incidence of use in the United States during the 1960s and 1970s. Despite a decline following this period, it is reported that there was a slight increase in use during the late 1990s. Hallucinogens are used most by individuals between the ages of 26 and 34 years. Environmental factors, along with the personality and expectations of the person using the drug, may contribute to the decision to use these substances. The prevalence of PCP use is more common in men 20 to 40 years of age. It is reported that about 3% of drug-related emergency room visits and deaths are related to PCP use. The highest percentage of initial use is seen in the 12- to 17-year-old age group.

Inhalant-Related Disorders

Most drug compounds containing nitrous oxide that are inhaled can produce psychoactive effects. Tolerance is reported with heavy use, although withdrawal patterns that meet the criteria for an assigned disorder have not been documented. Because inhalants are inexpensive, legal, and easily accessible, they tend to be used over a longer time. This may result in the person spending more

time recuperating and giving up important social, occupational, or recreational activities. Substance use often continues despite the person's awareness of both physical and psychological problems caused by the chemicals.

Signs and Symptoms

Behavioral or psychological changes include confusion, belligerence, aggression, apathy, and impaired judgment and social functioning. Hallucinations, delusional thinking, and perceptual changes may develop during periods of confusion and intoxication. These changes are usually accompanied by dizziness, visual disturbances, unsteady gait, tremors, and euphoria. Higher doses can lead to lethargy, slowed psychomotor response, muscle weakness, and stupor. People who use inhalants usually have an odor of paint or solvent on their breath or clothing with a residue "glue-sniffer's rash" evident around the nose and mouth. There may be redness of the eyes, respiratory distress, rales or rhonchi, coughing, sinus discharge, headache, weakness, and abdominal pain with nausea or vomiting. Inhalants can cause permanent damage to both the central and the peripheral nervous system. Death can occur from cardiac arrhythmias or respiratory failure, commonly referred to as "sudden sniffing death." Box 15.8 provides interventions for the person who is inhaling or huffing.

Just the Facts

"Sudden sniffing death syndrome" can occur with the use of inhalants, on the first incident or any time. Death is the result of acute cardiac arrhythmias, hypoxia, or electrolyte imbalances as the inhaled substance sensitizes the heart muscle to the body's own adrenaline, leading to a fatal heart rhythm disturbance.

BOX 15.8

Interventions for the Person Who Is Inhaling or Huffing

- Use a calm approach—do not excite or argue with the person (can become aggressive)
- Try to determine what substance was used (aerosol cans, bags, rags, etc. can provide clues)
- Keep person calm in a well-ventilated environment (may have respiratory difficulty)
- Avoid stimulation (can cause hallucinations or violence)
- Get help for the user as quickly as possible!

During adolescence, the use of inhalants may first be noticed because of school-related problems such as truancy, a drop in grades, or dropping out of school. Most adolescents use inhalants under the influence of peer pressure in a group setting. However, heavy usage tends to be a solitary pattern.

Incidence and Etiology

Because of the easy accessibility of these drugs, it is difficult to track the actual number of inhalant users. However, there tends to be a pattern of usage beginning in the 9- to 12-year-old age group with peak usage during adolescence. It is more prevalent in males than in females. Over the past 10 years, the prevalence of sniffing glue and aerosols such as whipped topping and spray paint has increased. There is also a rise in reports of lighter fluid inhalation, with a higher incidence in deprived populations, especially in children and adolescents.

Opioid-Related Disorders

Heroin, which may be injected or snorted, is the most abused drug in this class. In addition, opioid drugs are regularly prescribed treatments and are contained in analgesics, anesthetics, antidiarrheal agents, and cough suppressants. Heroin is synthesized from morphine, a natural substance extracted from the seed pod of the Asian opium poppy plant. It usually appears as a white or brown powder or as a black sticky substance, known as "black tar heroin."

Two commonly prescribed opioids are oxycodone and hydrocodone. Like morphine, oxycodone is generally prescribed as an analgesic. Hydrocodone is effective as a cough suppressant and analgesic. All oxycodone products (OxyContin, OxyIR, Percodan, Percocet) are Schedule II drugs. They are abused orally, crushed and sniffed, or dissolved and injected. Hydrocodone is usually prescribed for pain relief in combination with acetaminophen (Vicoden and Lortab), but is also combined with aspirin (Lortab ASA), ibuprofen (Vicoprofen), and antihistamines (Hycomine). As of February 2013, all strengths, formulations, and combinations of products of hydrocodone are Schedule II controlled substances. Included also in this stricter control is a prohibited automatic refill of these products. The hydrocodone products are the most frequently prescribed drug agents for pain in the

United States. Despite this medicinal advantage, these are among the most abused pharmaceutical drugs and are associated with drug trafficking, diversion, and addiction. Law enforcement documentation of diversion by theft, doctor shopping, fraudulent prescriptions, phony "called-in" prescriptions, and internet fraud is widespread. Research now suggests that abuse of the prescription opioid pain medications such as Vicoden and Lortab may lead to subsequent heroin abuse.

Opioid dependence is evident by compulsive, prolonged self-administration of these substances for no legitimate medical reason. The drugs are usually purchased through illegal channels or by faking medical conditions to acquire multiple prescriptions from different physicians. Health care professionals with opioid dependence may resort to drug diversion in their place of employment or to prescription forgery to obtain the drug (see the section "Substance Abuse by Health Care Professionals in this chapter).

Signs and Symptoms

With opioid intoxication there is an initial high followed by apathy, depressed mood, inability to coordinate motor functioning, and impaired judgment. These changes are accompanied by drowsiness, slurred speech, inattention, memory lapses, and pupil constriction. Severe intoxication can lead to respiratory depression, unconsciousness, and death. Opioid dependence is commonly associated with a history of drug-related crimes and unprofessional conduct among health professionals who have access to controlled drugs. Periods of depression are common after repeated use of the drug.

Incidence and Etiology

The incidence of opioid drug use has increased among white middle-class people, especially in women. There is an increased risk in medical and other health professionals. The prevalence for opioid use tends to decrease after age 40. Men are three times more likely to use heroin than women. Use most commonly begins during late teens or early 20s. According to the National Council on Drug Abuse, a 2011 survey showed approximately 4.2 million Americans aged 12 or older had used heroin at least once. Estimates show that approximately 23% of individuals who use heroin develop substance dependence. Heroin use is more common among men, with a 3:1 ratio over women. Survey reports from 2003 show the highest rate of heroin use among high school seniors since the 1970s. Use most commonly begins during the late teens or early 20s. Family members of people with opioid dependence typically have an increased incidence of other substance-related disorders or antisocial personality disorder.

Stimulant-Use Disorder

The amphetamine and amphetamine-type stimulants include both those sold on the illegal market and those that may be obtained by prescription for the treatment of obesity, attention-deficit/hyperactivity disorder (ADHD), and narcolepsy. Most of the effects of these drugs are similar to those of cocaine, although the risk for inducing cardiac arrhythmias and seizures is lower.

Crack cocaine is the most common form of cocaine used in the United States today. It is easily vaporized and inhaled, making the onset of effects particularly rapid. Cocaine has extremely potent euphoric effects, which increases the potential for dependence after the drug has been used for a very short time. An early sign of dependence is that the person is unable to resist using the drug when it is available. Because of the 30- to 50-minute half-life of the drug, the user must use the drug frequently to maintain the high. This short effect and the craving for more lead users to spend thousands of dollars in a short time, with devastating personal and financial consequences. Most people with dependence have signs of tolerance and withdrawal at some point.

Methamphetamine is a powerful chemical substance similar to the neurotransmitter dopamine. Because of this similarity, methamphetamine can change the function of any neuron that contains dopamine. It can also affect neurons that contain the neurotransmitters serotonin and norepinephrine. Methamphetamine is able to trick the neurons into taking it up just like they would dopamine. For this reason, the person feels an initial "high" that eventually stops and ends in a surge of unpleasant feelings called a "crash." This leads the person to use more of the drug with less and less chance of obtaining the pleasurable feeling.

Amphetamines are used medically as an aid in treating narcolepsy, some forms of depression, obesity, and ADHD. Adderall and Ritalin, commonly prescribed brand names for ADHD, are the most commonly abused prescription stimulants. They are often abused by high school and college students as a means to keep them awake in school or for test preparation. The drugs are typically crushed and snorted or dissolved in water and injected.

Signs and Symptoms

Common mental and physical complications of chronic cocaine use are paranoid ideation, anxiety, and weight loss. There may be rambling speech, headache, ringing in the ears, and tactile (coke bugs) and auditory hallucinations. The withdrawal symptoms are likely to enhance craving and the likelihood of reusing the drug. Because of its powerful effects on the CNS, it is common to see erratic and aggressive behaviors. Mood changes such as depression with suicidal ideation, irritability, anhedonia, emotional swings, and inattentiveness are also seen. The substance takes over the person's life to the point of social isolation.

The psychoactive effects of most amphetamine-type stimulants last longer than those of cocaine, and the stimulating effects on the autonomic nervous system may be more potent. The person may develop mood changes, weight loss, and malnutrition. Chronic abuse produces a psychosis that resembles schizophrenia with paranoia, picking at the skin, delusions, and hallucinations. Violent and erratic behavior is frequently seen among chronic abusers. It is common for users of amphetamine to also use alcohol and benzodiazepine antianxiety drug agents to calm the jittery feelings caused by the stimulant.

Incidence and Etiology

Most data that have been collected are based on usage patterns rather than disorders. The actual percentage of those who use or abuse cocaine and have diagnosed disorders is not known. Cocaine use is seen in all races and socioeconomic, age, and gender groups. Although the overall prevalence of cocaine use in the United States has decreased, the highest rate increase in 2003 was in 18- to 25-year-olds. There is a tendency for men to be more commonly affected than women.

The pattern of amphetamine and methamphetamine usage fluctuates by geographic location, with a greater concentration in heavily populated areas. The peak use of these drugs is between 26 to 34 years of age. High school students represent about 16% of users. Chronic use often leads to decreased effectiveness. Some move on to other addictive substances, whereas others decrease or stop using amphetamines after 8 to 10 years.

Caffeine-Use Disorder

Caffeine is found in many different sources including coffee, caffeinated soda, tea, over-the-counter pain relievers, cold remedies, antidrowsiness aids, and weight-loss agents. Chocolate and cocoa have a lower caffeine content than the other sources listed. There is no link between the intake of caffeine and a clinical picture that meets the criteria for substance dependence or abuse. There is evidence that caffeine intoxication and withdrawal may be clinically significant.

Just the Facts

The average consumption of caffeine in the United States is approximately 500 mg/d. Intake in excess of 10 g can cause grand mal seizures, respiratory failure, and death.

Signs and Symptoms

Mild sensory alterations, such as ringing in the ears or flashing lights, have been reported by those who are heavy users. Physical symptoms from excessive intake may include anxiety, agitation, restlessness, sweating, flushed face, and diarrhea. There are some reports of cardiac arrhythmias and gastrointestinal discomfort.

Incidence and Etiology

The use of caffeine and caffeine-related products is seen across all cultural groups. Consumption is much greater in Sweden, Norway, Denmark, Great Britain, and other European countries. Intake tends to decrease with age and is greater in men than in women. Caffeine is used more among those who smoke or use alcohol and other substances. The prevalence of caffeine-related disorders is unknown.

Nicotine-Use Disorder

Although not considered a maladaptive drug by most users, nicotine is included in the *DSM-5* substance category for abuse and dependence. The health dangers related to cigarette smoking are well publicized, with warning labels related to these health hazards printed on all tobacco products. Nicotine dependence can develop with use of all forms of tobacco (cigarettes, cigars, chewing tobacco, snuff, and pipes). The nicotine content of tobacco, added to the repetitive nature of its use, contributes to its ability to produce rapid dependence. Tolerance to nicotine is demonstrated by a more intense effect

the first time it is used without producing adverse effects such as dizziness or nausea.

Signs and Symptoms

The most common signs of dependence are tobacco odor, cough, excessive skin wrinkling, and chronic pulmonary disease. Tobacco use markedly increases the risk of lung, oral, and other cancers and increases the risk for cardiovascular and cerebrovascular conditions.

Nicotine withdrawal symptoms are experienced within 24 hours of cessation or reduction in usage. Symptoms include a depressed mood, insomnia, irritability, frustration, anxiety, decreased concentration, restlessness, bradycardia, and increased appetite with weight gain. These symptoms usually peak in intensity between the first and fourth days with considerable improvement by 3 to 4 weeks. The hunger and weight gain may persist for 6 months or more.

Incidence and Etiology

Nicotine use usually begins in the early teens, and about 95% of those who continue to smoke become daily users. People often use nicotine to relieve or avoid symptoms of withdrawal early in the morning or after prolonged periods where use of the drug is not permitted. Those who spend a considerable amount of time using the substance are considered chain-smokers. Research since 2000 indicates the gap between men and women narrowing with the prevalence of smoking only slightly higher in men than women. Studies also show that women are less likely to quit smoking and more likely to relapse if they do quit.

Sedative-, Hypnotic-, or Anxiolytic-Use Disorders

Sedative, hypnotic, and anxiolytic drugs include the benzodiazepines, carbamates, barbiturates, and other sedative agents. All prescription sleeping medications and antianxiety drugs also fall into these categories. These agents are all brain depressants and are particularly lethal when mixed with alcohol. These drugs are available both by prescription and on the illegal street market. The medications with a rapid onset are more likely to be abused by those who obtain them by prescription.

Signs and Symptoms

Craving during use or after a period of abstinence is a typical feature of this category of drugs.

Significant levels of tolerance can develop to any of the sedative, hypnotic, or anxiolytic agents. The clinical picture is usually one of maladaptive behavioral and psychological changes such as mood lability, impaired judgment and functioning, and inappropriate sexual or aggressive behavior. Other indicators may be slurred speech, unsteady gait, nystagmus, and impaired mobility or coordination. Physiological effects may include tachycardia, tachypnea, hypertension, hyperthermia, diaphoresis, tremors, insomnia, anxiety, and nausea.

Dependence and abuse of these agents is often associated with abuse of other substances such as alcohol, cannabis, cocaine, heroin, methadone, or amphetamines. The sedatives may be used to counteract the adverse effects of the other substances. Habitual users are usually in search of the original feeling of euphoria and take increased doses trying to achieve this end. Accidental overdose and acute respiratory arrest that result in death are not uncommon.

Incidence and Etiology

Most people take these drugs as directed by their physician for legitimate medical reasons with no intent of misuse. Approximately 6% of those surveyed acknowledge using the drugs illicitly. Those who originally obtained the prescription for medical reasons and have continued to increase doses often justify the continued use by claiming the original symptoms. They often go to multiple physicians in different locations to acquire the prescriptions to continue their habit. Use of this group of drugs to get an intentional "high" is most common among teenagers and young adults in their 20s. The prescription pattern of increasing dosage is more prevalent in adults 40 and older, with a 2:1 female-to-male trend.

Substance Abuse by Health Care Professionals

People who work in the health care professions are entwined in a fast-paced and demanding environment. The decision to use alcohol or other drugs as a means of tolerating and coping with the pressure is alarmingly prevalent within the health care industry. There are many who believe that the chaotic and stressful climate in which doctors, nurses, and other health care providers' work leads some to give in to the relief that the drugs offer. The easy accessibility of sedative, hypnotic, anxiolytic, and opioid drugs to those who work

in health care professions has also contributed to the number of drug-impaired health care workers. Most of them do not start using a drug with the intention of abusing. However, once the cycle of abuse or drug diversion begins, the person is often powerless to control the need for the substance and dependence takes over.

Professional ethics and practice standards of these groups and a personal set of values are the reasons why most people in the health-related fields refrain from ever falling into this trap. Most health care workers are able to provide care that includes medication administration with integrity and professionalism. However, the vulnerability of health care workers who experience the stresses of physical exertion, family demands, and the emotional strain of caregiving is all too real. The availability of medications together with a perceived false justification that drugs can enhance performance set the stage for diversion.

Substance abuse among health care workers is usually noted first by coworkers. In most states, it is an ethical and legal mandate of the Nurse Practice Act for a licensed nurse to report an impaired nurse to the regulatory division of the Board of Nursing. An obligation to protect the patient from unsafe nursing actions is a responsibility concurrent with licensure to practice nursing. Table 15.3 provides some indicators that a nurse may be impaired or engaging in drug diversion along with reporting guidelines. To address the numbers of health care workers who fail in keeping these standards, many states have formed professional help groups for impaired health professionals. These groups work closely with professional licensing boards to develop guidelines by which the person may seek and receive treatment. There are very strict and specific compliance rules and regulations governing the status of the license to practice in these situations. The stipulations as to whether the person may or may not return to practice varies with the situation. The license may be suspended and reinstated once the requirements for treatment have been proven, or the license may be revoked.

Treatment of Substance-Related Disorders

Drug addiction is a disease of serious consequences and adverse effects that do not seem to deter the user from a compulsive craving and seeking of the

TABLE 15.3   The Impaired Nurse or Health Care Provider

CLUES—DRUG-RELATED PROBLEMS	WHEN TO REPORT
Alcoholic	At least two people witness smell of alcohol on breath, hair, or clothing
Moody and irritable	A positive blood alcohol level
Unkempt appearance	Displays a pattern of poor nursing judgment or repeated medication errors
Numerous excuses for behavior	Slurred speech, falling asleep, or staggering while on duty
Smell of alcohol on breath or hair	DWI while driving to work or on duty (home health)
Excessive use of mouth fresheners	Positive urine drug screen result for which a legitimate prescription cannot be produced
Social isolation	Falling asleep at work, staggering gait, or slurred speech
Slurred speech, motor incoordination	Forgetfulness, poor performance, frequent errors
Bloodshot eyes	Drug diversion evidence
Flushed face	Giving drugs without doctor's order
	Signing out drugs to discharged or deceased patients
Drug-Impaired	
Changes jobs frequently	
Pinpoint pupils	
Rapid mood swings or changes in performance	
Social isolation	
Frequent breaks or use of bathroom	
Repeatedly volunteers for extra shifts, overtime	
Offers to give medications for other nurses	
Consistently signs out for vial or ampoule of controlled drugs so wasting is necessary	
Discrepancies in signing for controlled substances and on medication record	
Patients complain of ineffective pain medication	
Always wears clothing with long sleeves	
Befriends doctors who may prescribe medications	
Multiple family problems	

drug. Many become chronic users with relapses common even after long periods of abstinence. The **relapse**, or return to using the drug after apparent recovery, is a factor in the approach to treatment-based programs. Although this cycle is a complex problem, treatment can enable the individual to change their behavior and assume a more wholesome lifestyle.

Ultimately, the long-term goal of treatment programs is for the person to attain complete abstinence. However, the bumps in this road to recovery are far too evident. Because successful recovery depends on the length of time an individual remains in treatment, it becomes critical to find a treatment that is suited for each individual client.

Intensive efforts must be used to retain the client in order for the plan to be effective. Incentives must be established to encourage sobriety and behavior changes during the treatment process. Short-term goals of reducing drug abuse, decreasing the negative medical and social effects of drug use, and helping the individual find meaningful employment with a more productive life are the integral ingredients in reaching abstinence.

Whether treatment is voluntary or court ordered, the chronic nature of the disorder and potential for relapse limits the chance that a single short-term treatment plan will be enough. In addition, coexisting medical and mental illnesses together with specific social, marital, and family issues complicate the overall picture. This is the reason for ongoing multiple support methods and therapy to help the individual during the rough spots in this long road to recovery.

A combined approach of behavioral therapies together with medications and other services has proven the most effective in drug-abuse treatment programs. A continuum of interventions that emphasize life changes often use the 12-step recovery program such as that used in Alcoholics and Narcotics Anonymous.

Detoxification

Detoxification is the first phase of dependency treatment and consists of immediate withdrawal from the physical and psychological effects of the drug that usually last from 3 to 5 days. For those individuals who are severely dependent

Case ⊘ Application 15.1

"Suspicious Behavior"

Judy is a licensed practical nurse who works the day shift in an oncology center. Patrick, a registered nurse who lives across the street from her, works the night shift on the same unit. He often works with only one night off and fills in for other nurses who want time off. His wife stays home with their five children, three of whom are under the age of 6 years. Judy has noticed that for the past few weeks, Patrick has been less social and more distant when she tries to talk to him. He seems so tired and sluggish; sometimes his speech is even slurred in the morning during shift report. There have been several times that Judy has asked him to complete charting that he leaves undone. She is concerned that maybe he is working too much and mentions the change in behavior to the unit supervisor.

The unit supervisor asks Judy if she has been giving more unit doses of injectable morphine to the unit patients. She states that the unit supply of morphine has been refilled almost daily for the past few weeks. Judy states that the majority of the patients with increasing doses are on PCA (patient-controlled analgesia) pumps and that she is administering about the same number of single injections each day. When they check the sign-out register for controlled drugs, they note that most of the injectable doses are being given during the night shift. Some of the doses are signed out for patients who have PCA pumps who would not be receiving routine single doses of the drug. Judy senses that she and the unit supervisor are thinking the same thing.

What are the indicators for a problem in this situation?

_____

_____

What symptoms does Patrick demonstrate that may explain the increased need for stock refills?

_____

_____

What factors may have led to Patrick's situation?

_____

_____

on a drug or drugs, the withdrawal can produce life-threatening symptoms that include delirium, seizure activity, and coma. Unsupervised, the withdrawal from drug dependence can result in death. For example, if street drugs are used to self-medicate the withdrawal symptoms, the result may be a lethal drug interaction and overdose. To provide a safe and humane withdrawal, the use of appropriate medications can help in minimizing the withdrawal symptoms by aiding to restore normal brain functioning and diminish cravings during the treatment process. Medications are currently available for detoxification of clients with opioid, nicotine, cocaine, methamphetamine, and marijuana addiction. Psychoactive medications such as antidepressants, antianxiety agents, mood stabilizers, and antipsychotic medications may be crucial to the treatment of those with coexisting mental conditions. The specific medications used will vary depending on the individual needs and severity of the person's disease.

Treatment Programs

Both inpatient and outpatient programs are available for drug-abuse treatment. Once detoxification has taken place, continued treatment may be provided by medical and nonmedical services. Length of stay in residence facilities is dependent on the needs of the individual with the average being 6 to 12 months. Outpatient programs are designed to follow up the more intensive inpatient treatment. Cognitive-behavioral therapy is used in treatment centers for alcohol, marijuana, cocaine, and methamphetamine abuse. Both individual and group therapy are utilized to assist the client in identifying and understanding their maladaptive patterns of thinking and drug-seeking behaviors. A core element in the approach of therapy is to help the individual to anticipate the reality of relapse and ways to cope with desire for the drug. They are taught ways to avoid situations where relapse is more likely and to engage in new social support systems that are drug free.

Realizing that addiction is a complex problem that has devastating effects on the entire life of the individual offers some insight into the difficulty seen in their ability to maintain abstinence. Incentives and multiple means of encouragement must be provided as the client takes steps toward a more positive and productive lifestyle. Individual and family education groups, relapse prevention groups, follow-up drug testing, and 12-step programs are some of the approaches for continued support during the recovery process. Reversing the addictive behaviors is difficult and relapse is common but hope for recovery and abstinence remains the ultimate goal.

Application of the Nursing Process

Assessment

When assessing the client who abuses substances, remember that underneath the surface of denial and rationalization are the feelings of fear, insecurity, anxiety, and low self-esteem. Some people who are frightened by the effects of the substance or their behaviors while under the influence of the substance may present voluntarily for treatment, whereas others are reprimanded to treatment subsequent to a substance-related arrest.

The assessment interview should be directed toward identifying the type of substance the person has been using, the amount and frequency of use, the last time substance was used, the method of administration, and the length of time the substance has been abused. Also obtain a description of any attempts to decrease or discontinue using the substance and any previous treatment. Remember that most substance abusers underreport the amount they ingest. The CAGE questionnaire is often used to screen for alcohol dependency. CAGE is an acronym that includes the following questions:

1. Have you ever felt you should **C**ut down on your drinking?
2. Have people **A**nnoyed you by criticizing your drinking?
3. Have you ever felt **G**uilty about your drinking?
4. Have you ever had a drink first thing in the morning (**E**ye-opener) to steady your nerves or get rid of a hangover?

A positive answer to two or more of these questions indicates that the client abuses alcohol.

This information is reported to the treating physician.

Also take note of any suicidal ideation or intent, along with the presence and character of any withdrawal symptoms. Withdrawal may be an issue especially if the person enters the hospital for another medical reason other than substance abuse. Knowledge of withdrawal symptoms for the various abused substances can help you recognize and report their occurrence.

Try to identify the client's motivation for treatment as it is crucial to the outcome. Reason for admission is often a determining factor in the client's willingness to comply with the terms of the treatment contract. If the client is seeking relief from the substance-related problems with a sincere recognition of the drug problem, an expectation of success is more realistic than if the client has been admitted involuntarily or for another medical reason not pertaining to the substance-related problem.

Mind Jogger

How might a drug user employ a surface attitude of sincerity and willingness to change as a manipulative means toward discharge?

Nurse–client interactions during the initial interview help to establish a trusting therapeutic relationship, in which the client is accepted and respected for who he or she is at the present time. Long-term recovery is often marked by periods of relapse with reoccurrence of substance using behavior after a significant period of abstinence. The nurse should refrain from judging the client or referring to this as failure. As a nurse, you act as a role model to demonstrate more effective problem-solving and coping skills. Active listening is used to embrace the person beneath the substance and to offer concern and support for the efforts to gain control over his or her life.

A baseline physical and emotional nursing assessment is done to determine admission status and provide a baseline from which to determine progress toward an expected outcome.

Nervous System

- Orientation
- Level of consciousness (LOC)
- Coordination, gait

- Short- and long-term memory (any difficulty following commands)
- Signs of depression or anxiety
- Tremors or decreased reflexes
- Pupils (constricted or dilated)
- Complexion (ruddy or pale, petechiae)

Cardiovascular and Respiratory
- Vital signs
- Peripheral pulses
- Dyspnea on exertion
- Abnormal breath sounds (an alcoholic client is susceptible to aspiration while intoxicated)
- Arrhythmias
- Fatigue
- Peripheral edema

Gastrointestinal
- Nausea or vomiting
- Changes in weight or appetite
- Time of last meal
- Signs of malnourishment
- General nutritional status
- Color and consistency of stool

Integumentary
- Location, size, and characteristics of any skin lesions
- Needle tracks or scarring on arms, legs, fingers, toes, under the tongue, or between gums and lips

Emotional Behavior
- Affect
- Rate of speech
- Suspiciousness, anger, agitation
- Occurrence of hallucinations, blackouts
- History of violent episodes
- Support system: Is anyone present with the client? How do they interact with each other? Are they willing to be involved in the treatment of the client?

Selected Nursing Diagnosis

Once the assessment data have been collected, the registered nurse determines problems that result from the person's substance dependence and its effect on the person's ability to function in activities of daily living. Potential nursing diagnoses applicable to the client with substance abuse or dependence are included in Table 15.4.

Expected Outcomes

During the acute stage of withdrawal, the client needs physical and psychological support to return to a more stable state of health. The detoxification is usually accomplished within 7 days, depending on whether it is a short-acting or long-acting drug and the time needed for it to be eliminated from the body. Once the drug is out of the system, the person may experience sleeping and eating difficulties along with varied levels of irritability and anxiety. Remember that the substance user without the drug is a person who is hungry, angry, lonely, and tired, whose mind and body will want the drug. During this stage of treatment the nursing goals will be to
- promote safety and protection of the client.
- promote adequate food intake to restore nutritional balance.
- promote and maintain fluid and electrolyte balance.
- promote a restful sleep pattern.
- decrease anxiety and promote relaxation.
- stabilize vital signs and general physical state.
- prevent seizures.

After the withdrawal period, nursing interventions contribute to the long-term treatment goals. Efforts are directed to help the client live a full and productive life as a member of society without the use of the substance. Expected outcomes that address the planning strategies for continued sobriety and abstinence from drug use are that the client
- identifies the drug as a problem and takes ownership of the problem.
- identifies changes in lifestyle that are necessary.
- acknowledges responsibility for own behavior and recognizes the association between the substance and personal problems.
- verbalizes understanding of substance abuse and dependence as an illness requiring continued treatment and support.
- identifies alternative coping mechanisms to use in response to stress instead of the substance.
- demonstrates increased feelings of self-worth by verbalizing positive statements about self.
- demonstrates efforts at positive change with interdependence on others and living 1 day at a time.
- begins to develop or reestablish a support system with family, employer, and non–substance-using friends.

TABLE 15.4 Potential Problems Resulting from Substance Dependence

NURSING DIAGNOSIS	RELATED RISK FACTORS
Risk for Injury	Impaired judgment
	Risk-taking behaviors
	Substance withdrawal
	Seizures
	Delirium
	Flashbacks
	Anger and agitation
Anxiety	Withdrawal symptoms
	Anticipated abstinence
Imbalanced Nutrition	Inadequate nutritional intake
	Impaired absorption
	Money used for drugs instead of food
	Drug chosen over food
Deficient Fluid Volume	Secondary nausea and vomiting
Ineffective Coping	Reliance on drug to solve problems
	Loss of family, income, job
	Excessive and ineffective denial of problem
	Underlying fears
Ineffective Health Maintenance	Drug-impaired health status
Noncompliance	Resumption of drug use after period abstinence
Impaired Social Interaction	Dysfunctional interpersonal relationships
Powerlessness	Dependence on drug
	Inadequate coping skills
	Dysfunctional family system
	Negative role models
	Self-destructive drug-related behaviors
Situational Low Self-Esteem	Weak underdeveloped ego
Altered Sensory Perception	Hallucinations, withdrawal syndrome
Disturbed Sleep Pattern	Drug interference with REM stage of sleep cycle
Risk for Self-Directed or Other-Directed Violence	Decreased inhibitions and inability to control anger
Deficient Knowledge	Drug effects and withdrawal process

- identifies available social support systems and how to access them.
- continues to abstain from substance use.
- verbalizes understanding of illness and the recovery process.
- demonstrates willingness to participate in a group recovery treatment program.

Mind Jogger

What support systems are available for referral in your area? What factors may contribute to a lack of success in these programs?

Interventions

Planned interventions during the acute withdrawal state are directed toward controlling the symptoms of withdrawal without oversedating the client. Benzodiazepines are usually the drug of choice for alcohol detoxification, starting with a relatively large dose with daily reductions until withdrawal is complete. Multivitamin therapy and thiamine replacement therapy are used to prevent neuropathy and encephalopathy from chronic alcohol use (Wernicke–Korsakoff syndrome), because chronic alcohol users are usually deficient in thiamine and niacin.

Antabuse (disulfiram) is a long-term alcohol-abuse treatment that inhibits alcohol ingestion by producing severe adverse effects if alcohol is ingested. Symptoms may include diaphoresis, flushing, throbbing headache, palpitations, severe nausea and vomiting, weakness, dyspnea, and hypotension. Severe cases may result in coma,

"Nowhere Else to Turn"

Frank is a 37-year-old unemployed mechanic who has been admitted for evaluation and treatment of polysubstance abuse with opioid and alcohol dependency. Following a motor vehicle accident while "wiped out" on cocaine and alcohol, Frank is voluntarily admitting himself for detoxification. He has been using heroin, cocaine, and alcohol constantly for the past week. He is unable to remember where he has been or how long it has been since his last meal. He states he has a $200- to $300-a-day drug habit and drinks at least a six pack of beer daily. He admits to doing many "bad things" to acquire the drugs. He is divorced and has not seen his three children in more than 2 years.

How would the nurse approach Frank on admission?

_____

_____

What questions would be important to ask Frank?

_____

_____

Frank states the last time he injected heroin and cocaine was 24 hours ago, shortly after which the accident occurred. He has had two previous admissions to treatment programs, but has not been successful in maintaining his abstinence. What criteria for substance dependency does Frank's case demonstrate?

_____

_____

The nurse assesses Frank's affect as appropriate and his mood as anxious and dysphoric. He remains isolated in his room with the curtains drawn. He states he is having some abdominal cramping and his legs are "knotting." He denies craving at this time but says his skin feels like it is "crawling." What nursing diagnoses would the nurse assign to Frank's symptoms?

_____

_____

The physician orders methadone tablets for the next 72 hours. The rationale for giving this medication is:

_____

_____

How does Frank's behavior indicate symptoms of withdrawal?

_____

_____

What other nursing interventions are important for Frank during the detoxification process?

_____

_____

Frank tells the nurse, "I have nothing to live for anymore." How should the nurse respond?

_____

_____

cardiac or respiratory arrest, and death. Additional anticonvulsants may be ordered if seizure activity is not controlled by the benzodiazepines. Antiemetic agents may also be used to control symptoms of nausea and vomiting.

Opiate withdrawal symptoms can be minimized with clonidine (Catapres) in a detoxification setting. This agent lowers blood pressure, so it is essential to monitor vital signs closely during the withdrawal period. This approach is not as effective as using an opioid substitute, but the benefit is that it is nonaddicting and can keep the client opiate free so that other therapies can be initiated. Methadone is typically the opioid substitute used in heroin withdrawal maintenance programs. It is a chemical relative of heroin and is taken once daily by mouth to prevent symptoms of heroin withdrawal and to reduce craving for the drug. The daily dose is titrated over 2 weeks to a maintenance dose. The client may be in a maintenance program for up to 2 to 4 years. A longer-acting drug called orlaam (LAAM) can be taken three times weekly and is used in some situations. In addition, the regimen for opioid withdrawal may include a muscle relaxant, antianxiety agent, and an anticholinergic for abdominal cramping.

Nursing interventions toward expected outcomes during acute substance withdrawal include the following:

Potential for Injury
- Remove hazardous articles and furnishings
- Seizure precautions every 15 minutes
- Assess for hypoglycemia and electrolyte imbalance
- Observe for respiratory depression, arrhythmias
- Identify and reduce seizure precipitating factors
- Monitor medication levels
- Initiate and administer withdrawal sedation

Neurological–Cardiovascular Compromise
- Determine level of intoxication and withdrawal stage
- Reorient as necessary
- Provide a quiet and safe environment
- Monitor vital signs every 1 to 2 hours during first 3 to 4 days of withdrawal
- Monitor neurological signs every hour until stable, then as needed

- Provide education about substance effects on body

Nutritional Imbalances
- Provide high-protein, high-vitamin (B and C) diet
- Provide pleasant and positive mealtime environment
- Provide frequent, small feedings with between-meal high-nutrient snacks
- Encourage oral hygiene
- Provide free access to alternative nutritious beverages
- Offer bedtime snacks
- Restrict caffeine intake
- Teach client importance of nutritional balance
- Record intake and output
- Weigh daily

Anxiety, Fear, Hopelessness
- Approach client in calm, reassuring, and nonjudgmental manner
- Encourage expression of feelings
- Reinforce client's value as a person
- Listen actively

Noncompliance and Denial of Illness
- Educate about illness and addiction process
- Listen to client's reasons for noncompliance
- Discuss importance of following treatment plan
- Help to identify alternatives to maladaptive coping strategies

Social Isolation and Ineffective Individual Coping
- Initiate a therapeutic one-on-one relationship
- Encourage client to talk about him or herself
- Demonstrate appropriate role-modeling behaviors
- Help client to identify reasons for social isolation
- Help client to set realistic interaction goals
- Teach problem-solving skills
- Encourage participation in all group activities
- Refer to therapist, counselors, and treatment programs
- Refer to social services or community support services
- Refer family members to Al-Anon or Al-Ateen as appropriate

"Cycle of Denial"

Tom is admitted for detoxification after his arrest for driving while intoxicated. He has been drinking for the past 3 days, with his last drink taken 12 hours ago. The following day Tom is hollering and anxious because, he says, "There are black bugs all over this bed!"

How should the nurse respond to Tom's comment?

_____

_____

While doing a physical assessment of Tom, the nurse notes adventitious breath sounds. What action should the nurse take?

_____

_____

Tom's wife, Anna, tells the nurse she shouldn't have gone to her mother's earlier in the week because he did not want her to go. She says he wouldn't have been drinking if she had stayed home. The nurse would describe this behavior as:

_____

_____

How should the nurse respond to Anna?

_____

_____

How can involvement in an Alcoholics Anonymous treatment program benefit Tom? What is essential to Tom's success at sobriety?

_____

_____

CLIENT TEACHING NOTE 15.1

 ### Sources of Information on Drug Abuse and Treatment

- Al-Anon Family Group
  National Referral Hotline
  800-344-2666
- Alcoholics Anonymous (AA)—Worldwide
  475 Riverside Drive
  New York, NY 10115
  212-870-3400
- Drug Abuse Information and Treatment
  Referral Line
  800-662-HELP; Spanish 800-66-AYUDA
- Narcotics Anonymous and Nar-Anon Family
  Group
  Nationwide Referral Line: 202-399-5316

- National Council on Alcoholism and Drug Dependence
  12 West 21st Street
  New York, NY 10010
  800-622-2255 or 800-475-4673
  http://www.ncadd.org
- National Institute on Drug Abuse
  6001 Executive Blvd., Rm 5213
  Bethesda, MD 20892
  300-443-1124
  http://www.nida.nih.gov or http://www.drugabuse.gov
- National Clearinghouse for Alcohol and Drug Information
  1-800-729-6686
  http://www.health.org

BOX 15.9

Alcoholics Anonymous, Al-Anon, Narcotics Anonymous: Hope and Help for Drug Abusers and their Families

- Alcoholics Anonymous (AA) is an international fellowship of men and women who have a drinking problem. Anyone may attend open AA meetings, but only those with a drinking problem may attend closed meetings.
- Members share their experiences, provide anonymity to each other, and meet together to attain and maintain sobriety. AA is a program of total abstinence. Members stay away from one drink, 1 day at a time. Sobriety is maintained through sharing experience, strength, and hope through meetings and the Twelve Steps for recovery from alcoholism.
- Purpose of Al-Anon is to help families and friends of alcoholics recover from the effects of living with the problem of drinking of a relative or friend. Al-Ateen is a recovery program for young people and is sponsored by Al-Anon members. The only requirement for membership in these groups is that there be a problem of alcoholism in a relative or friend.
- Narcotics Anonymous (NA) was started from the AA concept for those for whom drugs have become a major problem. Membership is open to all drug addicts, regardless of the particular drug or combination of drugs used. When this group was formed, the word "addiction" was substituted for "alcohol" to reflect the disease concept of addiction. One of the keys to the success of this group is the therapeutic value of addicts working with other addicts, sharing their successes and challenges in overcoming active addiction. The Twelve Steps and Twelve Traditions of NA are the core principles of the recovery program.
- Web Sites:
  - http://www.alcoholics-anonymous.org
  - http://www.al-anon.org
  - http://www.na.org

Evaluation

The evaluation process will depend on the anticipated outcome. Acute withdrawal outcomes are achieved when the client no longer exhibits any signs or symptoms of substance intoxication or withdrawal and has sustained no injuries during the detoxification period. As the client gains insight into the illness and expresses a willingness to admit and take responsibility for his or her own substance problem, the treatment process can become a meaningful step toward a positive recovery phase. Acceptance of this responsibility is the first step toward a drug-free existence. Relapse is common, and recovery is an ongoing process of commitment toward a goal of abstinence.

Client Teaching Note 15.1 provides sources of information on drug abuse and treatment to include in patient teaching for the client and his or her family (Box 15.9).

Summary

- Substance abuse and dependency are among the most preventable of the mental disorders. Yet millions of people continue to use and abuse drugs each day, with alcohol being the drug most often abused by Americans.
- Substance-use disorders are divided into 10 categories by *DSM-5*. These substances include prescription and over-the-counter drugs, abuse of which is showing a steady increase. Most symptoms caused by abuse of these drugs will subside as the drug dosage is decreased or discontinued. Substances also include toxins, volatile substances such as gasoline or antifreeze and other chemicals used with the intent of intoxication.

- Various theories exist regarding why substance abuse and dependence occurs, including observational learning of maladaptive coping tools, the urge to conform to the group, and addictive behaviors demonstrate a chronic and generational pattern, supporting the theories of genetics and codependency.
- The substance-related disorders include substance-use disorders and substance-induced disorders. The characteristic feature of the disorders is the behavioral, cognitive, and physiological indications that the person continues to use the substance regardless of the negative effects it imposes on his or her daily life. There is also an intense craving for the substance leading to substance-seeking behaviors.

Addiction is a physiological and psychological dependence on alcohol or other drugs that affect the CNS in such a way that withdrawal symptoms are experienced when the substance is discontinued.

- Substance-induced disorders include intoxication and withdrawal, in which the symptoms may vary with the particular substance, although some have similar effects.
- Substance-specific related disorders include various conditions that are directly related to the effects of the specific substance. Although the drug groups share some commonalities, some associated features are specific for an individual substance. All of the drugs except caffeine are associated with psychoactive symptoms classifying them as mind-altering drugs.
- Treatment is twofold beginning with detoxification and withdrawal from usage, followed by intensive and monitored therapy. Therapeutic techniques may be part of an inpatient or residence program, or through a disciplined outpatient program. The ultimate goal of treatment is complete abstinence, which is difficult due to the chronic and addictive nature of the illness.
- The first step in recovery is for the person to admit that a problem exists. Success is often dependent on involvement in a recovery group such as Alcoholics Anonymous, where participants support each other in their continuing efforts of abstinence.
- Relapse is common in the long-term treatment process. Cognitive and behavioral changes along with lifestyle alterations that encourage a drug-free existence are necessary.
- During the acute stage following admission to treatment, the nursing assessment is first directed toward obtaining data regarding drug use that is then used for planning interventions for a safe withdrawal phase. The detoxification phase will leave the abuser free of the drug with the potential to confront the drug problem.
- Nursing diagnoses identify the problems created as a result of the substance dependence and its effect on the person's ability to function in activities of daily living.
- Nursing interventions during the acute withdrawal state are directed toward controlling the adverse symptoms of withdrawal without oversedating the client.
- Acceptance of the responsibility to remain in treatment long enough for a positive recovery is ultimately a choice the client has to make.

Bibliography

Alcoholics Anonymous World Services, Inc. (2004). *How it Works—Twelve steps and twelve traditions*. Retrieved March 21, 2014, from http://www.12steps.org/12stephelp/howitworks.htm

American Psychiatric Association. (2013). *Diagnostic and statistical manual of mental disorders* (5th ed.). Washington, DC: American Psychiatric Association.

Drug Enforcement Administration, U.S. Department of Justice. (2005). *Drugs fact sheets*. Published by the U.S. Department of Justice. Retrieved March 16, 2014, from http://www.justice.gov/dea/druginfo/factsheets.shtml

Elliott, D. Y., Geyer, C., Lionetti, T., & Doty, L. (2012). Managing alcohol withdrawal in hospitalized patients. *Nursing, 42*(4), 22–29.

Enoch, M. A., & Goldman, D. (2002). Problem drinking and alcoholism: Diagnosis and treatment. *American Family Physician, 65*(3), 441–450.

Gladding, S. T., & Newsome, D. W. (2010). *Clinical mental health counseling* (3rd ed.). New Jersey: Merrill Pearson Education, Inc.

Grohol, J. M. (2013). *DSM-5 changes: Addiction, substance-related disorders & alcoholism*. Retrieved March 15, 2014, from http://pro.psychcentral.com/2013/dsm-5-changes-addiction-substance-related-disorders-alc

Herdman, T. H. (2012). *NANDA international nursing diagnoses: Definitions & classification 2012–2014*. Oxford, UK: Wiley-Blackwell Publishers.

Kennedy A., Wood, A. E., Saxon, A. J., Malte, C., Harvey, M., Jurik, J., Kilzieh, N., Lofgreen, C., & Tapp, A. (2008). Quetiapine for the treatment of cocaine dependence: An open-label trial. *Journal of Clinical Psychopharmacology, 28*(2), 221–224.

McCrady, B. S., & Epstein, E. E. (2005). *Addictions, a comprehensive guidebook*. New York, NY: Oxford University Press.

Monroe, T., & Pearson, F. (2009). Treating nurses and student nurses with chemical dependency: Revising policy in the United States for the 21st century. *International Journal of Mental Health & Addiction, 7*(4), 530–540. Retrieved March 16, 2014.

National Council on Alcoholism & Drug Abuse. *Signs of drug use*. Retrieved March 15, 2014, from http://www.ncada-stl.org/addiction-information_signs.html

National Institute on Drug Abuse. (2006/08). *NIDA infofacts: Treatment approaches for drug addiction*. Retrieved May 03, 2014, from http://www.drugabuse.gov/infofacts/treatmeth.html

National Institute on Drug Abuse. (2011). *Research report series—prescription drugs: Abuse and addiction*. Retrieved March 16, 2014, from http://www.nida.nih.gov/ResearchReports/Prescription/Prescription.html

National Institute on Drug Abuse (NIDA). (2012a). *Drug facts: Bath salts*. Retrieved March 21, 2014, from http://teens.drugabuse.gov/drug-facts/bath-salts

National Institute on Drug Abuse (NIDA). (2012b). *Drug facts: Spice ("Synthetic Marijuana")*. Retrieved March 21, 2014, from http://www.drugabuse.gov/publications/drugfacts/spice-synthetic-marijuana

National Institute on Drug Abuse. (2013a). *Inhalants*. Retrieved March 16, 2014, from http://www.nida.nih.gov/drugpages/inhalants.html

National Institute on Drug Abuse. (2013b). *Marijuana abuse*. Retrieved March 16, 2014, from http://www.nida.nih.gov/infofacts/marijuana.html

National Institute on Drug Abuse (NIDA). (2013c). *Drug facts: Heroin*. Retrieved March 16, 2014, from http://www.drugabuse.gov/publications/drugfacts/heroin

National Institute of Drug Abuse. (2014). *Drug facts: Nationwide trends*. Retrieved March 16, 2014, from http://www.drugabuse.gov/publications/drugfacts/nationwide-trends

Polimeni, A., Moore, S. M., & Gruenert, S. (2010). Mental health improvements of substance-dependent clients after 4 months in a therapeutic community. *Drug and Alcohol Review, 29*(5), 546–550.

Publishers Group. (2011). *Street drugs; drug identification guide*. Reprints available at www.streetdrugs.org or info@streetdrugs.org

Rice, J. B., White, A. G., Birnbaum, H. G., Schiller, M., Brown, D. A., & Roland, C. L. (2012). A model to identify patients at risk for prescription opioid abuse, dependence, and misuse. *Pain Medicine, 13*(9), 1162–1173. Retrieved March 16, 2014.

Stewart, K. B., & Richards, A. B. (2000). Recognizing and managing your patient's alcohol abuse. *Nursing, 30*(2), 56–59.

Substance Abuse and Mental Health Services Administration. (2013). Results from the 2012 national survey on drug use and health: Summary of national findings and detailed tables. Retrieved October 12, 2014, from http://www.samhsa.gov/data/NSDUH/2012SummNatFindDetTables/index.aspx

Townsend, M. C. (2011). *Nursing diagnoses in psychiatric nursing* (8th ed.). Philadelphia, PA: FA Davis Co.

Varcolaris, E. M. (2011). *Manual of psychiatric nursing care planning* (4th ed.). St. Louis, MO: Saunders Elsevier.

Student Worksheet

Fill in the Blank

Fill in the blank with the correct answer.

1. The term _____ is used in reference to any drug, medication, or toxin that has the potential for abuse.

2. A pattern of either conscious or unconscious helping _____ maladaptive behaviors to continue.

3. _____ is a physiological or psychological dependence on a drug of abuse in which withdrawal symptoms are experienced if drug is discontinued.

4. The first phase of treatment is _____ or immediate withdrawal from the effects of drug use that usually lasts from 3 to 5 days.

5. Delirium tremens is _____.

6. A nutritional disease of the nervous system caused by a thiamin and niacin deficiency found primarily in alcoholics is _____.

Matching

Match the following terms to the most appropriate phrase.

1. _____ Form of amnesia for events during drinking period
2. _____ Early symptom of alcohol withdrawal
3. _____ Strong inner drive to use a substance
4. _____ Reversible behavior pattern caused by recent substance use
5. _____ Overly responsible behavior
6. _____ Develops as brain adapts to repeated use of drug with declining effects
7. _____ Marked symptoms of "crashing" following intense period of substance use
8. _____ Vitamin used in treatment of alcohol dependence
9. _____ Constant involuntary movement of eyeball
10. _____ Not admitting to having a drug problem

a. Shakes
b. Denial
c. Thiamine
d. Codependence
e. Withdrawal
f. Tolerance
g. Intoxication
h. Nystagmus
i. Blackout
j. Craving

Multiple Choice

Select the best answer from the multiple-choice items.

1. The nurse is assessing hourly vital signs on a client in acute alcohol withdrawal. The client's blood pressure and pulse were recorded as 132/68, 78 at 2200; 138/72, 84 at 1400; 148/86, 90 at 0200; and 160/94/94 at 0400. Which of the following actions would the nurse initiate?
   a. Increase fluid intake to 3,000 cc in the next 12 hours
   b. Initiate interventions for fall precautions
   c. Obtain a clean catch urine specimen
   d. Notify the physician

2. Jeff is admitted to the psychiatric unit with a blood alcohol level of 0.03%. He is disoriented with slurred speech and a staggering gait. The nurse would correctly assess that this client:
   a. Has symptoms of intoxication
   b. Has developed a tolerance to alcohol
   c. Is experiencing alcohol withdrawal
   d. Is probably using more than one substance

3. Ronald tells the nurse he is not an alcoholic. He states he drinks "two or three beers" with his buddies every day after work and maybe one or two after he gets home. He says, "I can handle it. I've never missed work because of it." The nurse would recognize Ronald is using the mental mechanism of:
   a. Denial
   b. Projection
   c. Displacement
   d. Rationalization

4. While the nurse is assessing a client to be admitted for treatment of alcohol dependency, the client says, "I suppose you think I am just another drunk." The nurse's best response to this statement would be:
   a. "We treat many people who have the same problem you do."
   b. "Why do you think you are a drunk?"
   c. "At least you are being honest about it."
   d. "We are most concerned that you receive treatment for your problem."

5. Emma is a licensed nurse who is admitted for treatment of prescription drug (oxycodone and lorazepam) dependency. Which of the following attitudes by the nursing staff would be considered an enabling behavior?
   a. Helping her to identify the issues in the nursing environment as a result and not the cause of her drug habit.
   b. Agreeing that the staff shortages and increasing pressures at work may have led to her drug-using behaviors.
   c. Supporting her as she acknowledges that this treatment is required by the State Board of Nursing.
   d. Encouraging her to participate in a drug-related support group.

6. The nurse is assessing a client who has been admitted from the emergency room after several days of inhaling spray paint. In addition to the odor of paint and a sinus discharge, the client who has been inhaling might display:
   a. Dilated pupils, masklike facial appearance, nystagmus
   b. Constricted pupils, drowsiness, attention deficit
   c. Lip-licking, nausea and vomiting, dyskinesia
   d. Coughing, dyspnea, watery eyes

7. A 59-year-old is admitted to the inpatient unit with a diagnosis of chronic alcoholism and Wernicke–Korsakoff syndrome. Which of the following will be included in this client's treatment plan?
   a. Methadone maintenance program
   b. Patient teaching in stress management
   c. Thiamine and niacin vitamin supplements
   d. Fifteen-minute-interval suicide precautions

8. Rex has admitted to the detoxification unit with a diagnosis of methamphetamine dependence. Which of the following is most necessary for Rex to remain drug-free after detoxification?
   a. Understanding how the drug is affecting him
   b. Admission that he has a drug problem
   c. Moving to a new geographic location
   d. Becoming involved in a community activity center

9. Andy is being examined in the emergency room after police aborted his attempt to jump from a 10-story building. His urine sample tests positive for LSD. Which of the following adverse effects is Andy most likely experiencing?
   a. Illusion
   b. Temporary insanity
   c. Perceptual changes
   d. Delirium tremens

10. Which of the following drugs has the potential to be detected in a urine sample for up to 4 weeks?
    a. Cannabis
    b. Cocaine
    c. Alcohol
    d. Inhalant

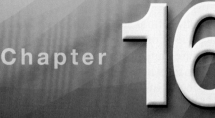

Chapter

16

Eating Disorders

⊙ Learning Objectives

After learning the content in this chapter, the student will be able to:

1. Describe signs and symptoms that characterize anorexia nervosa and bulimia nervosa.
2. Identify etiological factors in the development of severe disturbances in eating behaviors.
3. Assess indications of eating disturbances in the client with an eating disorder.
4. Formulate nursing diagnoses and anticipated outcomes for clients with eating disorders.
5. Plan effective nursing interventions for behaviors associated with abnormal eating patterns.
6. Define evaluation criteria to determine effectiveness of planned interventions.

⊙ Key Terms

anorexia nervosa
binge eating
bulimia nervosa

compensatory methods
purging

In a multicultural society where an abundance and variety of foods and established eating habits are fundamental to everyday life, it is customary to plan events and family happenings around food. In addition, the fast-paced "eat and go" phenomenon has made fast food a multibillion dollar industry. While food is certainly enticing to the mind and essential for the body, nutrition and dietary intake can also become a factor in the treatment of eating disorders. Numerous "dieting" approaches are advertised and sold as quick-fix remedies to curb an increasing trend in obesity. Although obesity is considered a medical condition with many health risks and possible contributing psychological factors, according to *DSM-5*, it has not been established that obesity is consistently associated with a behavioral or psychological syndrome. In the midst of a society in which the image of an "ideal" physique and appearance is associated with glamor and popularity, the desire to conform to this standard is set in motion. When "thin is in," the perceived need to conform often overshadows sensible and nutritionally safe food intake. People who have a preoccupation with obesity, weight reduction, and nutritional intake have a difficult time distinguishing between realistic ways of controlling weight and body image and what constitutes a severe disturbance and often a dangerous pattern of eating behaviors.

Mind Jogger

Does the media promotion of weight-loss programs and products increase the attention on "being thin?"

Research indicates that the incidence of eating disorders is related to genetic predisposition along with environmental risk factors. The exact cause, however, is unclear, with social, psychological, and physiological issues all contributing to the clinical challenge of understanding and treating the problem. People with these disorders have in common the misperception that individual self-worth is related to shape and weight and the ability to control them. Other symptoms tend to evolve out of this irrational thinking. As we discuss the disorders associated with eating patterns, you will gain an understanding of how food and its relationship to the view that a person has of self can become a negative and menacing threat to life.

Just the Facts

Studies show eating disorders are more common in the Western countries than in Asian countries.

Types of Eating Disorders

The three most common eating disorders included in the DSM-5 are anorexia nervosa, bulimia nervosa, and binge eating or compulsive eating disorder. Eating disorders are described by the DSM-5 as persistent behaviors related to food and food consumption and absorption that if left untreated, can have devastating and serious effects on the person's physical or psychosocial health.

Anorexia Nervosa

Anorexia nervosa is characterized by an individual refusal to maintain the least essential normal body weight. The *DSM-5* describes the person as "intensely afraid of gaining weight," and demonstrating a "significant disturbance in the perception of the shape or size of his or her body." Although the term "anorexia" means a loss of appetite with nervous origin, the absence of appetite is not used to describe this disorder. The primary symptom is the maintenance of subnormal levels of weight for age and height. When the disorder develops during childhood or adolescence, the problem may be seen as a failure to advance in a growth pattern rather than in weight loss. The guidelines suggest that for the diagnosis of anorexia nervosa to be assigned, the person should fall below 85% of the normal body weight for that person's age and height. Other specific criteria suggest a body mass index equal to or below 17.5 kg/m^2. These criteria, however, must be viewed with the person's body build and that of other family members in mind. Genetic tendencies for a smaller body frame and bone structure would need to be considered.

Just the Facts

Anorexia nervosa is characterized by an extreme fear of gaining weight that results in a relentless quest for thinness and refusal to maintain body weight that is normal for height and age.

Signs and Symptoms

The behaviors the client uses to achieve weight loss are categorized into two subtypes of anorexia nervosa. The restricting type includes those whose weight loss is achieved through dieting, starvation, or excessive exercise. Weight loss is often accomplished by reducing total food intake to only a few foods, with a drastic exclusion of both overall caloric intake and essential nutrients or food groups. The person may avoid food or meals, weigh his or her food, and methodically count every calorie in his or her food.

In addition, the person may attempt increased weight loss through **purging** (i.e., self-induced vomiting or excessive use of laxatives and diuretics) and increased compulsive exercise. The person with anorexia nervosa has an extreme fear of gaining weight or "becoming fat" that is not relieved by weight loss. This fear may actually intensify as weight loss accumulates.

People with the second subtype, the binge-eating/purging type, also restrict their food intake as described above, but they also regularly indulge in binge eating, purging, or both. **Binge eating**, or binging, is defined by the DSM-5 as eating in a discrete period of time (usually 2 hours) an amount of food that is definitely larger than most people would eat under similar circumstances. **Purging** involves evacuation of the digestive tract by self-induced vomiting or excessive use of laxatives and diuretics. Most people with anorexia who engage in binge eating also follow these episodes with purging methods.

> ### Just the Facts
> Anorexia may cause hair and nails to become brittle, fragile, and easily broken resulting from the lack of essential nutrients needed for body maintenance.

The person with anorexia nervosa exhibits a distorted view of body weight and shape. Because of this distorted perception, the fear of becoming fat may actually intensify as weight is lost. Some people may see their body as being "fat," whereas others may realize they are thin but see certain body areas such as the buttocks, arms, abdomen, or thighs as too fat. They may use methods such as repeated weighing, measuring of body parts, or viewing themselves in a mirror to reinforce their perceived self-image. The person's self-esteem is

> **BOX 16.1**
>
> ### Associated Medical Conditions of Anorexia Nervosa
>
> - Decrease in WBC
> - Anemia
> - Osteoporosis
> - Metabolic disturbances
> - Malnutrition
> - Constipation
> - Dry skin
> - Swollen salivary glands
> - Subnormal body temperature
> - Dehydration
> - Impaired kidney function
> - Dental problems
> - Elevated liver enzymes
> - Decreased thyroid functioning
> - Low levels of sex hormones (estrogen/testosterone)
> - Lethargy
> - Lanugo on trunk, face, upper arms, and shoulders
> - Calluses on dorsal hand surface from inducing vomiting (Russell's sign)
> - Arrhythmias, cardiac arrest, and death

dependent on body shape and size. Weight loss is seen as a major accomplishment of self-control, whereas weight gain is viewed as a failure. Distorted thinking is also seen in repeated denials of the dangerous medical implications of this condition, as described in Box 16.1. An indicator of physiological dysfunction in a female who is menstruating is decreased levels of pituitary hormones (FSH and LH) and ovarian estrogen secretion, which result in amenorrhea, or the absence of menstrual periods. Most of the physical conditions can be reversed as weight returns to normal.

> ### Just the Facts
> An indicator of physiological dysfunction in the woman with anorexia nervosa who is postmenarche is the presence of amenorrhea.

Other symptoms seen in people with this disorder include a depressed mood, social withdrawal, irritability, insomnia, swollen joints, lethargy, and a decreased libido. The person loses bone mass, and vital signs can dip to dangerously low levels, sometimes leading to cardiac arrest and death. Symptoms of depression may be secondary to the effects of starvation and lack of nutrition to body cells. People with anorexia nervosa also

BOX 16.2

Signs and Symptoms of Anorexia Nervosa

Restricting type—weight loss achieved by:
- Reduced total food intake and nutrition
- Compulsive exercise
- Obsessive preoccupation with food
- Intense fear of becoming fat, not relieved by weight loss
- Distorted view of body weight and shape
- Self-esteem dependent on body shape and size
- Weight loss seen as accomplishment
- Denial of potential medical problems
- Amenorrhea (female)
- Lethargy
- Depression and decreased libido
- Social withdrawal

Binge-eating/purging type:
- Binge eating
- Purging or self-induced vomiting
- Misuse of laxatives, diuretics, or enemas

exhibit an obsessive preoccupation with thoughts related to food. They may hoard food items or collect magazines and recipes related to food. Many actually prepare tasteful meals for their families but do not actually consume any portion of the food themselves. Some consider this a psychological response to the body's undernourished state (see Box 16.2).

Just the Facts

Anorexia nervosa most often begins between the ages of 13 and 18 years, with women accounting for more than 90% of the cases.

Incidence and Etiology

Anorexia nervosa most often begins between the ages of 13 and 18 years, with more than 90% of the cases occurring in women. Although this disorder primarily affects females, one in four pre-adolescent cases of anorexia occurs in boys. It is rare in women over the age of 40. Although some cultures may be more accepting of different body sizes, there is pressure within the United States to maintain a certain ideal of thinness that affects primarily females but is extending to males as well.

Symptoms commonly follow stressful life events, such as starting high school, moving to a new location, sexual abuse, or traumatic family relationships. Clients with this disorder are typically well educated, coming from middle- to upper-income families. Early appearance is one of a loving, cohesive family with model compliant, obedient, and perfectionist children who aim to please parents and teachers. However, further evidence usually reveals unresolved family conflicts with inconsistent patterns of overprotective and rigid parenting in which the child remains in a dependent state. The eating disorder may be a desperate attempt by the adolescent to separate from the family system, in particular, from a dominant and overcritical mother.

Mind Jogger

Considering their distorted view of self and compulsive need for perfection, in what type of occupational situations might the person with an eating disorder be employed?

People with anorexia nervosa are often shy, quiet, orderly, and oversensitive to rejection with heightened feelings of inferiority, self-imposed guilt, and unreasonable expectations for perfection. These personality characteristics of excessive self-criticism and sensitivity commonly lead to emotion-focused problem solving. A misperceived inability to overcome their lack of self-worth and value is addressed by an attempt to gain control of their lives by exercising control over their body.

A sense of worth and value becomes intertwined with the ability to shed pounds. The image seen in the mirror is not necessarily compatible with the image seen in the distorted thinking of people with anorexia. They believe that their need for autonomy and control of self is demonstrated by controlling what they eat, which is ultimately their body image. They have a distorted view of their body and perceive weight gain as a lack of control over themselves and failure to meet their unrealistic self-standards.

Mind Jogger

How might the peer pressure of adolescence contribute to the person with anorexia nervosa's sense of value in a thin appearance? How might the unmet needs of the person with anorexia nervosa be seen in terms of Erikson's theory of psychosocial development?

Bulimia Nervosa

The characteristics of **bulimia nervosa** are binge eating with repeated attacks to the self and self-induced destructive methods to prevent weight gain. Subgroups include both purging and non-purging types, depending on the use of the methods and regularity of their use.

Signs and Symptoms

There is a seeming lack of control or inability to stop eating during a binge episode. The type of food consumed varies, but typically is an indulged craving for high-calorie, sweet, or carbohydrate foods such as pastry, ice cream, cake, or pizza. The person with bulimia usually consumes more calories on a binge than those without the disorder consume in an entire meal. Clients are usually ashamed of their eating problem and attempt to hide their symptoms. Rapid hidden consumption of food is typical with continued eating despite an uncomfortable feeling of fullness. Binging usually follows a depressed mood state, individual stressors, periods of strict dieting, or negative self-talk about body image. The binge may temporarily relieve the dysphoric state; however, increased depression and self-dislike quickly emerge after the episode. A continued pattern of binge eating results in an impaired ability to refrain from indulging in the binge or to stop it once the eating begins (see Box 16.3).

The second primary symptom of this disorder is the repeated use of inappropriate and risky methods of preventing weight gain. The most commonly used method is induced vomiting after the binge. Purging is used by most people who present for treatment of the eating disorder. The person may feel a temporary sense of relief after the vomiting, both physically and psycho-

logically, indicating a distorted view of success in preventing weight gain. Purging is usually easily induced after repeated stimulation of the gag reflex by inserting fingers or other flat objects into the pharynx. A smaller percentage of people use laxatives, diuretics, or enemas as **compensatory methods**, but these are usually used in addition to induced vomiting. Fasting for a period of time may also be used in combination with excessive exercise to alleviate the guilt felt after binging. The person may engage in exercise during inappropriate times in unusual places regardless of any medical contraindications or complications (Box 16.4).

Incidence and Etiology

The client with bulimia nervosa is typically within a normal weight range for height and age. Behaviors center on a dissatisfaction with body size and shape that leads to an outward preoccupation with dieting and limited food intake but with little or no alteration in weight or appearance. The person may sneakily stash food or make excuses for spending extended time in the bathroom, usually after consuming a large amount of food. Many with bulimia nervosa have symptoms of depression, borderline personality disorder, anxiety and panic disorders, or posttraumatic stress syndrome. Substance abuse is also common, with some affected individuals engaging in theft and forgery. Social skills are inadequate, and interpersonal relationships suffer from the person's lying and hidden behaviors. The disorder usually follows a chronic pattern, with most cases lasting for an average of

BOX 16.4

Associated Medical Conditions of Bulimia Nervosa

- Loss of dental enamel—teeth appear ragged and "moth-eaten"
- Increased dental caries
- Swollen salivary glands
- Calluses or scars on dorsal surface of hand
- Menstrual irregularities
- Constipation
- Rectal prolapse
- Tears in esophageal or gastric mucosa
- Electrolyte imbalances
- Metabolic alkalosis (loss of stomach acid) or metabolic acidosis (frequent diarrhea)
- Gastric distress or bleeding
- Kidney failure

BOX 16.3

Signs and Symptoms of Bulimia Nervosa

- Binging with inability to stop eating
- Craving for high-calorie or sweet foods
- Consumption of many calories in a binge
- Shame over eating problem
- Attempts to hide food consumption
- Depression
- Negative self-image
- Repeated use of induced vomiting
- Use of laxatives, diuretics, or enemas
- Normal weight for age and height with little fluctuation
- Outward preoccupation with food
- Stashing of food
- Associated personality and anxiety disorders
- Inadequate interpersonal skills

3

5 to 10 years. Even after clinical recovery, many clients continue to experience considerably more body image problems and psychosomatic symptoms than those who have never had a binging and purging disorder.

Just the Facts

People with bulimia nervosa are more aware of their own eating disorder and more distressed by the symptoms than those with anorexia nervosa. Also, even after clinical recovery from bulimia nervosa, many clients continue to experience considerably more body image problems and psychosomatic symptoms than those who have never had a binging and purging disorder.

Mind Jogger

It is said that the person with bulimia nervosa replaces anxiety felt before the binge with guilt following the binge. How might this lead to other self-abusive behaviors?

Binge-Eating Disorder

Binge-eating disorder is recognized as a mental disorder in the DSM-5, a condition similar to bulimia, but with a slightly different pattern. An episode of binge eating is the ingestion of an amount of food in a limited time period (usually less than 2 hours) that is definitely larger than the ordinary person would consume in a similar period of time under the same circumstances. The variant characteristic is that recurrent binge-eating episodes during which the individual loses control over the eating compulsion are not followed by the destructive behaviors of purging by vomiting, laxative and diuretic use, or excessive exercise.

Signs and Symptoms

The person with this disorder tends to be overweight or obese as a result of the binge eating. He or she usually feels guilt and shame about their eating initiating a cycle of binge eating as a coping mechanism or compensation to relieve the distress. Food consumption is usually accomplished quickly and often by oneself, with the amount eaten in excess of 10,000 calories at one time. The fact that the person is full does not stop the binging. Restricting food in between

BOX 16.5

Signs and Symptoms of Binge-Eating Disorder

- Inability to stop eating or control food intake
- Rapid consumption of large amounts of food
- Eating continuously during day
- Hiding food to eat in secret
- Feelings of stress only relieved by food
- Eating even when feeling full
- Embarrassment and feelings of disgust over amount of food eaten

binges also seems to trigger more binging. Many clients also have a history of other psychological problems such as anxiety, depression, and obsessive–compulsive or other personality disorders (Box 16.5).

Incidence and Etiology

Binge-eating disorder often occurs in mid-life, with females and males equally affected. Although it is not known exactly what causes the binge eating, most individuals with the disorder tend to have a low self-image and impulsive behaviors. Media emphasis on weight and appearance is considered an underlying stigma that adds to the self-criticism, shame, and guilt.

Treatment of Eating Disorders

For clients with anorexia nervosa, the goals of treatment revolve around reversal of the restrictive or maladaptive patterns of eating and thinking about food. Individual planning is also centered on the reestablishment of healthy eating habits. Physical problems often correct themselves as weight is regained and normal nutritional intake is consistent. In addition to these issues, treatment of the client with bulimia nervosa also includes a focus on relinquishing the behaviors of binging and purging as normal eating patterns are restored. Cognitive-behavioral psychotherapy addresses the psychological issues of both disorders.

With the anorexic client, family therapy focuses on modifying the family dynamics to allow recovery to occur. Inclusion of the family in the treatment plan and counseling sessions assists family members to see how the maladaptive behaviors of the family are intertwined in the client's eating behaviors. The client must confront dysfunctional thoughts and irrational beliefs about self-image and food in realistic terms. Behavior therapy may involve a reward contract in which privileges are exchanged for increased food intake. Gradual increase in caloric intake may also be used to help the client overcome the fearful avoidance of food. Antidepressant medications (e.g., fluoxetine, nortriptyline, olanzapine, and mirtazapine) may be used in combination with psychotherapy. In some cases, antianxiety medications (e.g., lorazepam or chlorpromazine) may be useful to relieve anxiety associated with treatment.

In the client with bulimia nervosa, therapy is designed to help the person take a self-inventory of eating, binging, and purging behaviors. Education is provided about healthy nutritional habits along with efforts to reorganize the maladaptive thinking related to food, body image, and personal achievement. Behavioral methods include a means of exposing the person to foods that invite binging, but the action is prevented. With repeated exposures, the person gradually becomes less fearful of the foods that previously initiated the compulsive behavior. Anxiety-reducing relaxation techniques are used to decrease the need for compensatory action and introduce preventative strategies. Family therapy may help clients whose family dynamics are a contributing factor, but it has not been found to be as effective as in the client with anorexia nervosa. Antidepressant medications have been used successfully for clients with bulimia nervosa when combined with psychotherapy. Fluoxetine and desipramine are commonly used with careful monitoring for side effects.

The method of treatment program varies with the needs of the individual client. Care is often provided in outpatient therapy involving a psychotherapist, physician, and registered dietician. Inpatient programs are more intense and more structured than outpatient treatment can provide. Hospitalization may be necessary in severe cases that involve medical complications. Approximately 40% of anorexia clients may achieve a partial or full recovery within 5 years of treatment, while at least 50% of clients with bulimia nervosa and binge-eating disorder fully recover. Recovery support websites provided in Client Teaching Note 16.1 that offer information about treatment centers and help that is available.

CLIENT TEACHING NOTE 16.1

 Information Sources on Eating Disorders

- Recovery Connection 1-800-993-3869
- National Institute of Mental Health (NIMH)
  6001 Executive Boulevard
  Bethesda, MD 20892-9663
  Toll free: 1.866.615.NIMH (6464)
  E-mail: nimhinfo@nih.gov
  Website: www.nimh.nih.gov
  http://mentalhealth.samhsa.gov
- National Eating Disorders Association's 24-hour information and referral helpline at 1-800-931-2237
  http://www.nationaleatingdisorders.org
- National Association of Anorexia Nervosa and Associated Disorders P.O. Box 7
  Highland Park, IL 60035
  Hotline: 1-847-831-3438
  http://www.anad.org/site/anadweb

Research is ongoing toward finding the underlying causes and genetics involved in the eating disorders. Neuroimaging is also being used in an attempt to better understand how the person with these disorders processes information about food, food consumption, and self-image.

Application of the Nursing Process

Assessment

Many people with eating disorders deny their problem and maintain their maladaptive eating patterns for several years before treatment is sought, often by concerned family members. Behaviors such as binging and purging by the person with bulimia nervosa are done in secret and may not be detected until more objective symptoms are noted. It is difficult to gain insight into the problem unless it is viewed from the client's perspective. As the nurse, your attitude and approach when assessing the client, whether in an emergency room or other clinical situation, are essential to gaining the trust of the client. Many people with eating disorders are ashamed of their behaviors and may want to divulge the magnitude of their problem, but may refrain because of negative or blocking statements made by the nurse. It is important to examine your own feelings about food, dieting, and body image to maintain an objective view of the client's situation.

Information about dietary intake and eating patterns should be gathered with caution to avoid questions that may infer that the client has an eating disorder. Questions that ask how often the client induces vomiting after eating or inquire about feelings after binge eating would imply that a problem exists. A nonconfrontational and nonjudgmental approach is important to convey caring, compassion, and willingness to understand the extent of the client's problem. Because they are usually supersensitive to criticism and frustration, it is best to avoid asking clients questions that can be misinterpreted in this context. Use of active listening and open-ended techniques will aid in encouraging the client to communicate freely (e.g., "Tell me how you feel about your body. How do you feel after eating? or What happens after you eat?). This approach allows the client to provide clues that can lead to further assessment of the problem.

Other data to be collected include any reports of insomnia or fatigue, increased feelings of anxiety, and intolerance to cold temperatures. Determine any changes in bowel elimination or decreased urine output because they relate to laxative or diuretic use. Observe the body for general signs of inadequate nutrition, increased hair growth, brittle dry nails or skin, and erosion of tooth enamel. Look for abrasions or calluses on the back of the hands related to induced purging.

Selected Nursing Diagnoses

Because the effects of eating disorders may affect several body systems, outcome planning based on the individual assessment is necessary. Nursing diagnoses that encompass the usual problems encountered in the care of clients with eating disorders may include the following:

- Imbalanced Nutrition: Less than body requirements, related to eating patterns and excessive exercise
- Constipation or Diarrhea, related to laxative abuse and inadequate dietary intake
- Impaired Oral Mucous Membranes, related to frequent vomiting
- Disturbed Body, related to misperception of weight and shape
- Ineffective Coping, related to situational crisis

- Anxiety, related to feelings of hopelessness and lack of control
- Denial, ineffective related to behaviors that are detrimental to health
- Dysfunctional Family Processes, related to family dynamics and defined individual boundaries
- Deficient Fluid Volume, related to vomiting, diarrhea, diuretic or laxative use
- Post-Trauma Syndrome, related to sexual or physical abuse
- Powerlessness, related to lack of insight into self-destructive behaviors and irrational thinking about food and body image
- Impaired Social Interaction, related to psychological barriers and concealing behaviors

Expected Outcomes

Initial treatment is focused on decreasing the client's anxiety, stabilizing the weight loss pattern, and normalizing eating patterns. Outcomes for the client with an eating disorder may include the following:

- Verbalizes decreased fear and anxiety related to weight gain and inability to maintain control
- Consumes adequate nutritional intake to meet appropriate body requirements for height and age
- Verbalizes importance of appropriate eating pattern
- Verbalizes understanding of events or thoughts that precipitate anxiety
- Ceases engaging in self-destructive behaviors (binge eating or purging)
- Participates in activity level appropriate for health maintenance
- Verbalizes rational thinking processes and view of body image
- Expresses understanding of relationship between symptoms, distorted thinking, and behaviors
- Discusses present health problem with health care team members
- Identifies ways to maintain a healthy means of weight control
- Identifies family roles and boundaries, and modifies them as indicated
- Identifies strengths and makes positive self-statements
- Demonstrates improved interpersonal skills in social setting

It is also important for the client's family to verbalize an understanding of the relationship of the overall family dynamics to the client's disorder.

Interventions

The nurse may have multiple roles in working with a client who has an eating disorder. In addition to meeting the physiological needs of the client, the nurse may also function to provide psychotherapeutic interventions that include teaching, counseling, and being a group leader. Formulating a plan of care for the client with an eating disorder should include the following actions:

- Initiate a behavior modification plan with privileges and restrictions based on food intake and weight gain.

"Cassidy's Secret"

Cassidy is a 23-year-old college graduate recently married to Stan, a promising young banking associate. Stan has brought Cassidy to the outpatient clinic after he found her unresponsive when he arrived home from work. Cassidy is 5 ft 8 in tall and weighs 101 lb. Stan states he knew she was on a crash diet during the months prior to their wedding but had no idea that her weight loss was a serious problem. He relates that during their courtship she often found ways to avoid eating and would spend countless hours working out in the university gym. As he reflects on the past few years, Stan says that Cassidy often described herself as fat, even though she seemed to get thinner. He mentions that her college roommate told him Cassidy wasn't eating right, but he thought it was just the stress of finishing school. Stan tells the nurse that Cassidy is the oldest of three children from a single-parent family. Her mother worked many hours and left Cassidy to manage her two younger brothers. He says that she would often express ambivalent feelings about her mother, stating that her mother "needed" her but did not care about her. During family occasions, Cassidy's mother would show outward affection for her daughter and state how proud she was of her.

Cassidy is pale, thin, and somewhat emaciated, with sunken cheeks and dry mucous membranes. She hesitates to open her mouth, which when examined reveals numerous dental caries and brownish stained enamel. Cassidy states that she started self-induced vomiting when she was 9 years old. She had started getting "pudgy" and her mother told her she was going to be fat if she didn't stop eating. She also states that her mother told her she could keep herself from gaining weight by making herself vomit after she ate. Her mother told her she had been doing this for years to try to lose weight, but never seemed to change in size. Cassidy says she binges on things like pie, chocolate, and banana splits, after which she purges with vomiting and laxatives. She admits to taking as many as 8 to 10 laxative pills at a time to feel relief from the guilt she feels over her food intake and to ensure weight loss after the binge. She works out for as much as 4 hours daily at the gym to compensate for the food she eats. Cassidy relates a feeling of shame for her eating problem and is embarrassed that Stan has now found out the secrets she has tried so hard to conceal.

What approach should the nurse employ to help Cassidy at this point?

_____

_____

How do Cassidy's symptoms indicate an eating disorder?

_____

_____

Cassidy is diagnosed with anorexia nervosa and admitted for stabilization of her physical symptoms and for treatment to address the psychological issues underlying her eating problem. Cassidy expresses sadness because she and Stan want to have a baby, but she is afraid that her behavior will hurt her chances of having a normal pregnancy. What factors related to an eating disorder may affect the issue of pregnancy?

_____

_____

How can the nurse help Cassidy to view her self-image in a positive way excluding body appearance and weight?

_____

_____

Case ⊘ Application 16.1

- Weigh the client daily before breakfast using the same scale.
- Maintain a strict intake and output log.
- Monitor status of skin and oral mucous membranes.
- Stay with the client during meals and at least 1 hour following food intake.
- Restrict time for meals to 30 minutes to reduce focus on food and eating.
- Remind client that tube feeding may be employed if nutritional status deteriorates.
- Monitor amount and time of activity level.
- Monitor vital signs on a regular basis.
- Establish a trusting relationship conveying care, concern, and compassion.
- Use a firm and supportive approach to eating and related behaviors.
- Encourage the client to verbalize feelings of fear and anxiety related to achievement, family relationships, and intense need for independence.
- Help the client to achieve realistic view of his or her body by measurements and comparisons to norms for height and age.
- Assist the client in setting practical limits on expectations for self-standards.
- Promote independent decision making as appropriate to establish a sense of control.
- Provide ways to reinforce the client's strengths and positive attributes.
- Encourage family to participate in education regarding connection between family processes and the client's disorder.
- Encourage participation in group and social role-play activities.
- Avoid discussions that focus on food and weight.
- Role model appropriate ways of dealing with environmental stressors.
- Explore with the client ways of increasing autonomy and assertive behaviors.

Evaluation

Evaluation will focus on the established anticipated outcomes for the individual client. Normal weight for height and age and normal laboratory values and vital signs, with absence of previous abnormal physical findings, will demonstrate a successful health status outcome. Psychotherapeutic progress is seen as the client embraces a realistic self-image and sets reasonable expectations and standards for achievement. An improved sense of control over self and coping skills to confront environmental stressors with self-confidence will result in a more positive self-esteem. As the guilt and shame over previous behavior is released, the client is able to recognize the relationship between food, eating patterns, and the ill-fated journey of the disorder.

It is also important to evaluate family interaction patterns and progress of the client toward autonomy and independent decision making. Follow-up counseling and support toward continued abstinence from previous unhealthy behaviors is indicated in view of the high incidence of relapse. Referrals to support groups are helpful to reinforce treatment outcomes and prevent a return to maladaptive eating habits.

Summary

- Research indicates that both genetics and environmental risk factors play a role in the chances that a person may develop an eating disorder. The exact cause is not known, but many social, psychological, and physiological issues contribute to the clinical picture.
- Anorexia nervosa is characterized by an individual refusal to maintain normal body weight; guidelines suggest that for the diagnosis of anorexia nervosa to be assigned, the person should fall below 85% of the normal values for height and age. There is an accompanying disturbance in the person's perception of his or her body shape and self-image.
- Weight loss in anorexia is usually accomplished through a reduced food intake of calories and nutrients. The restrictive subtype is characterized by weight loss accomplished through dieting, starvation, or excessive exercise. The second subtype may also involve binge eating, purging, or both.
- An intense fear of becoming fat feeds the distorted view the person has of his or her body weight and shape.
- Research demonstrates that many clients with anorexia nervosa come from families with unresolved conflicts of parent–child relationships,

often with the client in the clutches of an overindulgent and controlling mother. A sense of worth becomes entwined in the ability to lose weight because the client's distorted thinking associates control of self with control over what is eaten.

- Bulimia nervosa is characterized by binge eating (i.e., eating in a short period of time an amount of food larger than most people would normally eat in the same situation). Despite an uncomfortable feeling of fullness, the person is unable to stop eating. After the binge, there is usually a feeling of shame and effort to hide the symptoms.
  - The client with bulimia nervosa is typically within a normal weight range for height and age. However, distorted thinking centers on a dissatisfaction with body size and shape that leads to an outward preoccupation with dieting. Despite the limited food intake, there is little change in the person's outward appearance.
- In binge-eating disorder, the episodes of binge eating relates to the ingestion of an amount of food in a limited time period of 2 hours or less that is larger than the ordinary person would consume in the same time period under the same circumstances. Clients lose control over their eating but do not follow with purging or other compensatory behaviors of laxative and diuretic use. Clients with this disorder often struggle with being overweight or obese.
- Treatment methods for individuals with eating disorders focus on reversing the restrictive or maladaptive patterns of eating and thinking about food and reestablishing healthy eating habits. Psychotherapy may employ education about healthy nutritional habits, behavioral methods and contracting, group therapy, and especially cognitive therapy to reorganize the maladaptive thinking related to food, body image, and personal achievement.
- The attitude and approach of the nurse are paramount to establishing a trusting relationship in which the client is willing to participate in treatment. To gain insight into the problem, it is important to hear the symptoms and perception of the illness from the client's perspective.
- As the client is able to release the shame and guilt over previous behaviors, there is a restored ability to recognize the relationship among food, eating patterns, and the eating disorder.

Bibliography

(2003). Anorexia nervosa–Part I. *Psychology and Behavioral Sciences Database Collection, 19*(8).

(2003). Anorexia nervosa–Part II. *The Harvard mental health letter/from Harvard Medical School, 19*(9): 5–7.

American Psychiatric Association. (2013). *Diagnostic and statistical manual of mental disorders* (5th ed.). Washington, DC: American Psychiatric Association.

Cockerham, E., Stopa, L., Bell, L., & Gregg, A. (2009). Implicit self-esteem in bulimia nervosa. *Journal of Behavior Therapy and Experimental Psychiatry, 40*(2), 265–273. Retrieved March 22, 2014.

Crow, S. (2014). Professionals' knowledge of and attitudes about eating disorders patients. *Eating Disorders Review, 25*(1), 2–5. Retrieved March 22, 2014.

Hay, P. J. (2013). Assessment and management of eating disorders: An update. *Australian Prescriber, 36*(5), 154–157. Retrieved March 22, 2014.

NANDA. (2012). *International nursing diagnoses: Definitions & classifications 2012–2014.* Oxford, UK: Wiley-Blackwell Publishers.

National Institute of Mental Health. (2011). *Eating disorders.* NIH Publication No. 11-4901. Retrieved March 22, 2014, from http://www.nimh.nih.gov/health/publications/eating-disorders/index.shtml

Oluyori, T. (2013). A systematic review of qualitative studies on shame, guilt, and eating disorders. *Counseling Psychology Review, 28*(4), 47–59. Retrieved March 22, 2014.

Orbanic, S. (2001). Understanding bulimia. *American Journal of Nursing, 3*(101):35–41.

Qian, J., Hu, Q., Wan, Y., Li, T., Wu, M., Ren, Z., & Yu, D. (2013). Prevalence of eating disorders in the general population: A systematic review. *Shangai Archives of Psychiatry, 25*(4), 212–223. Retrieved March 22, 2014.

Student Worksheet

Fill in the Blank

Fill in the blank with the correct answer.

1. The client with anorexia nervosa demonstrates a disturbance in the _____ of the shape and size of his or her body.
2. The anorexic client sees weight loss as a major accomplishment of _____, whereas weight gain is seen as _____.
3. The adolescent search for autonomy is often seen in the client with anorexia who makes a desperate attempt to separate from a _____ parent.
4. _____ is used by most persons with bulimia to achieve a temporary sense of relief after a binge.
5. The client with bulimia nervosa is typically within a normal _____ for height and age.
6. When caring for the client with an eating disorder, the nurse restricts meal time to _____ to reduce the focus on food and eating.

Matching

Match the following terms to the most appropriate phrase.

1. _____ Purging
2. _____ Binging
3. _____ Reward contract
4. _____ Amenorrhea
5. _____ Compensatory methods

a. Absence of menstrual periods
b. Privileges are exchanged for increased food intake
c. Self-induced vomiting or use of laxatives
d. Use of laxatives, diuretics, or enemas, and induced vomiting to prevent weight gain
e. Eating a large amount of food in a short time with inability to stop

Multiple Choice

Select the best answer from the multiple-choice items.

1. The nurse assessing a 17-year-old who is being evaluated for anorexia nervosa would recognize which of the following data as suggestive of this diagnosis?
   a. Periodic patterns of weight gain and loss over the past year.
   b. Refusal to talk about the subject of food and nutritional planning.
   c. Extreme weight loss from self-imposed restricted food and nutrient intake.
   d. Periods of overeating and self-induced vomiting with no change in weight pattern.

2. While implementing nursing interventions for the client with an eating disorder, it is important for the nurse to:
   a. Provide opportunities for independent decision making.
   b. Confront the client with the absurdity of his or her distorted thinking.
   c. Use an approach that conveys a sense of concern and sympathy.
   d. Encourage client to talk about the caloric value of various food items.

3. Medications that have been found to be effective in combination with psychotherapy to address the symptoms related to bulimia nervosa are:
   a. Antithyroid
   b. Antidepressant
   c. Anticholinergic
   d. Beta-adrenergic blockers

4. Kate is a 20-year-old teacher who has admitted herself for treatment of bulimia nervosa. The best initial approach for the nurse would be:
   a. "Why would you want to lose weight when you look so good already?"
   b. "I just don't understand why you make yourself vomit after you eat."
   c. "Tell me about the last time you did binge eating and what you did afterward."
   d. Would it not be easier to go on a weight-reduction diet instead of hurting yourself?"

5. While assessing a young woman admitted with a suspected eating disorder and electrolyte imbalance, the nurse notes poor oral condition and calluses on the index and middle fingers of her right hand. The nurse notes these symptoms as characteristic of:
   a. Purging behavior
   b. Starvation
   c. Binge eating
   d. Excessive stress

6. The nurse would recognize the behaviors of a client diagnosed with anorexia to include:
   a. Excessive craving for high-calorie, sweet, or high carbohydrate foods.
   b. Continued eating even though a feeling of fullness is felt.
   c. Frequent mirror-viewing and measuring of body parts.
   d. Stashing of food with hidden food consumption.

7. The nurse caring for a client with an eating disorder would anticipate interventions to address the nursing diagnosis:
   a. Fluid volume excess, related to purging behaviors
   b. Anxiety, related to feelings of hopelessness and lack of control
   c. Grieving, anticipatory related to potential loss of health
   d. Altered thought processes, related to distorted body image

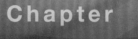
Sexual Disorders

⊙ Learning Objectives

After learning the content in this chapter, the student will be able to:

1. Define human sexuality and various modes of sexual expression.
2. Describe signs and symptoms of sexual dysfunction disorders.
3. Identify etiological factors in the development of sexual dysfunction disorders.
4. Discuss signs and symptoms of paraphilic disorders.
5. Identify etiological factors in the development of a paraphilic disorder.
6. Discuss current treatment available for people with a sexual disorder.
7. Perform an unbiased nursing assessment of the client with a sexual disorder.
8. Formulate nursing diagnoses and outcomes to address problems common to clients with sexual disorders.
9. Plan selected nursing interventions to address the needs of the client with a sexual disorder.
10. Describe evaluation methods for determining the effectiveness of planned interventions.

⊙ Key Terms

exhibitionism
fetishism
frotteurism
necrophilia
paraphilia
pedophilia
sexual dysfunction
sexual masochism

sexual orientation
sexual sadism
sexuality
telephone scatologia
transvestic fetishism
voyeurism
zoophilia

exuality is described as an innate part of human dynamics integral to our development throughout the life cycle. It is the blend of physical, chemical, and psychological functioning characterized by our gender and sexual behavior. The manner in which our parents and other adults interact with us during early psychosexual developmental periods is instrumental in the formation of a wholesome adjustment and attitude toward our body and our feelings about sexuality. This adjustment as a child leads to a healthy self-image and satisfying adult sexual relationships that respect the rights of others. The expression of sexual feelings is demonstrated throughout our life in various individual ways. It is important for the nurse to develop a self-awareness of his or her attitudes and beliefs toward sexual issues that may hinder the effective care of any client. This allows the nurse to be a client advocate, to present factual information about sexual development, and to promote an understanding of these human needs for all age groups.

Mind Jogger

How might the nurse's attitude toward sexuality affect his or her ability to initiate a therapeutic relationship with the client?

An individual preference or sexual attraction is referred to as one's **sexual orientation**. These modes of sexual expression fall into several categories. Heterosexuality is a sexual preference for members of the opposite sex. This is generally accepted as the usual attraction and is necessary for procreation of the species. Homosexuality is a preference for members of the same sex, whereas a bisexual orientation is an attraction to members of both sexes. Although the issue of sexual orientation continues to be one of debate and controversy, a healthy view of human sexual development and sexuality is a prerequisite to a healthy and satisfying sexual exchange between two people. A sexually intimate and fulfilling relationship is mutually satisfying for both partners. It must be emphasized that the feelings toward sexuality and sexual intimacy experienced by the adult are significantly affected by the feelings experienced as a child during early developmental years.

Sexual disorders include all mental alterations that prevent a person from functioning in a normal healthy relationship within societal norms. The origin of these disorders covers a wide array of factors including physiological, psychological/

emotional, and cultural issues. Relationships are strained and broken, and self-esteem is undermined by problems related to the various sexual disorders.

Mind Jogger

How do parents' attitudes about sexuality and sexual behaviors influence their children?

Types of Sexual Disorders

The DSM-5 addresses sexual disorders under the categories of sexual dysfunctions, paraphilic disorders, and gender dysphoria.

Sexual Dysfunction Disorders

Sexual dysfunctions are identified by abnormal sexual desire and psychophysiological changes that accompany the sexual response cycle. These disturbances cause marked discomfort and anxiety leading to troubled interpersonal relationships. The dysfunctions may include sexual interest/arousal disorder, female orgasmic disorder, delayed or premature ejaculation and erectile disorder in males, and pain/penetration disorder. The sexual difficulty may be present without a diagnosed sexual dysfunction disorder being assigned.

A sexual dysfunction can occur during any phase of the sexual response cycle or is characterized by pain associated with sexual intercourse. Phases of the response cycle consist of the desire to have sexual activity, subjective pleasures and physiological changes of excitement, peaking or sexual pleasure in orgasm, rhythmic release of sexual tension, and resolution or relaxation together with a general sense of contentment. A dysfunction in one or more of these phases is characterized by the degree of persistent or recurrent symptoms, the quality of sexual stimulation involved, and the level of distress indicated by the person. The problem may be present over the person's lifetime or may be acquired after a period of normal functioning and response. The dysfunction may be related to a particular set of circumstances or a problem that exists with some or all types of stimulation, situations, or partners.

Mind Jogger

What situation or circumstances within a relationship might lead to a sexual dysfunction?

General Signs and Symptoms of Sexual Dysfunction

- Decreased sexual desire
- Dislike and avoidance of sexual activity
- Lack of sexual arousal in women
- Failure to achieve or maintain erection during sexual act in men
- Failure to achieve orgasm during intercourse
- Premature ejaculation in men
- Pain during intercourse
- Involuntary perineal muscle contractions preventing vaginal penetration
- Medical conditions or medications that interfere with sexual functioning
- Sexual inhibition related to use and abuse of substances

Signs and Symptoms

Sexual dysfunction is a comprehensive term that covers a variety of different situations. The following sections describe characteristics and symptoms of each type of dysfunction. General signs and symptoms for sexual dysfunction disorders are found in Box 17.1.

Sexual Interest/Arousal Disorder

Hypoactive sexual desire disorder involves a low sexual interest with little motivation to engage in sexual activity. There is an absence of sexual fantasies with little frustration when the opportunity for sexual contact is not available. Occasionally, the decreased desire in one partner can reflect an increased need in the other partner.

In women with sexual arousal disorders, there is a recurring inability to attain or maintain adequate excitement response and vaginal lubrication to complete sexual activity. This results in painful intercourse and avoidance of sexual encounters.

In men, the continued inability to attain or maintain an erection until completion of the sexual act denotes an arousal disorder. In some situations, there is an inability to attain an erection anytime during intercourse. With others, the erection is accomplished but is lost on penetration or during the activity.

Just the Facts

Medications such as antihypertensives, antipsychotics, antidepressants, anxiolytics, and anticonvulsants can cause hypoactive sexual desire disorder.

Orgasmic Disorders

Women with orgasmic disorder experience a persistent delay or absence of orgasm following normal sexual activity. This may affect the person's body image, self-esteem, or satisfaction in the relationship. The disorder tends to be more prevalent in younger women during early sexual experiences. Once a female learns how her body reaches orgasm, it is uncommon for her to lose the ability to achieve a climax.

Men may feel aroused at the beginning of the sexual act but lose pleasure in the activity and fail to achieve orgasm. In other situations, the problem is premature ejaculation, in which there is recurrent onset of orgasm and ejaculation with minimal stimulation. The ejaculation occurs before the man is ready to do so. Age, type of sexual stimulation, and any prolonged abstinence from sexual activity can contribute to this problem.

Sexual Pain/Penetration Disorder

Dyspareunia is genital–pelvic pain in women associated with sexual intercourse. This may be superficial, or it may only occur during deep penetration. Vaginismus is the repeated occurrence of involuntary perineal muscle contractions that prevent penetration of the vagina. This is more common in younger women or those with a history of sexual abuse or trauma.

Sexual Dysfunction Due to a General Medical Condition

There are a variety of conditions that can lead to a sexual dysfunction. Medical conditions and prescription medications that can directly affect sexual functioning are listed in Box 17.2. A person's unfamiliarity with medications or medical situations that interfere with sexual response or performance may prevent the problem from being recognized.

Sexual dysfunction can also occur as a result of substance use. Depending on the substance used, the physiological effects may include decreased desire and arousal, inability to achieve orgasm, or sexual pain.

Incidence and Etiology

People frequently deny the need for treatment of sexual dysfunctions or are unaware that treatment may be available. The person often avoids the issue, adding to the resulting interpersonal friction and disturbance within his or her relationship. Some may be reluctant to discuss sexual problems with health care workers, or in other cases, the problem may be reported by a spouse, partner, or friend. Other contributing factors could be a lack

---

BOX 17.2

Medical Conditions and Medications That May Contribute to Sexual Dysfunctions

- *Localized diseases:* Endometriosis, cystitis, vaginitis, uterine prolapse, pelvic inflammatory disease, testicular disease, genital injury or infections, atrophic vaginitis
- *Systemic diseases:* Hypothyroidism, diabetes mellitus (most common in men), adrenal cortical malfunction, pituitary dysfunction, hypogonadal secretions, hypertension, arteriosclerotic cardiovascular disease
- *Peripheral/CNS disorders:* multiple sclerosis, spinal cord injury, neuropathy, brain lesions, muscular dystrophy
- *Other:* Prostatectomy complications, oophorectomy without hormone replacement therapy, mastectomy, chemotherapy, and radiation
- *Medications:*
  - Alcohol
  - Anticholinergics
  - Antidepressants
  - Antihypertensives
  - Antipsychotics
  - Barbiturates
  - Benzodiazepine
  - Calcium channel blockers
  - Digitalis
  - Dilantin
  - Diuretics
  - Flagyl
  - Lithium
  - Marijuana

"Nail in His Shoe"

Esther and Martin have been happily married for more than 30 years. Martin states their sexual relationship has been very good and satisfying for most of that period. Recently, however, Martin has been experiencing impotence and a decrease in his sexual drive. He feels he is letting his wife down and is becoming depressed. Rather than feeling like a failure, he has become distant and the relationship is deteriorating. Martin adds that this is just another "nail in his shoe." He states the doctor can't seem to get his blood pressure under control and has added another drug. He feels defeated and worthless.

What factors might be contributing to Martin's sexual dysfunction?

What further information should the nurse obtain from Martin?

What information should be provided for Martin regarding his medication?

In addition to medication adjustment, what other type of treatment may be needed for Martin and his wife?

Case Application 17.1

of understanding about anatomic functioning and effective sexual stimulation techniques. Because sexual desire is a mind and body process, a person's past experiences can sabotage the arousal and response cycle. This inhibition to arousal can arise from deep psychological fears or feelings of guilt and shame associated with the sexual act.

Studies show that for people between the ages of 18 and 59, most sexual dysfunction is related to orgasm, hypoactive sexual desire, and arousal problems in women. Erectile dysfunction in men tends to increase after age 50, whereas premature ejaculation tends to be most prevalent in younger men.

Paraphilic Disorders

According to the DSM-5, the term **paraphilia** refers to any extreme and persistent sexual interests other than typically normal sexual interests that are experienced between two consenting human individuals. The paraphilias include those sexual behaviors involving unusual objects, activities, or situations that may impose clinically significant anxiety or problems in social, occupational, or other areas of functioning. Most people with unusual sexual interests do not necessarily have a mental disorder. A paraphilic disorder is a paraphilia that "causes distress or impairment to the individual," or a paraphilia whose satisfaction involves "inflicting personal harm, or risk of harm to others." (DSM-5, p 685) Included in this category are eight conditions: voyeuristic disorder, exhibitionistic disorder, frotteuristic disorder, sexual sadism disorder, sexual masochism disorder, pedophilic disorder, fetishistic disorder, and transvestic disorder (Table 17.1).

TABLE 17.1   Categories of Paraphilias

PARAPHILIA	CHARACTERISTICS OR SYMPTOMS
Exhibitionism	Focus is on exposure of genitals to a stranger; this may include masturbation, often with no further attempt at sexual activity with that person. The surprise or shock observed during the exposure is often part of the stimulus for arousal
Fetishism	Use of inanimate objects (fetish) such as women's lingerie, shoes, or negligee with sexual activity involving these objects. Contact or view of the apparel is usually required for orgasm
Frotteurism	Activity that involves touching or rubbing contact with a nonconsenting person. Men often carry out the behavior in an area where a crowd or dim lighting will obscure the action. Activity will involve rubbing of the genitals against a woman's thigh or buttocks or fondling these areas while fantasizing intimacy with the woman
Pedophilia	Sexual activity with a prepubescent child 13 years of age or younger. The person with the disorder must be at least 16 years of age or older, and the child must be at least 5 years younger than the perpetrator. Victims are of both genders, although a preference is often displayed by the behaviors. Activities may involve undressing the child, exposure and masturbation in front of the child, touching and fondling, performing oral sex acts on the child, or penetration of the mouth, vagina, and anus with fingers, foreign objects, or penis
Sexual masochism	Recurrent strong sexual urges, behaviors, or sexually stimulating fantasies involving the actual act of being beaten, bound, humiliated, or otherwise made to suffer. These acts may be fantasized or the urges may be enacted during sexual encounters. Acts may include physical restraint, blindfolding, paddling, whipping, electric shock, cutting, or humiliating with human urine or feces. Forced cross-dressing may occur. Hypoxyphilia is a dangerous form of masochism that involves oxygen deprivation by noose, plastic bag, chemicals, or other means of causing peripheral vasodilation that can result in accidental death
Sexual sadism	Person receives sexual excitement from observing psychological or physical suffering by the victim. While relishing the terror inflicted, the perpetrator receives additional satisfaction from the accompanying feelings of complete control over the victim. Whether consensual or inflicted, it is the suffering by the victim that causes the sexual arousal
Transvestic fetishism	Cross-dressing by a man in women's clothing. Sexual arousal is the result of fantasies where he imagines himself as a woman (autogynephilia).The man usually keeps a collection of women's garments with preference for certain items for arousal
Voyeurism	Act of visual observation (window-peeping) of a stranger undressing, naked, or engaging in sexual behavior without the victim's knowledge. The act is done to achieve sexual arousal with orgasm achieved by masturbation. Generally, no further sexual contact is pursued
Telephone scatologia	Obscene phone calls that lead to sexual arousal
Necrophilia	Sexual arousal by physical contact or sexual relations with a deceased human or animal
Zoophilia	Arousal by sexual contact with animals

Signs and Symptoms

These disorders include intense, sexually arousing fantasies, urges, or atypical and unrestrained behavior with other human or nonhuman objects that may cause suffering or degradation to the person or his or her partner, to children, or to nonconsenting adults over a period of at least 6 months. For some individuals, these activities are required for erotic arousal and are consistently included in each sexual encounter. For some disorders, the acting out of the fantasy or urge causes the person marked distress. If the paraphilic act causes injury to a partner, as in sexual sadism or pedophilia, the person may be arrested and incarcerated. In other instances, the person may be referred to treatment after some unusual behavior has brought the person in contact with law enforcement. The person with a paraphilic disorder may use the services of a prostitute to obtain a partner with whom sexual fantasies can be performed. Some may secure employment in settings where contact is made with the desired stimulus for arousal (e.g., a *pedophile* may work in a day-care center or with a scout troop, or a *fetishist* may create displays of women's underclothing). Others collect articles, books, videos, and pictures that represent their particular sensual obsession. Not all people express anxiety or discomfort with their disorder despite being viewed by society as having a perverted and unacceptable character. Others will experience significant guilt and anguish over their unacceptable sexual functioning and desire for degrading activity. Symptoms of depression or a coexisting personality disorder may be present.

There are several common characteristics of these compulsive sexual behaviors that tend to interfere with the ability of the person to form intimate relationships. A conflicting sense of powerlessness and hidden anger create a state of internal anxiety. The person responds to this inner turmoil with a compulsive need to carry out the aversive sexual acts. The person may act to fill a void or to escape the stressful situation with or without recognition of the sexual dysfunction. An attempt is made to overpower another human being, which offers a challenge to get away with the forbidden. People who commit sexual offenses receive a charge from seduction, conning, or intimidation of another to achieve their goal. Values are self-centered and power oriented, with secrecy offering an advantage and source of control. There is frequent use of denial and rationalization as the person attempts to justify the behavior by concealing both the problem and the shame experienced as a result of the actions. Despite arrest, serious penalties, or reprisal, the sexual acts tend to continue with no attempt to control them. The person usually experiences a weak sense of self, accompanied by a feeling of deception and self-dislike for the dual standard portrayed by their behavior. These feelings are reinforced by the subsequent exclusion and isolation from the acceptable and lawful standards of society.

Just the Facts

Sexual abuse of a child is defined as sexual activity imposed upon a child by an adult with greater power, knowledge, and resources.

Mind Jogger

What factors do you think contribute to the high relapse rate of sexual offenders?

Incidence and Etiology

Paraphilic disorders are not often seen in the clinical setting, nor do people typically seek treatment for them on their own. Treatment for these disorders is most commonly connected to entanglements with law authorities over sexual offenses, pornography, and possession of paraphernalia associated with the acts. Recognition is sometimes complicated by the fact that certain types of behavior are more acceptable in some cultures than in others. Paraphilias are most prevalent among men and are rarely diagnosed in women. The disorders tend to be chronic and lifelong, although the behaviors may subside with age.

Exhibitionism and fetishism are usually evident by late adolescence and tend to be chronic. Frotteurism is most common from age 15 to 25, with a gradual decrease in events as the person ages. Acts of sexual sadism tend to increase in severity over time and will most likely continue until the person is apprehended by the law. Voyeurism is usually present before age 15 and tends to be chronic.

The perpetrator who exhibits pedophilia usually portrays the actions to the child as "educational" or "enjoyable," and the child often receives threats or warnings of harm if anyone is told of the indiscretions. The child responds to this bribery and secrecy with a sense of guilt and confusion over the forced seductive sexual acts and submission to the perverted passions of the adult. Forced to accept something distasteful and painful, the child develops feelings of powerlessness, helplessness,

"A Professional Duty"

When picking up her child from a daycare center, a nurse observes a 6-year-old boy standing close to a female worker rubbing his genitals against her leg. The worker tells him to go and play, but he continues his behavior.

What actions should the nurse take in this situation?

_____

_____

What category of paraphilia does this situation describe?

_____

_____

and rejection by those who ironically should be their "protectors." Perpetrators victimize their own children, those within the family system, and strangers. These acts are considered criminal behavior by a civilized society and are punishable by the law. This disorder usually begins in adolescence and tends to be chronic in nature.

Just the Facts

Basic lack of trust, low self-esteem, a poor sense of identity, little or no pleasure in sexual activity, and promiscuity are common characteristics of the adult who was sexually abused by a parent (incest) as a child.

Gender Dysphoria Disorder

For a diagnosis of gender dysphoria disorder to be assigned, the person must have a strong and persistent cross-gender identification and insist that he or she is, or has the desire to be, of the other sex. The person must also have continual discomfort with his or her sexual role. Unlike nonconformity to the stereotype of a boy or girl, the disorder includes a profound problem in the person's sense of sexual identity.

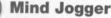

Mind Jogger

In what ways might a person demonstrate nonconformity to the assigned gender role of society?

Signs and Symptoms

People with gender dysphoria disorder are usually preoccupied with a desire to live as a member of the opposite sex. They may, to varying degrees, adopt the dress, habits, and appearance of the alternate sex. This behavior usually leads to social isolation, particularly in the adolescent who is subjected to teasing and distress by peers. Relationship difficulties result and functioning may be impaired.

In boys, cross-gender identification is shown by a preoccupation with feminine activities. They exhibit a preference for dressing in female clothing and enjoy play that is characteristic of girls, such as playing with dolls or being the "mother" when playing house. They tend to avoid toys and boisterous play that are considered typical for boys. They may express a wish to be a girl and exhibit a dislike for their male genitalia.

Girls usually demonstrate strong negative feelings toward attempts to have them dress or act

"Pain in Disguise"

Alex is a 39-year-old unemployed man who is admitted to the inpatient unit after ingesting a number of prescription drugs in a suicide attempt. While doing the initial interview, the nurse is distracted by the client's long fingernails and toenails painted in a flashy red color. Shoulder-length red hair encircles distinct attractive facial features accented with modest makeup. As Alex removes his jacket, it is noted he is wearing a shirt with lace, ruffles, and pearl buttons.

What is important for the nurse to do at this point?

_____

_____

What nursing approach is necessary for Alex to receive the appropriate treatment for his attempted suicide?

_____

_____

What sexual disorder is indicated by the appearance of this client?

_____

_____

Alex tells the nurse he hates himself as he is, that he has felt different all of his life, and wishes he were dead. He states, "The only time I feel real is when I am a woman, but I am only a fraud." What further information should the nurse obtain at this point?

_____

_____

Suggest some ways that Alex might be included in group activities without being a victim.

_____

_____

What outcomes are realistic for Alex?

_____

_____

in a feminine fashion. They usually prefer short haircuts and boy's clothing. They may ask to be called by a boy's name. There is a preference for rough and tumble play with boys, whereas little interest is shown for dolls or activities typical for girls. The girl may exhibit a desire for a penis and a dislike for developing breasts or beginning menstrual periods.

Adults with this disorder tend to be preoccupied with their desire to live as a member of the opposite sex. They may seek ways to adopt the appearance and social role of the other sex through hormonal or surgical means. They are usually uncomfortable in situations where they are functioning as a member of their designated sex.

Incidence and Etiology

Onset of this disorder tends to begin between the ages of 2 to 4 years. Parents typically become concerned when the child enters school if the "phase" of cross-gender interests has not changed. By late adolescence or adulthood, many of those with a childhood disturbance will report a homosexual or bisexual orientation but without an actual disorder. The disorder tends to occur more commonly in males than in females. Some people will also have a history of other sexual disorders.

Just the Facts

About 75% of boys with a history of gender dysphoria disorder report a homosexual or bisexual orientation as an adult.

Treatment of Sexual Disorders

Treatment of sexual dysfunction disorders in both genders varies by disorder and cause. Some of the disorders overlap and may require more than one particular treatment method. Hormonal therapy may be indicated in some cases. In others, a medication change can improve the sexual response. Active empathetic listening is vital to individual psychotherapy that is usually necessary to address underlying psychological factors such as sexual abuse and lack of arousal or desire for intimacy.

Treatment for the paraphilic disorders most often occurs after the individual is arrested. In some situations, as in pedophilia, the treatment is court ordered. Treatment consists of long-term cognitive-behavioral therapy, social skills training, support groups, antidepressants, and drugs that alter the sex drive by reducing testosterone levels. A coexisting physical or mental disorder may require additional treatment. Results, however, are not consistent. When treatment is sought voluntarily, the outcome tends to be better. When initiated only after mandated by the judicial system, the treatment process tends to be less effective. Incarceration of the person with paraphilia does not seem to change their behavior.

The psychological treatment of gender dysphoria disorder early in the individual's life can help the person to adjust and function in his or her biological body as much as possible. Therapy usually involves the family or partner of an adult. Hormonal therapy and sex-change surgery are available if the person chooses to pursue this option.

Application of Nursing Process to the Client with a Sexual Disorder

Assessment

The nurse can assist in gathering information related to a problem the client may be experiencing with sexual functioning. An interview for psychosexual dysfunction as described in Box 17.3

BOX 17.3

Interview for Psychosexual Assessment—Sexual Dysfunction

- Is your present sexual relationship a satisfying one?
- Tell me about the difficulties you are experiencing in your sexual performance.
- How long has this been a problem for you?
- Describe any negative sexual experiences you may have had.
- Do you experience any difficulty with sexual arousal?
- How often does this occur?
- Do you have any discomfort with sexual intercourse?
- What changes do you think might help your sexual relationships?

may be done to assess the particular areas that may be involved. All efforts should be made to ensure confidentiality and to respect the private content of the issues being discussed. The client should be encouraged to share feelings and concerns so that appropriate information and treatment can be provided. Referrals for specialized counseling or psychological treatment may be indicated if medical or drug-related problems are ruled out.

A multidisciplinary approach is used to cover the full range of sexually deviant behaviors. The assessment consists of a complete social and sexual history, psychosexual and psychological testing, and physiological studies of sexual arousal patterns. A psychiatric evaluation may also be performed.

Selected Nursing Diagnoses

Nursing diagnoses that are applicable individuals with sexual disorders may include the following:
- Sexual Dysfunction
- Ineffective Sexuality Pattern
- Chronic Low Self-esteem
- Anxiety
- Dysfunctional Family processes
- Disturbed Personal Identity
- Ineffective Coping
- Social isolation

Expected Outcomes

Once nursing problems have been assigned, realistic and measurable outcomes for the client with a sexual disorder may include: the following
- Acknowledges and accepts responsibility for compulsive and deviant acts without feeling extreme guilt and shame.

- Expresses anger and shame in an appropriate manner.
- Refrains from deviant sexual behavior by conscious control of arousal and sexual impulses.
- Confronts and resolves traumatic developmental issues.
- Confronts distorted sexual fantasies and thought processes.
- Develops an awareness of the feelings and rights of others.
- Develops insight into the effect that deviant behavior has on the victim.
- Develops more adaptive and effective coping and decision-making skills.
- Develops healthy interpersonal and sexual relationships.
- Participates and cooperates in a treatment plan to change behavior.

Interventions

It is suggested that there are often traumatic influences in the sexual and emotional development of the person leading up to the onset of the deviant sexual behaviors. Rehabilitation programs focus on cognitive-behavioral, psychodynamic, and trauma-based methods of therapy. Behavioral reconditioning may be used in an attempt to change sexual arousal patterns. A nurturing and caring milieu provides a safe shelter in which the person can acknowledge the past trauma and learn ways to control self-destructive sexual behaviors. Relapse is common during treatment of the paraphilia disorders, and a 12-step program is often initiated in the treatment process. Despite treatment, the perpetrator's personality does not change. Change is only possible when the offender makes a choice to participate in a treatment program. Behavior is directly related to the person's thoughts, so it is only when the person consents to expose inappropriate patterns of thinking and feels self-disgust that rehabilitation can begin. The person must engage in a daily inventory of thought processes and will never reach a point when this is not necessary.

The nurse is integral to planning and implementing the treatment process. Interventions may include the following:

- Develop self-awareness regarding feelings about own sexuality and relationships (dis-

comfort can be perceived by client as disapproval).
- Initiate a therapeutic relationship using an empathetic and nonjudgmental attitude.
- Encourage the client to verbalize feelings and perception of the sexual problem.
- Utilize communication techniques to guide client to discuss self-esteem and guilt issues.
- Ensure privacy and confidentiality during disclosure and treatment.
- Encourage group and self-help activities with referrals that support rehabilitation.
- Collaborate with mental health team to facilitate behavioral change.
- Report any knowledge of sexual offenses or abuse to appropriate authorities.

 Mind Jogger

How might the "thinking errors" influence other areas of the person's social functioning?

Evaluation

Although treatment is not often initiated by people with a sexual disorder, it is essential for the person to develop an awareness of the problem and the stressors that contribute to the dysfunction.

Through an understanding of the consequences of the disorder, the person can identify and work to develop satisfying, acceptable sexual practices with alternative ways of dealing with sexual feelings. It is anticipated that the person will demonstrate a willingness to make changes in patterns of thinking and engage in realistic problem solving.

As the person becomes aware of the underlying motives for his or her actions, a verbalized improvement in self-worth is anticipated. With a reduced level of anxiety and improved coping skills, the person is better equipped to communicate and interact in an appropriate manner. Given the chronic nature of many sexual disorders, it is important that a measure of self-control is evident through active participation in the treatment plan and ongoing demonstration of the desire to handle the situation in a way that results in satisfying and appropriate sexual experiences.

Summary

- Human sexuality is a blend of physical and emotional responses that combine to generate our sexual identity and behavior. Sexuality is integral in human development throughout the life cycle.
- A healthy sexual relationship is one that respects the rights of others and is mutually satisfying for both partners.
- Through self-awareness of his or her own sexuality, the nurse is able to promote an understanding of sexual needs and responses in the client.
- The sexual disorders are classified under the categories of sexual dysfunctions, paraphilias, and gender identity disorders.
- Sexual dysfunctions may be the result of psychological trauma, medical problems, or medication side effects.
- The paraphilia disorders encompass all altered mental processes related to sexual expression that prevent functioning within the laws and morals of society.
- An identification with our own gender begins at an early age. A resulting sexual orientation develops with an individual preference or mode of sexual expression. A crisis may develop in which the person has difficulty knowing or accepting the identified gender and may feel uncomfortable with his or her body parts.
- Deviant sexual behaviors tend to be compulsive and chronic in nature, leading to deceit and denial in an attempt to conceal the problem and avoid reprisal, social isolation, or arrest. Unable to form intimate relationships, a distorted thinking process leads the person to compensate for the anxiety and weak sense of self by performing deviant sexual acts. Despite attempts to hide the behavior, the person's unconscious demands gratification that can only be satisfied by repetition of the actions.
- A multidisciplinary approach is most effective in helping the person with a sexual disorder to confront and change or control the dysfunctional behavior.
- The quality of nursing intervention for clients with a sexual disorder is dependent on the empathetic and nonjudgmental attitude and approach of the nurse.

Bibliography

American Psychiatric Association. (2013a). *Diagnostic and statistical manual of mental disorders* (5th ed.). Washington, DC: American Psychiatric Association.

American Psychiatric Association. (2013b). *Paraphilic disorders*. Retrieved March 23, 2014, from http://www.dsm5.org/Documents/Paraphilic%20Disorders%20Fact%20Sheet.pdf

Balon, R., Segraves, T., & Clayton, A. (2007). Issues for DSM-V: Sexual dysfunction, disorder, or variation along normal distribution: Toward rethinking DSM criteria of sexual dysfunctions. *The American Journal of Psychiatry, 164*(2), 198–200. Retrieved March 23, 2014, from http://ajp.psychiatryonline.org/article.aspx?articleID=97829

Brown, G. R. (2013a). Sexuality and sexual disorders. *The Merck manual* (19th ed.). Rahway, NJ: Merck & Co. Retrieved March 23, 2014, from http://www.merckmanuals.com/professional/index.html

Brown, G. R. (2013b). Paraphilias. *The Merck manual* (19th ed.). Rahway, NJ: Merck & Co. Retrieved March 23, 2014, from http://www.merckmanuals.com/professional/index.html

Clayton, A. H., Reddy, S., Focht, K., Musgnung, J., & Fayyad, R. (2013). An evaluation of sexual functioning in employed outpatients with major depressive disorder treated with Desvenlafaxine 50 mg or Placebo. *Journal of Sexual Medicine, 10*(3), 768–776. Retrieved March 23, 2014.

Garcia, F. D., & Thibaut, F. (2011). Current concepts in the pharmacotherapy of paraphilias. *Drugs, 71*(6), 771–790. Retrieved March 23, 2014.

Hendrickx, L., Gijs, L., & Enzlin, P. (2013). Distress, sexual dysfunctions, and DSM: Dialogue at cross purposes? *Journal of Sexual Medicine, 10*(3), 630–641. Retrieved March 23, 2014.

NANDA International nursing diagnoses definitions and classifications 2013–2014. Oxford, UK: Wiley-Blackwell Publishers.

Student Worksheet

Fill in the Blank

Fill in the blank with the correct answer.

1. A disturbance in sexual desire or response leading to increased anxiety and interpersonal difficulty is termed a _____.
2. A systemic endocrine disorder that often causes sexual dysfunction in men is _____.
3. Deep psychological fears or feelings of guilt and shame associated with the sexual act can lead to a(n) _____.
4. Regardless of the required treatment for the person with a paraphilia, the perpetrator's _____ does not change.
5. The person with a paraphilia disorder must expose errors in _____ for rehabilitation to occur.

Matching

Match the following terms to the most appropriate phrase.

1. _____ Exhibitionism
2. _____ Fetishism
3. _____ Frotteurism
4. _____ Pedophilia
5. _____ Sexual masochism
6. _____ Transvestic fetishism
7. _____ Voyeurism

a. Having sexual activity with a child
b. Enjoyment of inflicting pain during a sexual act
c. Cross-dressing by a man in women's attire
d. Sexual gratification by rubbing against a stranger
e. Intentional exposure of one's genitals in public
f. Unsolicited visual observation of a stranger undressing
g. Sexual arousal using inanimate objects

Multiple Choice

Select the best answer from the multiple-choice items.

1. The nurse is doing patient teaching for a 45-year-old male client newly diagnosed with diabetes mellitus. The client tells the nurse, "I really don't want to talk about my sexual life. That is my business." The nurse can best meet the needs of this client by which of the following responses?
   a. "That is fine if you prefer not to discuss this issue. I will make a note to that effect on your record."
   b. "I understand. I would not want to tell someone about that part of my life either."
   c. "I know it must be difficult for you to talk with a stranger about such a private matter. We can discuss it at a later time."
   d. "We can't help you if you choose not to give us information. There are lots of people with your condition who have problems."

2. The nurse is talking with a 31-year-old female client who is experiencing dyspareunia. Tearfully, the client states her husband "expects me to have sex even though it hurts." Which of the following is the best response for the nurse to make at this time?"
   a. "We will be glad to refer you to a counselor who works with victims of sexual assault."
   b. "Tell me more about what happens when you have sexual intercourse."
   c. "After the doctor does a physical exam, we will try to help you with your problem."
   d. "I don't know how you put up with that. It must be very difficult."

3. The nurse is admitting a male client with a diagnosis of polysubstance abuse to the inpatient unit. The client is also a registered sex offender. In establishing a basis for treatment of this client, which of the following nursing interventions is most important?
   a. Using an empathetic and nonjudgmental approach
   b. Warning other clients about his sexual behavior
   c. Separating him from other clients on the unit
   d. Gathering information about his sexual behaviors

4. Josh is a 26-year-old who is mandated by the court to undergo therapy sessions for a charge of sexual indecency with a child. Which of the following will contribute most to success in his treatment process?
   a. Accepts a restriction of supervised-only visits with his son
   b. Allows a parole officer to attend each of his therapy sessions
   c. Admits that he has sexual fantasies about children
   d. Consents to expose the errors in his thinking

5. The emergency room nurse is assessing an 11-year-old girl who has reportedly been sexually abused by her grandfather. Which of the following most likely describes the objective emotional assessment of the child?
   a. Willingness to talk about the incident
   b. Anger toward her grandfather
   c. Fear and withdrawal when touched
   d. Clinging behaviors toward the nurse

6. A client is being followed in an outpatient clinic for treatment of depression and anxiety. Which statement by the client would indicate a possible sexual disorder related to medication side effects?
   a. "I really want to respond to my husband, but the feeling just isn't there."
   b. "Nothing seems to matter anymore. I don't even want talk to anyone."
   c. "I know I am not the best company, but my husband is supportive."
   d. "It takes all my energy just to get out of bed in the morning."

Chapter **18**

Disorders and Issues of Children and Adolescents

◉ Learning Objectives

After learning the content in this chapter, the student will be able to:

1. Describe common signs and symptoms for the various mental disorders in children and adolescents.
2. Identify etiological factors most implicated in the development of childhood mental disorders.
3. Discuss treatment options for the child or adolescent with a mental disorder.
4. Perform a nursing assessment of the child with a mental disorder.
5. Formulate nursing diagnoses with expected outcomes to address problems common to clients with these disorders.
6. Plan selected nursing interventions to address the needs of the child and adolescent with a mental disorder.
7. Determine criteria for evaluating the effectiveness of nursing implementation.

◉ Key Terms

copropraxia
dyslexia
echopraxia
encopresis

enuresis
intellectual disability
stuttering
tic

Although the disorders discussed in this chapter are typically first diagnosed or occur during childhood and adolescence, there is no defined line to distinguish between childhood and adult mental disorders. Many of the disorders first diagnosed during early developmental years will prevail throughout the individual's lifetime. Some disorders diagnosed during adulthood may have actually been present during earlier developmental periods. Therefore, it is difficult to draw a distinct division between the classifications. There are, however, those disorders that tend to occur first in childhood or adolescence as supported by studies that show as many as one in three children will have one or more mental disorders by the age of 16 years. There is a higher incidence between the ages of 9 and 10 years, with acceleration of the risk by age 16. Anxiety, panic, depression, and substance abuse disorders tend to increase with age, whereas the disorders discussed in this chapter are more common among younger children.

Numerous genetic and environmental factors may contribute to the incidence of mental disorders in children and adolescents. The chance of psychiatric symptoms is increased in individuals with multiple risk factors. Having a first-degree biological relative with the disorder is the most common underlying predictor of a similar disorder occurring in the child or adolescent. There is overwhelming evidence that many children who are diagnosed with a psychiatric disorder have a significant family history of mental issues. Environmental factors, including the socioeconomic status of the neighborhood in which the child lives, family income, and educational level of family members, all have an important impact on the child's behavior. It has been shown that youth from families living in extreme or moderately deprived neighborhoods tend to exhibit a significant increase in behavioral problems over those in less deprived areas. Parental divorce in situations where none of the other factors exists can also trigger problems for children and adolescents. When genetic predisposition and environmental factors are present in the same situation, the risk is compounded. In contrast, it must be said that not all children or adolescents who experience living in underprivileged circumstances develop a psychiatric disorder. Despite the inadequacy of their living conditions, many of these youth grow into well-adjusted, mature, and responsible adults.

Mind Jogger

What factors might contribute to situations where children emerge from a deprived environment to become responsible and secure adults?

Types of Mental Disorders in Children and Adolescents

Neurodevelopmental Disorders

The neurodevelopmental disorders include those conditions in which the child demonstrates symptoms of deficit before the age of 18 years. Typically, the deficits are seen early in the child's development prior to school age. These disorders are characterized by performance testing of mentality, skills, coordination, or activity that is substantially below that anticipated for the child's chronological age and education level.

Intellectual Developmental Disability

According to *DSM-5*, intellectual disability (intellectual developmental disorder) is "characterized by deficits in general mental abilities, such as reasoning, problem solving, planning, abstract thinking, judgment, academic learning, and learning from experience" (p. 31). **Intellectual disability (ID)** causes significant limitations in both intellectual functioning and adaptive behavior including the social and practical skills that are learned behaviors and used by people in their daily functioning. The impairments in adaptive functioning are seen in the individual's failure to meet expected standards of personal growth, independence, and social adaptation in all areas of daily functioning.

Signs and Symptoms
The individual with ID typically has intellectual functioning that is significantly below average or by having an IQ score of around 70 to 75 or lower. Significant limitations in adaptive behavior demonstrated by the Diagnostic Adaptive Behavior Scale (DABS), a standardized diagnostic assessment of adaptive behavior developed by the American Association on Intellectual and Developmental Disabilities, is also one of the measures of ID. The severity of the intellectual deficit is categorized by mild, moderate, severe, and profound levels of disability. These levels of severity are defined on the basis of the adaptive

functioning and not on IQ scores, because the deficits in adaptive functioning are what determine the level of support needed (DSM-5).

The cognitive impairment is seen in the delay of the child's conceptual skills of language and reading, time, numbers, money, and self-care skills. The interpersonal skills necessary for social interactions and relationships is lacking, along with the ability to follow rules and obey laws of society. Practical skills such as personal hygiene and care, attending to health care needs, transportation, daily routines and schedules may be difficult or neglected. Some individuals may be unable to use communication devices such as the telephone leading to safety issues and vulnerability to being victims of both physical and sexual abuse.

Some children with ID are passive, serene, and compliant, whereas others may be more aggressive and impulsive in their actions. The aggressive tendencies may stem from the child's inability to communicate in a meaningful way, which leads to frustration. Individuals with ID often are unable to take advantage of certain opportunities afforded to their typically developing peers, such as educational and job opportunities. One of the purposes of establishing a diagnosis of ID is to assist the individuals with special education services, home- and community-based waiver services, and government Social Security Administration and health care benefits.

Children and adolescents with neurodevelopmental ID are three to four times more likely to have a coexisting mental disorder than typically developing peers. Because communication is often limited for individuals with ID, objective symptoms such as depressed mood, irritability, anorexia, or insomnia may be the basis for determining that an additional problem exists. Those with co-occurring mental disorders are at risk for suicide and should be screened for suicidal thoughts or attempts (Box 18.1).

Incidence and Etiology

The causes of ID are primarily biological, psychosocial, or a combination of these factors. Prenatal damage related to toxins, maternal alcohol intake, infections, or genetic abnormalities account for the largest percentage of cases. Birth trauma and childhood illnesses largely account for the remainder of cases. In many individuals, there is no clear cause that can be determined. Children usually are brought for treatment with impaired functioning or the inability to cope with the demands

---

BOX 18.1

Signs and Symptoms of Intellectual Developmental Disability

- IQ 70 or below
- Decreased ability to adapt to daily living
- Impaired ability in reasoning, problem solving, judgment, and comprehension
- Impulsiveness, irritability, and aggressive behaviors
- Possible victim of abuse or ridicule
- Decreased social skills
- Depression

---

of everyday life. Although the intellectual deficit usually remains unchanged, interventions can provide some improvement of functional life skills in most cases of mild to moderate ID. Those with mild ID make up about 85% of clients with this disorder. This group can often be educated to approximately the sixth-grade level, in addition to learning the adaptive skills for semi-independent living. ID has a prevalence of approximately 1% of the general population, with severe disability averaging about 6 per 1,000 (Fig. 18.1).

Mind Jogger

How might the presence of a child with ID affect home life or siblings? What adjustments might be necessary as the child reaches school age?

Language and Communication Disorders

Children with language disorder have impairment in both verbal and sign language as evidenced by standardized testing. Children with this disorder

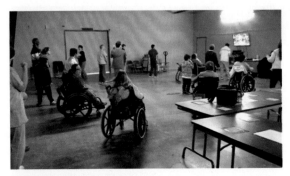

FIGURE 18.1

Group exercise activity at Mental Health Dayhab Center for individuals of all ages with Intellectual Developmental Disability.

have difficulty acquiring and using language due to deficits in comprehension or production of vocabulary, sentences, and speech. The language difficulty interferes with the child's performance in school and social functioning. Social communication disorder addressed deficits in using communication in an appropriate social context for interactive exchange.

Signs and Symptoms

The child with language disorder may have limited speech and vocabulary with difficulty learning new words or applying grammar concepts. Children with an expressive disorder (e.g., gestures, verbal animation) usually begin talking later than usual and progress at a slower rate than that which is considered age-appropriate. The child with a mixed language disorder also has a problem in understanding words and sentences that require complex thinking such as cause and effect or comparison of two concepts. There is a decrease in the ability to process incoming sounds or associate and organize words and sentences. Structural areas of language in which a deficit is seen are defined in Table 18.1. The inability to comprehend may be less apparent than the ability to speak effectively. The lack of comprehension is often seen when the child does not follow commands correctly or respond appropriately to questions. The ability to complete a thought process or follow rules of a game may also indicate the lack of understanding (Box 18.2).

Incidence and Etiology

Children with language and communication difficulty are often younger than 3 years of age when diagnosed. Delays are seen in approximately 10% to 15% of children. This number drops signifi-

---

BOX 18.2

Signs and Symptoms of Language Disorder

- Limited speech and vocabulary
- Difficulty learning new words
- Difficulty applying grammar concepts
- Delayed talking
- Slow progress in speech
- Difficulty in understanding words and sentences that require complex thinking
- Decreased ability to process incoming sounds
- Difficulty associating and organizing words and sentences
- Inability to speak effectively
- Lack of comprehension
- Failure to follow commands
- Inappropriate responses to questions
- Inability to follow rules of a game

---

cantly by school age, and most respond well to treatment. The incidence of a mixed language disorder is less common, with less than 5% of preschool children having this impairment.

Mind Jogger

What implications might the difficulty in comprehension and expression have for a child who is hospitalized?

Speech Sound Disorder

A failure to utilize sounds or articulate syllables intelligibly during speech is the essential feature of the child diagnosed with speech sound disorder. In many cases, the child also has a hearing impairment that contributes to the speech problem.

Signs and Symptoms

A common characteristic of this disorder is **stuttering**, which is characterized by repetitive or prolonged sounds or syllables that include pauses and monosyllable broken words. Stuttering causes considerable discomfort for the child in both academic and social situations but may be absent when the child is singing or reading aloud. There may be accompanying motor movement such as jerking, twitching, or tremors. Increased levels of anxiety and stress will often initiate the problem, which leads to further anxiety, frustration, and low self-esteem (Box 18.3).

TABLE 18.1	Structural Areas of Language
STRUCTURE	**DESCRIPTION**
Phonemes	Basic sounds of a spoken language used in phonics (sounding out to pronounce words)
Prefixes, suffixes, and root words	Give meaning to language (e.g., friend, friendly, unfriendly)
Syntax	System of rules that specify how words can be arranged into phrases and sentences (grammar) that underlie all language use

BOX 18.3

Signs and Symptoms of Speech Sound Disorder/Fluency Disorder

- Stuttering or problem with articulation or making sounds and sound patterns
- Repeating of sounds, words, or phrases
- Pauses during sentences or words
- Sounds of some word letters may be omitted or changed
- Eye-blinking or head movements while talking
- Increased anxiety
- Increased tension in voice
- Frustration and low self-esteem
- Raspiness or pitch changes in voice

Incidence and Etiology

Speech sound problems are more prevalent in boys and tend to be mild. The development of a stuttering problem is typically seen between 2 and 7 years of age, with a peak at 5 years. It is seen in less than 2% of children in this age group.

Autism Spectrum Disorder

The autism spectrum disorder (ASD), refers to a range of complex neurodevelopmental disorders that involve a delay in the development of various basic skills, including communication and socializing with others. The children with ASD have difficulty processing and understanding input from the world around them. The child may have specific areas in which problems exist and other areas of normal functioning. The DSM-5 no longer includes Asperger's syndrome which is now included in the broader category of ASD.

Autistic Disorder

Autistic disorder is characterized by severe abnormal development of the ability to socially interact and communicate with the outside world. Symptoms usually appear before 3 years of age. Children with this disorder are withdrawn and live in a fantasy world with little interest in their environment.

Signs and Symptoms

Early indicators that a problem may exist may be no babbling by age 1, no single words by 16 months, or no two-word phrases by age 2. The child does not respond to his or her name, and nonverbal behaviors such as eye contact, facial expression, and gestures used to communicate are profoundly deficient in children with autism. The child fails to develop age-appropriate peer relationships from lack of interest in or enjoyment from peer relationships and play activities with other children or from a lack of communication skills. Unusual patterns of playing with toys and other objects may be demonstrated, such as arranging their toys in a certain way or repetitious banging of an object. Time is occupied with an inflexible and consistent routine of nonpurposeful behaviors and rituals. Children with autism often have accompanying ID, ranging from mild to profound. Verbal skills and the ability to comprehend written words are usually below the level appropriate for the child's age.

Children with autism may exhibit other behaviors such as hyperactivity, impulsivity, aggressiveness, and inattention to the world around them. The child may demonstrate unusual or exaggerated responses to sensory stimuli, such as screaming when touched, or exhibit a lack of anticipated response to painful stimuli. The child may be very sensitive to some noises, but ignore others. Some children exhibit a fascination with certain colors, objects, or music. Eating patterns may be stereotyped, such as repeatedly eating the same food. The child may awaken during sleep and engage in rocking movements, head banging, or other self-injurious behaviors. Mood instability often occurs with sudden outbursts of laughing or crying. The adolescent who is able to understand his or her disorder may experience depression over this mental deficit. Autism is a lifelong disorder that affects not only the individual, but family and those around them (Boxes 18.4–18.6; Figs. 18.2 and 18.3).

BOX 18.4

Signs and Symptoms for Autism Spectrum Disorder

- Lack of responsiveness to others
- Unusual play behavior with toys
- Temper tantrums
- Severe impairment in communication
- Repetitive routines
- Does not like to be touched or held
- Withdrawal from social contact
- Unusual responses to environmental stimuli (e.g., head banging, hand flopping, rocking, clinging to inanimate objects)

BOX 18.5

Malachi—Autism Early Diagnosis: From a Mother's Perspective

"Malachi's early development seemed normal. He crawled and walked at the usual milestones, he was even trying to talk. But when he was 18-month-old, he stopped talking, he stopped looking at me when I talked to him, and wouldn't respond to me or to other children. At the encouragement of family members, he was taken to a clinic that specialized in autism and behavior issues with children, where at the age of 3 years he was diagnosed with autism. He attended special classes for autistic and intellectually disabled children and was given speech therapy. His teacher took a special interest in Malachi and worked tirelessly to engage him in social interaction and play with other children. She still calls to see how he is doing.

His special education teachers have been so helpful in working with him and teaching me as his mother, how to handle his behaviors and to help him adjust to the world around him. At times, his behavior has been violent. This is usually at times when he cannot handle his emotions—the most recent was when his maternal grandmother died. He was very close to his grandmother and called her frequently. He couldn't handle the sadness and grief which led to destructive behaviors and admission to a behavioral inpatient unit for stabilization. Most of the time, he does very well. He rocks and paces constantly, always in some sort of motion. He loves his camera and his pictures downloaded on the computer. He has hundreds of pictures that he loves to show to anyone who will look at them."

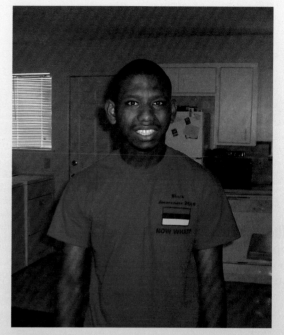

FIGURE 18.2

Malachi—age 16 years. (Permission granted by mother of individual.)

Malachi is now 16 years old, lives with his mother and is a happy young man who loves to take pictures and have his picture taken. He has a very special and bonded relationship with his mother. He is in the Big Brother–Little Brother program, likes to participate in athletics at his school, and attends church regularly with his mother.

Incidence and Etiology

The symptoms of autistic disorder are difficult to distinguish in the child under the age of 2 years because social and communication skills are in an early stage of development. Some parents indicate seeing early signs of developmental lag, whereas others report no obvious indicators of a problem. The incidence of this disorder is rising in the United States, with new data from the Centers for Disease Control and Prevention reporting that 1 in 68 children or 14.7 per 1,000 8-year-olds were identified with ASD. Boys are affected almost five times more often than girls. There is an increased risk of autism in siblings of children with the disorder, with the risk being in the range of 5%, or 1 in 20. Most children identified with ASD were not diagnosed prior to age 4, although it can be diagnosed as early as age 2 (Box 18.6; Fig. 18.3).

Attention Deficit/Hyperactivity Disorder

In attention deficit/hyperactivity disorder (ADHD), a persistent pattern of inattention, hyperactivity, or impulsive behaviors is more frequently exhibited than would be considered normal for a child of comparable age and developmental level. Some display of these symptoms must be present before the age of 12 years, often appearing between ages of 3 and 6. Many children are diagnosed after the problematic behaviors have been present for some time.

Just the Facts

Attention involves the filtering of incoming sensory stimuli to screen out most information. This allows only a select few stimuli to pass into conscious awareness.

BOX 18.6

Phillip—Autism for a Lifetime: From a Mother's Perspective

"When Phillip was diagnosed with autism at age 11, I grieved at the loss of 'what might have been...' We knew he had mild retardation and learning disability, but the label of autism seemed so hard to accept.

Parenting a child with autism is stressful but full of surprises. Autism can be overwhelming; no road map, no rule book, and no one to tell you how to handle it best. Phillip did not talk until he was almost 3 years old which was a struggle for me in communication to say the least. As a toddler, he was very high maintenance. But the older he got, we learned to adjust to his 'ways' and it got easier.

School was a challenge. Phillip went to a special education class most of the day, though he did join other classes in recess and choir. Most of his teachers were very good and adjusted to his 'learning style.' But sadly, we did encounter a few teachers who just didn't connect with his needs. His sister had to deal with people laughing at him or bullying him. Phil graduated with his class at age 19, walked the stage and received a modified diploma. It was a wonderful day for all our family.

My biggest concern now is what happens when we die?"

Phillip is now 43 years old and lives in a group home with four other individuals. He attends a Mental Health Center Dayhab during the week, and has a part-time job that provides the routine, ritual, and structure that he needs for his functioning. He often goes with his parents to family events, church, and other activities, and participates in Special Olympics.

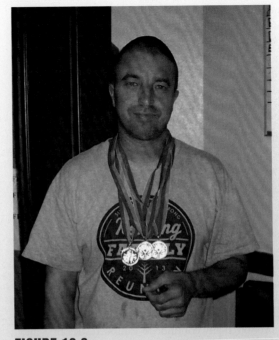

FIGURE 18.3

Phillip at age 43 years with his Special Olympics medals. (Permission granted by mother of individual.)

"From Martina's World"

Martina, a 3-year-old with flaming red hair and bright blue eyes, is admitted to the pediatric unit with asthmatic bronchitis. In addition to her medical condition, Martina has autistic disorder. Martina does not seem aware of the nurse's presence in the room but is intensely occupied with a blue stuffed dog. The nurse is preparing to administer scheduled oral medications to the child. Martina's mother is present in the room.

What approach would help the nurse to establish a trusting relationship with Martina?

_____

_____

What purpose will eye contact serve in helping Martina to communicate with the nurse?

_____

_____

What other behaviors might the nurse anticipate as Martina attempts to deal with her unfamiliar surroundings and activities?

_____

_____

Case & Application 18.1

Signs and Symptoms

Primary symptoms of inattention, hyperactivity, and impulsive actions are the key behaviors seen in children with ADHD. The behavior causes significant difficulty for the child when adapting in home, school, or social settings. There is usually an obvious pattern of disruption and inappropriate functioning as a result of the behavior. To be diagnosed with ADHD, the symptoms must be present for a period of 6 months or longer.

The symptoms of hyperactivity may not be the same at all developmental age levels. Toddlers and preschool children with ADHD usually exhibit more exaggerated activity than other children of the same age. Continual and often destructive physical activity is seen, along with an inability to remain seated for activities such as a television show or story-telling session. In school-age children, these behaviors may be minimized in intensity although fidgeting, noise-making, and other disruptive behaviors increase. The child often gets up from the table during meals or seated activities in the classroom. Although symptoms of the disorder often diminish in late adolescence or adulthood, many continue to exhibit restlessness and difficulty with activities requiring quiet attentiveness or concentration. This results in an unorganized approach to school work and work-related activities with minimal ability to follow through on task-oriented projects. Risk-taking behaviors are common, with little regard for the potential consequences of these actions. Impulsivity, which can occur in any age group, is demonstrated by impatience, the inability to refrain from interrupting, and discourteously intruding on the rights of others. Children with ADHD lack the self-control to delay their responses. The impulsive and fearless nature of physical activity often leads to accidental injury and destruction of property. Because children have different personalities and temperaments, and mature at varying rates, it is important that the child's behavior is observed during different situations and activities.

Additional symptoms may include a low tolerance or frustration with accompanying temper tantrums, mood changes, low self-esteem, stubbornness, demanding behavior, and poor parent–child and peer relationships. These behaviors tend to be labeled as willful, leading to conflict within the family and school systems. Family maladjustment and poor parent–child interaction are usually present. These relationships may improve with successful intervention and therapy. The intelligence level of individuals with this disorder ranges from lower than average to gifted (Box 18.7).

BOX 18.7

Signs and Symptoms of Attention Deficit/Hyperactivity Disorder

- Inattention to close detail or careless errors in homework or assigned tasks
- Inability to maintain focus on a task or play activity
- Often seems preoccupied and inattentive to the person who is speaking
- Repeatedly moves focus from one activity to another, failing to follow directions
- Failure to follow a task to completion
- Dislikes tasks that require maintained mental concentration and effort (e.g., reading, mathematics, mental games), often avoiding them
- Marked disorganization and careless handling or loss of materials necessary to perform a task or complete homework
- Easily distracted by irrelevant external stimuli such as a lawn mower or car honking
- Fidgety and frequent squirming with inability to remain seated when requested to do so
- Difficulty following instructions or taking turns in games or classroom activities
- Excessive and spontaneous talking and interruptions of others at inappropriate times
- Difficulty in playing quietly, appearing as a perpetual wheel in motion
- May engage in potentially dangerous or destructive activity, oblivious of the possible consequences
- Poor parent–child relationships
- Low tolerance to frustration
- Temper tantrums, low self-esteem, stubbornness, demanding
- Poor peer relationships

Mind Jogger

In what ways would the problem behaviors of a child with ADHD impact siblings and family life?

Incidence and Etiology

ADHD is more commonly seen among first-generation biological relatives of those with the disorder. In addition, the child's family and school environment along with peer influence also play a part in the development of problematic behavior. Many children with ADHD come from families in which members have a higher incidence of substance abuse and other mental disorder. It is most commonly diagnosed in school-age children, with a higher incidence seen in boys. According to the CDC, as of 2011, approximately 11% of children between the ages of 4 and 17 years have been diagnosed with ADHD with the numbers continuing to increase. The success of treatment varies, with the largest percentage of children continuing to demonstrate at least one of the disabling essential symptoms into adulthood.

Just the Facts

In addition to genetics, other possible links to ADHD include brain injury, environmental exposure, premature birth, low-birth weight, nutrition, or substance use during pregnancy.

Specific Learning Disorder

Learning disorders include situations in which the individual's performance on standardized testing in the skills of reading, mathematics, and written expression are much below the expected norm for that person's age, intelligence level, and educational standing. Children learn to use verbal communication skills and express themselves by observation and listening to those around them. Deficits may be seen in the ability to both interpret and utilize language skills.

Just the Facts

Learning refers to a relatively durable change in behavior or knowledge that is acquired by experience.

Dyslexia or Impairment in Reading

The most common type of learning disorder is **dyslexia**, or difficulty in the reading domain. In this disorder, there is a difference between the child's intellectual ability and their success in reading and spelling. Even though these children are of normal or higher intelligence, they may be behind in the level of reading expected for their grade level. The problem seems to stem from an inability to process incoming sensory stimuli with the correct interpretation.

Signs and Symptoms

The child with dyslexia usually does not read for pleasure. Spelling and writing by hand may be difficult, with a consistent pattern of letter confusion. Letter reversal is common; for example, "p" may be used for "g" or "b" used for "d." The child often reads from right to left with failure to see similar or different characteristics of words. For instance, instead of seeing "cat" the child sees "tac." There may also be a problem with sounding out words phonetically. Individuals who have dif-

---

BOX 18.8

Signs and Symptoms of Specific Learning Disorder

- Difficulty in learning and using academic skills of mathematics, reading, or written expression
- Difficulty with spelling of words
- Inaccurate or slow reading
- Effort is required to understand meaning of content that is read
- Difficulty with mathematical reasoning
- Written expression lacks clarity or content

ficulty learning may exhibit accompanying signs of discouragement, low self-esteem, and inadequate social skills. Evidence shows that early delays in language development are also associated with communication and developmental coordination problems. Signs and symptoms for specific learning disorder are found in Box 18.8.

Incidence and Etiology

Dyslexia is more frequently seen among boys than girls, and is often not diagnosed until the fourth grade or later when reading skills are more complex and increased comprehension is required. The fact that it is normal for some fluctuation to occur in a child's motivation in the academic setting must be considered as well. The quality and number of educational opportunities that are available to the child may also be a factor in the child's progress and skill. Hearing loss or visual impairment must be ruled out as a primary cause of the learning deficit. The prevalence is higher in first-generation relatives of those with learning deficits. Prognosis is good in a large percentage of cases in which diagnosis and intervention are made early in the learning process.

Just the Facts

The way children think about their successes or failures determines what effects these will have on their motivation and attitude toward learning. Children who attribute their failures to a lack of effort may try harder the next time, whereas those who attribute them to a lack of ability often quit trying.

Mind Jogger

How is the support of parents important in helping the child with a learning disorder?

Disruptive, Impulse-Control, and Conduct Disorders

The disruptive and conduct disorders include conditions that involve problems in the self-control of emotions and behaviors that violate the rights of others, or bring the child or adolescent into conflict with the norms of society or authority figures.

Oppositional-Defiant Disorder

Oppositional-defiant disorder is a repetitive pattern of angry mood, negative/defiant and hostile behavior toward authority figures typically beginning in the home.

Signs and Symptoms

Children with oppositional-defiant disorder demonstrate the tendency to argue incessantly with adults, lose their temper, and actively defy or refuse to comply with rules and requests imposed upon them. There is a pattern of deliberately acting in a way that annoys others, while blaming others for the behavior. Children with this disorder are usually vindictive, spiteful, and resentful in their interpersonal relationships and usually exhibit resistance to compromise or negotiation with peers or adults. The problematic behaviors may lead to suspension or expulsion from school and frequent encounters with law enforcement officials. There is an increased incidence of sexually transmitted diseases and teenage pregnancy reported in these clients. The tendency for suicidal ideation and suicide attempts increases and may be the factor in seeking treatment (Box 18.9).

BOX 18.9

Warning Signs for Suicide Risk in Children and Adolescents

- Verbal threats or behavior hints about suicide
- Decline in quality of schoolwork
- Truancy from school or running away from home
- Sudden withdrawal from friends or family
- Withdrawal from previously enjoyed activities
- Drug or alcohol abuse
- Giving away prized possessions
- Excessive fatigue or physical complaints
- Prolonged expression of sadness or uselessness
- Lack of response to praise and rewards
- Neglect of personal appearance or hygiene
- Unusually rebellious behaviors

BOX 18.10

Signs and Symptoms of Oppositional-Defiant Disorder

- Arguing without compromise
- Willful defiance of rules
- Hostility and anger
- Low tolerance to frustration
- Argumentative, angry, irritable mood
- Use of drugs or alcohol
- Physical violence
- Violation of curfews
- Spiteful or vindictive acts

Parental rejection and neglect with harsh and abusive physical punishment or sexual abuse are often cited as predisposing factors for this disorder. The child may have been removed to a foster or group home situation with a frequent shift in caregivers. Rejection by peers may lead the child to an association with those who engage in delinquent antisocial behaviors, violence, and drug-related activity (Box 18.10).

Incidence and Etiology

Oppositional-defiant disorder tends to be more prevalent in preschool children who demonstrate early difficulty with temperament or hyperactivity. It is more commonly seen in young boys and is seen equally among older boys and girls. These children have a low tolerance for frustration with frequent angry outbursts and conflict with parents and teachers. It is usually evident before the age of 8 years, with onset not often occurring later than early adolescence. A familial pattern of psychiatric problems is often pre-existent in the child. It is also seen more often in families where there is serious marital conflict between parents. A thorough evaluation of the child is important, because many of the behaviors seen in this disorder may normally be seen in children of preschool age through adolescence.

Mind Jogger

What factors in the family and social environment do you think contribute most to the incidence of the conduct disorders? What comparisons do you see between these factors and the rate of crimes against society?

Intermittent Explosive Disorder

Intermittent explosive disorder is characterized by angry, aggressive outbursts that have a rapid onset,

"Too Much for Anthony"

Anthony is a 14-year-old client who has been admitted to the adolescent psychiatric center after repeated incidents of suspension from school for disruptive and defiant behaviors toward his teachers and peers. He is an only child from a single parent family. His father died when he was 3 years old, leaving his mother with minimal employment skills to support her young son. Anthony was born with the congenital anomaly of imperforate anus, in which there is no anal opening for elimination of feces from the bowel. Surgery was performed to make an opening; however, without sphincter control, Anthony has had to endure the incontinence and embarrassment that accompanies this condition.

His mother relates that Anthony was always a hyperactive child. When he started school, the teachers were calling several times a week to tell her that they could not manage him in their classroom. He was given time-out suspensions from class in addition to receiving many failing grades in his academic learning. Anthony was placed in an alternate class situation for children with learning disabilities. In addition to being easily distracted, Anthony cannot sit still nor concentrate on any one task long enough for its completion.

Anthony's mother says that she is afraid he is going to end up in jail if something isn't done. She says, "He has been a hassle for me ever since he was born. Sometimes I really wish he had never been born. Maybe he would be better off in jail—then I wouldn't have to deal with him."

He is given a diagnosis of ADHD with oppositional-defiant disorder. It is also determined that Anthony has an intelligence level in the gifted range.

What psychological factors may be underlying his disruptive behavior?

_____

_____

What may have contributed to his performance in the school setting?

_____

_____

What feelings may Anthony be having related to his mother's attitude toward him?

_____

_____

What approach might be used to help Anthony's mother to deal with her son's illness?

_____

_____

Case Application 18.2

typically lasting less than 30 minutes. These outbursts are usually in response to a minor situation and may involve damage and/or physical aggression toward another person, animal, or property.

Signs and Symptoms

Onset of intermittent explosive disorder is typically during late childhood or adolescent years, and accounts for many incidents of school-based violence. The impulsive, aggressive response is significantly out of proportion to the psychosocial stressor that seemingly triggers the behavior. The impulsive aggressive behavior typically occurs in recurrent episodes that follow a chronic pattern over the individual's lifetime. The outbursts are usually unplanned and do not have ulterior motives attached (e.g., money, power, or property) (Box 18.11).

Incidence and Etiology

Intermittent explosive disorder is more prevalent in younger individuals and occurs more frequently in males. The disorder appears to be more common in individuals with family history of mood disorders or substance abuse. The onset of the disorder is frequently unexpected with no warning period of behaviors leading up to the time of diagnosis.

BOX 18.11

Signs and Symptoms of Intermittent Explosive Disorder

- Recurrent verbal or physical aggression that involves damage or destruction of property
- Physical violence that causes harm to animals or another person
- Impulsive assaultive behavioral outbursts
- Feeling of relief from the tension immediately after the explosive behavior
- Assaultive behavior is out of proportion to the precipitating stressor
- Tends to see the motives of others as malicious and directly targeting him or her
- Blames others for provoking his or her violence
- May experience racing thoughts or heightened emotions during an assault

BOX 18.12

Signs and Symptoms of Conduct Disorder

- Repeated disruptive and destructive behaviors
- Willful defiance of family rules
- Violation of age-appropriate and societal norms
- Aggressive behavior
- Truancy from school or running away from home
- Sexual promiscuity
- Substance use and abuse
- Vandalism and physical violence
- Cruelty toward animals
- Bullies and initiates physical fights
- Deliberate destruction of property belonging to others
- Intentional setting of fire with property damage
- Lying and deceit
- Running away from home

Conduct Disorder

Conduct disorder is defined as a pattern of repetitive and continuous behavior that either infringes on the basic rights of others or defies the rules of society that would be appropriate for the child's age level. This behavior may have an onset prior to the age of 10 years, with many also having a history of other disruptive disorders. Individuals with adolescent-onset type tend to demonstrate conduct problems in group situations, although their behaviors may be less aggressive.

Signs and Symptoms

Children with this disorder demonstrate aggressive actions that result in or threaten harm to other people or animals. They tend to initiate hostile and bullying-type behavior, using threats and fighting with or without weapons that can inflict serious physical injury. They may steal, rape, mug, assault other people, or seriously abuse animals. It is common for these children to lie and "con" by asking personal favors with no intention of repayment. Other behaviors may cause damage or loss of property, such as setting fires or vandalism. The behaviors usually exist in several situations such as the home, school, or community setting. There is usually a pattern starting before the age of 13 years. Defiance of home and family rules and curfews with a pattern of "running away" from home overnight or truancy from school is common.

Preschool children with conduct disorder usually exhibit aggressive behaviors in their home situation and toward other children. They often deliberately destroy other people's prop-

erty. School-age children continue the deliberate aggressive behaviors, both physical and verbal. In the adolescent, there may also be an early onset of sexual promiscuity, substance use, and physical violence that accompany the earlier behavioral pattern (Box 18.12).

Incidence and Etiology

Conduct disorder may have an early onset, before age 10, or during adolescence. The disorder tends to be more common among boys than girls, and may be associated with other risk-taking behaviors, school problems, substance use, and bullying. Conduct disorder is influenced by both genetics and environmental factors, with the risk increased in children with a first-degree biological relative with the disorder or families with a history of substance use and other mental disorders.

Anxiety Disorders

As a child learns to adjust to the world and form a separate identity, many situations create anticipated anxiety or fears that are realistic and normal. The manner in which the child's behavior is viewed and reinforced by others can contribute to an intensified feeling. Reinforcement of the distress felt in these situations also leads to a learned response of excessive and unwarranted anxiety.

Separation Anxiety Disorder

During early childhood development, it is expected that the stages of separation anxiety will be seen in response to new and strange encounters with unfamiliar objects or people. In comparison, the child with separation anxiety disorder experiences excessive anxiety related to separation from home or attachment figures. The disturbance must occur before the age of 18 years and cause significant distress or impairment in functioning for a period of at least 1 month. Symptoms may become evident following a stressful period in the child's life such as starting school, parental divorce, a neighborhood move, or death of a pet or close relative.

Signs and Symptoms

The child with separation anxiety disorder is uncomfortable to the point of misery when separated from the person with whom a love attachment is formed. When the separation is necessary, as in attending school, the child may feel the need to stay in constant touch with the person or be preoccupied with the need to return home. The child may experience somatic complaints such as abdominal pain, nausea and vomiting, or headaches during or before the separation. Excessive worry about the event or of losing the loved ones during a separation may become persistent. There may be a fear of going to sleep without the loved one present or worry that something terrible is going to happen to that person. The degree of anxiety can range from uneasiness to panic and depression. Depending on the age of the child, fears and concerns may vary. The younger child may have fears of the dark, monsters, burglars, fires, water, or other situations that could pose a danger to the family or self. Apathy, sadness, depression, and feelings of being unloved or unwanted are common. These children are often described as demanding of attention, leading to frustration and resentment within the family circle.

Treatment is aimed at reducing the anxiety and reinforcing a sense of security in both the child and the family during periods of separation. Although some children are successful in accomplishing these goals, others go on to develop a chronic anxiety disorder, panic disorder, or depression (Box 18.13).

Incidence and Etiology

This disorder is more common in children of parents with anxiety or panic disorders. The incidence is fairly common, with approximately 4% of children and adolescents affected by this level of anxiety. The symptoms tend to decrease as the child reaches adolescence.

> **BOX 18.13**
>
> ### Signs and Symptoms of Separation Anxiety Disorder
>
> - Severe anxiety about separation from attachment figure
> - Worry about something harmful happening to attachment Figure or self
> - Refusal to attend school or related activities
> - Somatic complaints
> - Fear of going to sleep without the attachment figure present
> - Apathy, depression, sadness
> - Attention-demanding behavior

Tic Disorder (Tourette's Disorder)

A **tic** is defined as a sudden, repetitive, arrhythmic, stereotyped motor movement or verbal speech that occurs before the age of 18 years. There is never a symptom-free period of more than 3 months.

Signs and Symptoms

Simple tics may involve such movements as blinking of the eye, wrinkling of the nose, jerking of the neck or shoulder, or grimacing. More complex movements may include hand gestures, contortions of the face, or physical actions such as jumping, retracing steps, hopping, and skipping over lines. Occasionally, the person may assume unusual positions or posturing. **Copropraxia**, or a sudden tic-like obscene gesture, along with repetitive movements (**echopraxia**) can also occur. Vocal tics are meaningless recurrent sounds such as sniffing, snorting, and throat clearing. More complex behaviors include verbal outbursts of words or phrases, speech blocking, or meaningless changes in tone or volume of speech.

The person with a tic disorder usually experiences an irresistible urge to perform the tic and feels relief once the behavior has occurred. Tics tend to occur in spells that may last from seconds to hours. The severity or frequency of the spells usually changes during the course of the day or as environmental location changes. Some children may be able to suppress tics during a school session, but return to the behavior during recess. Tics generally tend to decrease during sleep or during concentrated activity such as reading or playing the piano. The incidence may increase during periods of stress or demanding and competitive activities. The emotional discomfort, shame, and self-consciousness caused by the

---

BOX 18.14

Signs and Symptoms of Tic Disorder (Tourette's Disorder)

- Eye blinking, wrinkling of nose
- Jerking of neck and shoulder
- Grimacing
- Copropraxia
- Echopraxia
- Imitation of body movements
- Involuntary vocal and verbal utterances
- Sniffing, snorting, throat clearing

BOX 18.15

Signs and Symptoms of Elimination Disorders

- Repeated passage of incontinent feces or urine in inappropriate places
- Feelings of shame and embarrassment
- Social isolation and avoidance
- Psychological issues related to harsh toilet training
- Physical factors such as ineffective straining or pain with defecation

---

behavior may lead to social isolation or personality changes (Box 18.14).

Incidence and Etiology

Tic disorders tend to be genetic. Tourette's disorder tends to occur at an early age, with a prevalence in boys. Many more children than adults are affected with this condition. Tics tend to occur in all cultures and ethnic groups.

Elimination Disorders

Although some cases of elimination problems may be related to physiological causes, most are psychological in origin. Learning to control bowel and bladder functions is integral to the growth and development of the child. Problems can arise from the approach or methods used to assist the child in achieving this control, or it may be a delay in development that may resolve with time.

Encopresis is characterized by a repeated passage of feces into inappropriate places such as clothing, trashcans, or the floor. The child with **enuresis** has repeated episodes of urine incontinence during the day or night.

Signs and Symptoms

The elimination behaviors are usually involuntary but may be intentional. In encopresis, the child must be at least 4 years of age or have attained normal physiological control over defecation. The symptoms must occur at least once a month over a period of at least 3 months. The problem of constipation or impaction may stem from either physiological factors such as ineffective straining or painful defecation or psychological issues such as anxiety related to place or surroundings

at the time the child feels the urge to defecate. In the case of enuresis, the symptoms must occur at least twice a week for at least 3 months to be categorized as a disorder. The child must be at least 5 years of age or have control over urine continence. The symptoms may occur only during the day or night, or both.

Most children with these disorders tend to feel ashamed and embarrassed to the point of social isolation, and they avoid any activities that would predispose them to these feelings (Box 18.15).

> **Just the Facts**
>
> Predisposing factors for elimination disorders include delayed or lax toilet training, psychosocial stress, physical abnormalities, medication side effects, and fluid intake.

Incidence and Etiology

Encopresis is only seen in a small percentage of 5-year-olds and occurs more commonly in boys. Enuresis is common in as many as 5% to 10% of children in the same age group. The incidence decreases as the child gets older, with most becoming continent by adolescence. Most children with elimination disorders have a first-generation biological relative who has had the disorder. The risk is much higher for children if one of the parents has a history of either of these problems.

Treatment of Child and Adolescent Disorders

It is often the parents who suspect the behaviors of their child may be abnormal. It is important for families who feel their child may have a problem to seek treatment options as quickly as possible. The symptoms of a possible emotional, behavioral, or developmental problem can mimic other conditions and should be evaluated by a physician as early as it is suspected.

Neurodevelopmental Disorders

These disorders are typically treated with a combined approach of various therapies and behavior management interventions that key in on the major symptoms of impaired social skills, communication deficits, and the repetitive dysfunctional actions. Therapy sessions are used to help the child develop social and communication skills to foster the ability to form peer relationships and improve family situations. Cognitive therapy is an attempt to help children with explosive behavior to manage their emotions in an appropriate manner, and reduce repetitive actions. Antidepressant or antianxiety medications can be used to minimize the anxiety the child experiences as he or she attempts to control behavior patterns. Parents are taught the techniques in order to give the child continuity in management of the behaviors. Special education may be needed to provide for the individual needs of each child.

ADHD can be successfully managed using a combination of medication and behavior therapy. Medication can be used to better control behavior problems. While not one particular medication works successfully for every child, it is important to find one that works best. Stimulants are the most commonly used treatment with most children responding favorably to their effects. The benefits of these medications result in improved attention, less disruptive behaviors, and improved peer relationships. Improvements in the child's academic functioning are also seen. Most children do not experience side effects in response to these drugs. However, some may experience insomnia, stomach aches and anorexia, headaches, drowsiness, irritability, or nervousness. Some nonstimulant medications are available for treating the disorders with fewer reported side effects. Parents should be taught not to alter the established dose regimen or abruptly discontinue the medication. Withdrawal symptoms can be induced with sudden interruption in the drug levels. Common stimulant medications and nonstimulant drugs used in children with ADHD are listed in Box 18.16.

In addition to medication, behavioral therapy is a vital part of the treatment program. The inter-

---

BOX 18.16

Medications Used in Treatment of ADHD

Stimulants: (Some are approved for use in children over 3, others approved for children over 6 years of age)
- Methylphenidate (Ritalin, Concerta)
- Amphetamine sulfate (Adderall and Adderall XR)
- Dextroamphetamine sulfate (Dexedrine)
- Pemoline (Cylert)
- Methylphenidate transdermal (Daytrana)
- Dexmethylphenidate (Focalin and Focalin XR)
- Metadate CD and Metadate ER
- Methylin

Nonstimulants:
- Strattera
- Intuniv (*children/teens between ages 6 and 17*)

Others:
- Desipramine (Pamelor)
- Bupropion (Wellbutrin)
- Venlafaxine (Effexor)

---

ventions are designed to help the child create a structured routine that centers on behavior modification, goals and rewards, and discipline using consequences for inappropriate conduct. Parents are trained in parenting skills to maintain consistency in the approach to behavior change.

Learning and Communication Disorders

It is currently felt that keeping the child with a learning or communicative disorder in the mainstream of the educational system can best benefit the child's development. Teachers work together with speech and language therapists, learning specialists, and parents to schedule the school curriculum to meet the goals for each child.

Anxiety Disorders

Cognitive-behavioral therapy and group therapy are utilized in addition to antianxiety medications to help the child or adolescent to cope with their fears and uncertainties. Parents or families may be included in the therapy sessions to assist them in understanding the nature of the disorder and how to support their child.

Elimination Disorders

Most children tend to outgrow the problem at some point. A thorough medical exam is first done to rule out any physical cause. Once it is determined that it is a mental disorder, various behavioral approaches can be utilized. These methods gradually train the brain to respond to elimination signals during sleep or at controllable intervals.

⟳ Application of the Nursing Process

Assessment

The mentally or emotionally disturbed child is usually referred for evaluation and treatment by parents, teachers, other health care professionals, or the judicial system. Parents are often concerned and frustrated with the child's actions and inability to adapt to daily living. To assess all factors that may contribute to the child's disturbed behavior, information is collected regarding the child, the family, and related environmental factors. These data assist the health care team to determine if there are any relevant extended family issues. It is important that family members be included in identifying areas of concern. Once the family is aware of the existent issues, they are able to reflect on the situation and actively participate in planning strategies necessary to help the child.

Parents, teachers, and other social contacts of the child are the usual sources of information regarding the child's troublesome behavior. A history should include the time at which the problematic behaviors began and any significant occurrences (e.g., treatment of pets, disruptions at school, discipline by parents) at that time that may have precipitated the symptoms. A thorough physical and emotional assessment is completed. The child's ability to communicate and interact with others is usually assessed and observed using play activities. A thorough assessment is also made of the child's feelings, self-image, distorted thinking, or other subjective symptoms such as abuse, depression, or suicidal ideation. It is not unusual for the child to reveal problems related to familial relationships, such as abuse, that are not divulged or known by others within the family circle. In addition, it is important to assess communication and interaction patterns between family members. Determine the degree to which the child's behavior and actions are disrupting the family functioning or other social settings in which the child participates.

Selected Nursing Diagnoses

Selection of the appropriate nursing diagnoses may vary according to the mental disorder to address the needs of the individual child. Selecting appropriate diagnoses is especially difficult because the child is in a period of constant growth and development, with unpredictable behavior that is influenced by both genetics and environmental factors. Because many of these disorders may overlap and coexist in the same child, planning may identify multiple problem areas. Nursing diagnoses that can be applied to all children and adolescents with mental conditions include the following:

- Risk for Injury, related to altered physical mobility or aggressive behavior
- Impaired Verbal Communication, related to verbal expression or inability to speak or form words and sentences
- Impaired Social Interaction, related to disruptive or inappropriate behaviors and decreased self-esteem

In addition to these common nursing diagnoses, others may include the following:

- Self-Care Deficit, related to cognitive processing or maturity level
- Delayed Growth and Development, related to genetic or environmental factors
- Risk for Injury, related to neurological deficits and indifference to the environment
- Disturbed Personal Identity, related to inability to recognize self as separate being
- Risk for Violence, Self- or Other-directed related to dysfunctional family environment, poor impulse-control, or aggressive and self-destructive behaviors
- Ineffective Coping, related to low self-esteem, disorganized and maladaptive environment, or immature and inadequate coping strategies
- Compromised Family Coping, related to disruptive or destructive child behavior, and maladaptive family system
- Anxiety, related to unmet needs and dysfunctional social relationships
- Noncompliance, related to low frustration level and negativism
- Disturbed Sleep Pattern, related to anxiety and fears of separation

Expected Outcomes

Once appropriate nursing diagnoses have been selected, planning includes determining anticipated outcomes toward which the individual client may be able to accomplish progress in resolving the identified problems. Realistic time frames will depend on the individual client and the nature and extent of the problem. Expected outcomes for the child or adolescent may include the following:

- Remains free of self-harm and does not harm others
- Establishes effective alternative communication with staff and family
- Chooses and initiates appropriate social interactions with peers
- Demonstrates consistent progress in self-care development toward maximum potential and independence
- Demonstrates increased autonomy and reliance on self
- Expresses positive feelings about self
- Exhibits ability to control impulsivity and take turns with others
- Describes possible consequences of behavior
- Participates in planning and implementation of behavior improvement program
- Tolerates overnight separation periods from attachment figure
- Verbalizes decreased anxiety during separation from parent or love figure
- Exhibits decreased complaints of somatic symptoms
- Identifies precipitating factors for anxiety
- Applies improved alternative coping strategies

Expected outcomes for parents and family members may include the following:

- Identify strengths and weakness of the child
- Participate in planning and implementation of behavior improvement program
- Establish and maintain consistency in boundaries for acceptable behavior
- Provide reinforcement of child's positive behaviors
- Describe appropriate ways to express feelings of frustration regarding child's inappropriate behaviors
- Develop appropriate ways to cope with anger and feelings toward the child

Interventions

Implications for nursing care of the child or adolescent with a mental illness will vary based on the individual needs of the child and the disorder being addressed. Interventions may overlap in the child with more than one diagnosis. General nursing approaches may include the following:

- Maintain a safe physical environment.
- Identify any suicide risk, ideation, or actions.
- Keep sharp or hazardous items out of reach or in a locked area.
- Intervene to prevent injury from aggression or acting-out behaviors.
- Redirect and channel aggressive behavior into a controlled activity.
- Maintain consistency of caregivers and approach to behavior issues.
- Identify capabilities of the child or adolescent related to self-care.
- Provide encouragement for the child toward independent self-care.
- Provide simple explanations for behavior boundaries.
- Establish a consistent pattern of reward for positive behavior and aversive stimuli response for negative behaviors.
- Identify association between nonverbal communication patterns and the child's individual needs.
- Use headgear such as a helmet or hand coverings to prevent self-inflicted injury during behaviors such as head banging, scratching, or hair pulling.
- Attempt to determine precipitating factors that lead to agitated and self-injurious behavior.
- Establish a trusting relationship by first using eye contact reinforced with a smile.
- Use a slow approach when introducing tactile stimuli such as touch or hugs.
- Use positive reinforcement for child's attempts at interaction with others.
- Provide familiar security objects such as a favorite toy, pillow, or blanket.
- Provide adequate supervision and limits for the child's activity.
- Use a matter-of-fact approach in explanation of consequences for negative behaviors.
- Plan activities that provide a chance for the child to succeed.
- Provide a distraction-free environment for task-oriented activity.
- Help the child or adolescent to recognize and accept anger as a feeling.
- Teach the child or adolescent ways to channel anger into socially appropriate physical outlets.

**Information Sources for Parents
of Children and Adolescents
with Mental Disorders**

- Autism Society of America
  7910 Woodmont Ave., Suite 300
  Bethesda, MD 20814-3067
  http://www.autism-society.org
  Tel: 301-657-0881/800-3AUTISM (328-8478)
- MAAP Services for Autism, Asperger Syndrome,
  and PDD
  P.O. Box 53
  Crown Point, IN 46308
  http://www.maapservices.org
  Tel: 219-662-1311
- National Institute of Mental Health (NIMH)
  6001 Executive Blvd. Rm. 8184, MSC 9663
  Bethesda, MD 20892-9663
  http://www.nimh.nih.gov
  Tel: 301-443-4513/866-415-8051
- National Resource Center on AD/HD:
  A Program of CHADD
  8181 Professional Place, Suite 150
  Landover, MD 20785
  1-800-233-4050
  www.help4adhd.org
- Learning Disabilities Association of America
  4156 Library Road
  Pittsburgh, PA 15234-1349
  Tel: 412-341-1515

- Include parents in discussions regarding events that trigger overwhelming fears and somatic symptoms in the child.
- Provide sources of information and support groups for parents (Box 18.17).

Evaluation

Criteria for evaluating the desired outcomes in the child will depend on the problematic behavior being addressed. It is anticipated that children with developmental disorders will increase their ability to interact and communicate with others. This can be measured by progress in their ability to trust others and initiate social contact with another person. Progress is also evaluated in the child's ability to control negative and self-harming behaviors.

Evaluation of the child with ADHD will include a consistent decrease in disruptive and dangerous behaviors along with the ability to function in a social or structured learning environment. Goals for the child with a conduct disorder are centered on the development of self-control and a decrease in impulsive behaviors. The outcome is measured by improvement in the ability to have satisfying relationships with both peer and family groups. Positive steps in developing self-esteem and feelings of self-worth should also be noted.

It is vital in each type of child or adolescent disorder that careful evaluation is given to the participation of parents and other family members in the treatment program. Take note of interactions between the child and family with emphasis on whether they are coping effectively with the child's behavioral symptoms. Evaluate the support given to the child and whether there is positive reinforcement of positive behaviors. A positive outcome is demonstrated in the child's ability to function and adapt appropriately to the environment around them.

Summary

- The most prevalent factor that may contribute to the incidence of a mental disorder in the child or adolescent is the genetic component with a familial history of mental disorders.
- This risk is compounded when environmental issues such as poverty, violence, substance abuse, and poor family relationships provide a dysfunctional system in which the child lives.
- Disorders may exist in various developmental areas including neurodevelopmental and intellectual level, interactive and communicative skills, and coordination or activity. Deficits may range from mild to profound, and may interfere with the child's ability to adjust and interact with the world around them.
- Children and adolescents with neurodevelopmental disorders have limited social skills and lack of enthusiasm involving their environment. They do not develop mentally or socially to a level consistent with their chronological age or education level.
- Learning disorders and language impairment interfere with the child's performance both socially and academically. The frustration experienced by these children often leads to decreased motivation and premature exit from the school system.

- Because both society and academic advancement require basic skills in reading, mathematics, writing, and communicative language, it is difficult for children and adolescents with learning and communication disorders to adjust and function as they grow older.
- Early intervention and treatment can help the child with a learning or communication disorder to adapt and accommodate for the deficit.
- Perhaps the most difficult situation for both clients and parents is the child or adolescent with a disruptive, impulse-control, or conduct disorder. Because of the disruptive and destructive nature of the behaviors, these children often become entangled with law enforcement officials early in their lives. The child is unable to understand or control the erratic episodes of behavior, which leads to frustration and ambivalent feelings in parents, teachers, and others who come in contact with the child.
- Family maladjustment and poor parent–child interaction are common among children and adolescents with disruptive, impulse-control, or conduct disorders. If the child's conduct is aggressive or hostile in nature, the likelihood increases that the behavior will lead to arrest and disciplinary action by the judicial system. There is often a familial pattern of psychiatric problems in children who are diagnosed with conduct or defiant disorders of this level.
- Other disorders in children are often the result of stress-related symptoms that manifest themselves in the form of anxiety, repetitive tic movements, or inappropriate elimination.
- Children and adolescents with mental disorders often have a poorly developed self-concept that is further eroded by the embarrassment and lack of understanding about the disorder.
- Therapeutic intervention includes helping the child to understand the relationship between the psychological symptoms and the condition.
- Many of the mental disorders seen in children and adolescents continue to manifest symptoms into the adult years. Some are not diagnosed until adulthood but may have been present since childhood, while others are not symptomatic until adolescence and beyond.
- Early intervention is necessary to assist both the child and family to develop the adaptive skills to encourage a functional level of existence.

Bibliography

American Psychiatric Association. (2013). *Diagnostic and statistical manual of mental disorders* (5th ed.). Washington, DC: American Psychiatric Association.

Andersen, S. L., & Navalta, C. P. (2011). Annual research review: New frontiers in developmental neuropharmacology: Can long-term therapeutic effects of drugs be optimized through carefully timed early intervention? *Journal of Child Psychology and Psychiatry, 52*(4), 476–503. Retrieved December 28, 2013.

Arabgol, F., Pahaghi, L., & Hebrani, P. (2009). Reboxetine versus methylphenidate in treatment of children and adolescents with attention deficit-hyperactivity disorder. *European Child and Adolescent Psychiatry, 18*(1), 53–39. Retrieved April 1, 2014.

Bellanti, C. (2009). Fostering social skills in children with ADHD. *Brown University Child and Adolescent Behavior Letter, 25*(1), 1–6. Retrieved April 1, 2014.

Centers for Disease Control and Prevention. (2014). 10 things to know about new autism data. Retrieved March 30, 2014, from http://www.cdc.gov/features/dsautismdata/

Childres, J. L., Shaffer-Hudkins, E., & Armstrong, K. (2012). Helping our toddlers, developing our children's skills: A problem-solving approach for parents of young children with autism spectrum disorders. *Journal of Early Childhood and Infant Psychology,* (8), 1–19. Retrieved March 29, 2014.

Elbe, D., & Reddy, D. (2014). Focus on Guanfacine extended-release: A review of its use in child and adolescent psychiatry. *Journal of the Canadian Academy of Child and Adolescent Psychiatry, 23*(1), 48–60. Retrieved March 28, 2014.

Goldstein, S., Naglieri, J. A., Rzepa, S., & Williams, K. M. (2012). A national study of autistic symptoms in the general population of school-age children and those diagnosed with autism spectrum disorders. *Psychology in the Schools, 49*(10), 1001–1016. Retrieved March 29, 2014.

Greene, R. W., Biederman, J., Zerwas, S., Monuteaux, M. C., Goring, J. C., & Faraone, S. V. (2002). Clinical significance of oppositional defiant disorder. *American Journal of Psychiatry, 159*(7), 1214–1224. Retrieved April 1, 2014.

Hosenbocus, S., & Chahal, R. (2012). A review of executive function deficits and pharmacological management in children and adolescents. *Journal of the Canadian Academy of Child and Adolescent Psychiatry, 21*(3), 223–229. Retrieved March 28, 2014.

Mulligan, A., Anney, R. J., O'Regan, M., Chen, W., Butler, L., Fitzgerald, M., Buitelaar, J., Steinhausen, H. C., Rothenberger, A., Minderaa, R., Nijmeijer, J., Hoekstra, P. J., Oades, R. D., Roeyers, H., Buschgens, C., Christiansen, H., Franke, B., Gabriels, I., Hartman, C., Kuntsi, J., Marco, R., Meidad, S., Mueller, U., Psychogiou, L., Rommelse, N., Thompson, M., Uebel, H., Banaschewski, T., Ebstein, R., Eisenberg, J., Manor, I., Miranda, A., Mulas, F., Sergeant, J., Sonuga-Barke, E., Asherson, P., Faraone, S. V., & Gill, M. (2009). Autism symptoms in Attention-Deficit/Hyperactivity Disorder: A familial trait which correlates with conduct, oppositional defiant, language and motor disorders. *Journal of Autism and Development Disorders, 39*(2), 197–209. Retrieved March 19, 2014.

NANDA International nursing diagnoses definitions and classifications 2013–2014. Wiley-Blackwell Publishers.

National Institute of Mental Health. (2006). Intermittent explosive disorder affects up to 16 million Americans. Retrieved March 19, 2014, from http://www.nimh.nih.gov/news/science-news/2006/intermittent-explosive-disorder-affects-up-to-16-million

National Institute of Mental Health. (2013). Autism spectrum disorder. Retrieved March 29, 2014, from http://www.nimh.nih.gov/health/publications/attention-deficit-hyperactivity-disorder/index.shtml

National Institute of Neurological Disorders and Stroke. (2013). Autism fact sheet. Retrieved March 29, 2014, from http://www.ninds.nih.gov/disorders/autism/detail_autism.htm

Pardini, D., & Frick, P. J. (2013). Multiple developmental pathways to conduct disorder: Current conceptualizations and clinical implications. *Journal of Canadian Academy of Child and Adolescent Psychiatry, 22*(1), 20–25. Retrieved March 28, 2014.

Reichow, B., Servili, C., Yasamy, M. T., Barbui, C., & Saxena, S. (2013). Non-specialist psychosocial interventions for children and adolescents with intellectual disability or lower-functioning autism spectrum disorders: A systematic review. *PLoS Medicine, 10* (12), 1–27. Retrieved March 28, 2014.

Rispoli, M., Lang, R., Neely, L., Camargo, S., Hutchins, N., Davenport, K., & Goodwyn, F. (2013). A comparison of within-and across-activity choices for reducing challenging behavior in children with autism spectrum disorders. *Journal of Behavioral Education, 22*(1), 66–83. Retrieved March 19, 2014.

Ruchkin, V., Koposov, R, Vermeiren, R, & Schwab-Stone, M. (2003). Psychopathology and early conduct disorder explain persistent delinquency. *Journal of Clinical Psychiatry, 64*(8), 913–920. Retrieved April 4, 2014.

Steensel, F. J., Bogels, S., & Bruin, E. (2013). Psychiatric comorbidity in children with autism spectrum disorders: A comparison with children with ADHD. *Journal of Child and Family Studies, 22*(3), 368–376. Retrieved March 29, 2014.

Stevanovic, D. (2013). Impact of emotional and behavioral symptoms on quality of life in children and adolescents. *Quality of Life Research, 22*(2), 333–337. Retrieved March 31, 2014.

Townsend, M. C. (2011). *Nursing diagnoses in psychiatric nursing* (8th ed.). Philadelphia, PA: F.A. Davis Co.

Vacca, J. T. (2013). The parenting process from the father's perspective: Analysis of perceptions of fathers about raising their child with autism spectrum disorder. *Best Practice in Mental Health, 9*(2), 79–93. Retrieved March 29, 2014.

Varcolaris, E. M. (2011). *Manual of Psychiatric Nursing Care Planning* (4th ed.). St. Louis, MO: Saunders Elsevier.

Weiss, J. A., Viecili, M. A., Sloman, L., & Lunsky, Y. (2013). Direct and indirect psychosocial outcomes for children with autism spectrum disorder and their parents following a parent-involved social skills group intervention. *Journal of the Canadian Academy of Child and Adolescent Psychiatry, 22*(4), 303–309. Retrieved March 29, 2014.

Wilson, B. A., Shannon, M. T., & Shields, K. M. (2013). *Prentice hall nurse's drug guide 2014.* Upper Saddle River, NJ: Pearson Prentice Hall.

Student Worksheet

Fill in the Blank

Fill in the blank with the correct answer.

1. _____ is the most common underlying contributor to the probability of a mental disorder in children.
2. _____ is the most common type of learning disorder.
3. Individuals with mild ID can be educated to approximately the _____ in addition to learning skills for adaptive living.
4. Speech that is characterized by repetitive or prolonged sounds or syllables that include pauses and monosyllable broken words is _____.
5. The filtering of sensory input to allow a select few to pass through into conscious awareness is termed _____.
6. Repetitive movements that occur in tic disorders are referred to as_____.

Matching

Match the following terms to the most appropriate phrase.

1. _____ ADHD
2. _____ Developmental coordination disorder
3. _____ Enuresis
4. _____ Conduct disorder
5. _____ Intellectual developmental disability
6. _____ Oppositional-defiant disorder
7. _____ Language disorder
8. _____ Autism
9. _____ Speech sound disorder

a. Repetitive and continuous behavior that infringes on the rights of others or defies rules of society appropriate for age level
b. Deficits in general mental abilities, problem solving, and learning from experience
c. Failure to utilize sounds or articulate syllables intelligibly during speech
d. Repeated episodes of urine incontinence during day or night
e. Clumsiness in motor activities with significant delays in developmental milestones
f. Persistent patterns of inattention, hyperactivity, or impulsive behaviors, more frequent than those seen in the average child
g. Repetitive pattern of negative, defiant, disobedient, and hostile behavior toward authority figures
h. Marked abnormality in the development of ability to socially interact and communicate with the outside world
i. Difficulty acquiring and using language due to deficits in comprehension or production of vocabulary, sentences, and speech

Multiple Choice

Select the best answer from the multiple-choice items.

1. Miguel is a 6-year-old who has been diagnosed with enuresis after tests show no physical reason for the symptoms. Miguel's mother is visibly upset and says, "It is his father's fault. He had the same problem." Which of the following would be the nurse's best response?

   a. "Why would you blame his father?"
   b. "This problem is not usually someone's fault."
   c. "You seem quite upset about your son's problem."
   d. "What is it in his father's background that makes you say that?"

2. Justin is a 7-year-old child who is having difficulty with reading and writing assignments in school. His teacher has suggested he be tested for a learning disorder. Which of the following categories would apply to Justin's problem?
   a. Stuttering
   b. Dyslexia
   c. Attention deficit
   d. Vocal tic

3. Amanda, a 6-year-old whose parents divorced 6 months ago, begins to cry and vomits each time her mother brings her to school. Her mother is asked to take her home each day. Which of the following is most descriptive of Amanda's behavior?
   a. Conduct disorder
   b. Separation anxiety disorder
   c. Oppositional-defiant disorder
   d. Pervasive developmental disorder

4. School officials have contacted the parents of John, a 14-year-old who has been truant from school four times in the past month. John set fire to his grandmother's garage when he was 10, assaulted his father for telling him to clean his room at age 11, and was suspended from school for writing graphic language on the school sidewalk with spray paint. When John is admitted to the psychiatric center for adolescents, which of the following nursing diagnoses should receive priority?
   a. Risk for violence, directed at others
   b. Self-esteem, disturbance
   c. Dysfunctional family processes
   d. Social interaction, impaired

5. Monica is a 16-year-old who has been admitted to the psychiatric unit with severe depression. Monica is placed on suicide precautions. Which of the following signs might be suggestive of suicidal behavior?
   a. Limits her visitors to four people
   b. Asks the nurse for shampoo so she can wash her hair
   c. Sleeps during the day in between therapy sessions
   d. Gives her charm bracelet to her best friend

6. The child with a language and communication disorder would most likely have a problem with which of the following tasks?
   a. Following rules for a game
   b. Being touched or held by another person
   c. Staying overnight with a relative
   d. Compromising during an argument

7. Beth is a 5-year-old who has difficulty articulating syllables in a way that her speech can be understood. She often has repetitive or prolonged sounds separated by pauses that make her anxious and upset. Which of the following describes the speech problem that Beth is experiencing?
   a. Syntax
   b. Copropraxia
   c. Stuttering
   d. Echopraxia

8. Richard is a 7-year-old who exhibits characteristic signs of delayed mental development. Upon testing, Richard is found to have an IQ level of 54. Which of the following situations would be a realistic outcome for Richard?
   a. Institutional care to provide adequate supervision
   b. Independent living with ability to provide own income
   c. Simple job with supervised independent living
   d. Self-care needs of feeding and toileting only

9. Bobby is a 7-year-old who is being evaluated for a learning disorder. While talking to his mother, the nurse receives the following information. Which of the following factors is most likely a contributing factor to the child's performance?
   a. Turns up the TV to volume that is uncomfortable for others
   b. Likes to play on swings and gym equipment at school
   c. Tends to pick on his little brother and sister
   d. Is afraid of the neighbor's dog

10. A 15-year-old is verbally aggressive toward the principal of his school after being reprimanded for breaking a school rule. He tells him, "You don't own me. Nobody owns me. I don't have to keep your silly rules." This type of behavior is characteristic in which of the following disorders?
    a. Mental retardation
    b. Oppositional-defiant disorder
    c. Separation anxiety disorder
    d. Tourette's disorder

Disorders and Issues of the Older Adult

⊙ Learning Objectives

After learning the content in this chapter, the student will be able to:

1. Describe characteristics of older adult clients.
2. Describe psychosocial issues relating to the mental health of the older adult.
3. Assess and differentiate between delirium and three types of dementia.
4. Describe the symptoms and stages in the progression of dementia due to Alzheimer's disease.
5. Discuss treatment approaches to mental disorders in the older adult.
6. Identify appropriate nursing diagnoses for clients with delirium and dementia.
7. List expected outcomes for clients with delirium and dementia.
8. Identify nursing interventions for clients with delirium and dementia.
9. Evaluate the effectiveness of implemented planned nursing care.

⊙ Key Terms

ageism
aging
agnosia
Alzheimer's disease (AD)
anomia
aphasia
apraxia
catastrophic event

confabulation
delirium
dementia
disorientation
Lewy body
primary aging
secondary aging
sundowning syndrome

ging is defined as a manifestation of changes that advance in a continuous and progressive manner during the adult years. The older adult population typically exhibits physical symptoms of aging such as graying of hair, a decrease in subcutaneous supportive tissue with wrinkling of the skin, and presbyopia (decline in the ability to focus on close-up objects). It is important to recognize the flexible nature of health and functioning among those older than 65 years. There are effects of **primary aging**, or those changes that occur as a result of genetics or natural factors, and those of **secondary aging**, which are influenced by the environment. A pattern of coping with environmental stressors is often established as a result of social learning early in life. Successful adaptation to the process of aging is encouraged by the ability to give meaning and perspective to life experiences. This is reflected in findings that most older adults, despite coexisting chronic medical conditions or disabilities, rate their physical or mental health as good or excellent (Box 19.1). Although the changes that accompany aging are inevitable, it is recognized that older adults who can adapt to these changes with relative acceptance experience the highest level of satisfaction with their lives.

Mind Jogger

What implication do these demographics have for nursing? In what way do childhood experiences influence how a person adapts to the aging process?

BOX 19.1

Chronic Medical Conditions Most Common in People 65 Years and Older

- Arthritis
- Visual disturbances
- Hypertension
- Peripheral vascular disease
- Congestive heart failure
- Urinary dysfunction
- Parkinson's disease
- Hearing loss
- Stroke
- Chronic obstructive pulmonary disease (COPD)
- Thyroid disease
- Diabetes mellitus

Mental Health Care for Older Adults

Chronic disease, memory impairment, and depressive symptoms affect large numbers of older adults, and the risk of these problems occurring typically increases with age. Social and behavioral aspects of life and the link of loss to age can have a great influence on a person's mental status and the prevalence of mental health disorders in late life. Losses that occur more frequently among the older population include loss of:

- Health
- Retirement and work
- Spouse or loved ones
- Income
- Status
- Friends
- Cognitive decline
- Home
- Independence
- Roles

Psychosocial Issues Related to Aging

Ageism is a commonly held belief that stereotypes and minimizes the worth of the aging person by indicating that senescence and mental health conditions are a part of the normal aging process. This promotes an assumption that older people are incompetent or senile and somehow an inferior population of society. Discrimination in the form of limited access to the funds and services of mental health resources is shown by a reluctance to separate these disorders as abnormal and treatable in all age groups. Unfortunately, many elderly people themselves accept as normal the coexistence of mental disorders and later life decline. Many symptoms are unreported by those who may see mental issues as a sign of weakness or loss of control, and there is also added fear of institutionalization. The person may be reluctant or unable to discuss feelings or emotions, preventing recognition of the problem. The cost of mental health care is in itself a factor that often decreases the chances that the older adult will seek treatment. Limited income and existing medical and pharmacological health care costs may also decrease the likelihood that mental health issues will be addressed.

Mind Jogger

How might this attitude of "normalcy" contribute to chronic medical illness?

Care of the older adult with mental illness has received some federal government attention with legislative regulation of both psychiatric treatment facilities and nursing homes. A high percentage of mental disorders are found among the residents of long-term care facilities. Specialized units and programs to address the needs of the mentally ill in these institutions have seen tremendous growth and are related to an increased focus on escalating inpatient hospital costs. Cost containment by Medicare, Medicaid, Health Maintenance Organizations (HMOs), and with mandates imposed by OBRA (Omnibus Budget Reconciliation Act of 1987) to regulate both pharmacological and physical restraints have brought about the emergence of supportive community care.

Mind Jogger

Does a subtle change in focus from "time lived to time left to live" have an impact on the mindset of the older adult? How?

Impaired Cognitive Functioning

Impaired cognitive functioning implies that there is some measure of deterioration in a person's ability to perform the activities of daily living (ADLs). The subtle mental decline attributed to the normal aging process is seldom evident in the day-to-day functioning of the older adult. Normal memory lapses such as misplacing an item, forgetting someone's name, or forgetting an appointment are considered typical as one ages. Changes may become more evident when there is an increase in anxiety produced by the need to perform under pressure. There is much variance among older adults and many continue to function at a very high level by compensating for their impairment with written reminders and lists. The greatest mental decreases with aging are seen in the areas of learning and retaining information. It is suggested that there is also some decline in abstract reasoning and complex problem-solving ability.

In contrast, cognitive impairment is a more defined problem centered on memory loss. There may be a significant loss in the ability to remember the content of what is read or descriptive details of what is seen or heard. Important events may be

repeatedly forgotten. This degree of impairment is quite different from that seen in normal aging. Memory is the basis for our thinking processes. The loss of memory leaves the affected person unable to remember past experiences, which are used to make current decisions and judgments. The person is left in a state of confusion, unable to understand present experiences.

Types of Mental Disorders in the Older Adult

The term *cognitive disorders* has replaced the previously used terms of *organic brain* or *mental disorders*. In these disorders there is a noticeable change in cognition from the former level of functioning. This category of conditions includes delirium, dementia, and amnestic disorders. Underlying these disorders is a medical condition, a substance that may be a medication or toxin, or a combination of the two. In other words, there is an underlying cause for the altered cognitive state.

Delirium

Delirium is characterized by a disturbance of consciousness and a change in cognition that develop over a short time. The disorders in this category all present with a disturbance in level of awareness and cognitive functioning, but they may have different etiologies such as a medical condition, trauma, infections, medications, or a combination of factors. The most common underlying causes in older people are listed in Table 19.1. Once the

TABLE 19.1	Common Causes of Delirium in Older Adult
DELIRIUM	**CAUSES**
Medical conditions	Systemic infections Metabolic disturbance Fluid and electrolyte imbalance Hepatic or renal disease Pathological conditions of brain
Substance induced	Medication toxicity Multiple drug interactions
Substance intoxication	High doses of narcotic drugs Alcohol Sedatives, hypnotics, or anxiolytics
Substance withdrawal	Abrupt discontinuation of any of the above drugs (any combination of pharmacological or physical causes)

cause is determined and treated, the condition is usually reversed and improvement in the mental state is seen.

Signs and Symptoms

The pattern of delirium is progressive. The deterioration in the level of consciousness and cognitive functioning is evident in the client's behavior and inability to carry out previously routine ADLs. Delirium develops rapidly with symptoms that may fluctuate depending on the time of day. There is a decreased level of consciousness with impaired thinking, concentration, and awareness of the surrounding environment. Speech becomes incoherent and motor coordination or activity rapidly deteriorates. The person may experience hallucinations and delusional thought processes. Appetite and sleep are disturbed as the mental decline continues (Box 19.2).

Mind Jogger

Does delirium have a rapid or insidious onset? What factors contribute to the development of delirium?

Just the Facts

Perceptual disturbance may include hallucinations (e.g., seeing and talking to a dead parent), illusions (e.g., seeing intravenous tubing as a rope), or delusions (e.g., may see injection as a threat of harm). Delirium is a disturbance in consciousness and cognition that occurs over a short period of time.

Incidence and Etiology

As noted previously, symptoms of delirium may be caused by different factors. Older adults are more at risk for delirium because of their higher incidence of chronic illness and their use of multiple medications to manage those disorders. The increased chance of hospitalization for acute infections, sepsis, and exacerbations of chronic illnesses such as congestive heart failure and chronic pulmonary disease adds to the risk. The combined use of both prescription and over-the-counter medications can contribute to the development of delirium. Significant risk factors for delirium are the body's decreased ability to metabolize and excrete drugs as the body ages, the smaller doses of some medications given to older people, and additional adverse drug reactions. In addition, other factors such as sensory deprivation, an altered sleep–wake cycle, and nutritional or fluid deficiencies can contribute to the onset of a delirious state.

Dementia

Dementia is characterized by irreversible, progressive declines in cognitive functioning, including a loss of memory, awareness, judgment, and reasoning ability. This decline in intellectual functioning is severe enough to interfere with a person's normal daily activities and ability to communicate or interact with others. Although not a specific disease in itself, dementia is a set of symptoms caused by a number of different disorders that affect the brain. Primary dementia does not result from any other disease, while secondary dementia occurs as a result of another condition. Most familiar is the progressive type of dementia in which cognitive ability gradually worsens over a period of time (Box 19.3).

There are several different types of progressive dementia, with Alzheimer's disease being the most common. In addition, vascular disease and

"Bertha's Behavior Speaks"

Bertha is an 86-year-old resident of the dementia unit in a nursing home facility. Her speech consists of irrational sentence fragments unrelated to any conversation directed to her. Her usual activity is ambulating down the corridor with her walker, going in and out of rooms at random. For the past 2 days, Bertha has resisted getting out of bed. She has been less responsive with few verbal utterances. Today the nurse finds her crying and restless. She has developed a fever and is shaking. The nurse notes a strong odor to the urine in the brief Bertha has been wearing. The nurse realizes that Bertha is unable to describe pain or the location of any discomfort.

What might the changes in Bertha's behavior indicate?

_____

_____

How might her behavior be related to other symptoms?

_____

_____

What action should the nurse take?

_____

_____

Case ❂ Application 19.1

Lewy body disease fall into this category and will be discussed in this chapter. Other conditions that may be associated with dementia are listed in Box 19.4.

Because memory impairment is common to both delirium and dementia, it is necessary to recognize that a person with delirium can also have a pre-existing dementia. One assessment that may help distinguish between them is that except in late dementia, most people with dementia alone are usually alert to the environment, whereas a person with delirium also has a disturbance in consciousness. This means that a person who is alert but disoriented and confused because of dementia may develop a deteriorating level of consciousness as a result of an acute state of delirium.

BOX 19.4

Other Conditions Associated With Dementia

- Pick's disease
- Frontotemporal lobar degeneration
- HIV infection
- Substance/medication use
- Traumatic brain injury
- Huntington's disease
- Creutzfeldt–Jakob disease
- Parkinson's disease
- Multiple sclerosis
- Amyotrophic lateral sclerosis
- Nutritional deficiencies
- Chronic alcoholism
- Infections
- Brain tumors
- Anoxia
- Chronic lung or heart disease

 Mind Jogger

What characteristics would distinguish an acute delirium in a client with dementia?

Dementia Due to Alzheimer's Disease

Alois Alzheimer, a German physician, first identified Alzheimer's disease in the early 20th century. A female client in her 50s was described as having the signs of what appeared to be a mental illness. Following her death, an autopsy revealed this woman had dense deposits, or neuritic plaques, outside and around the nerve cells in her brain. Inside the cells were twisted strands of fiber, or neurofibrillary tangles. Today, a definite diagnosis of Alzheimer's disease is still only possible when an autopsy shows these classic signs of the disease.

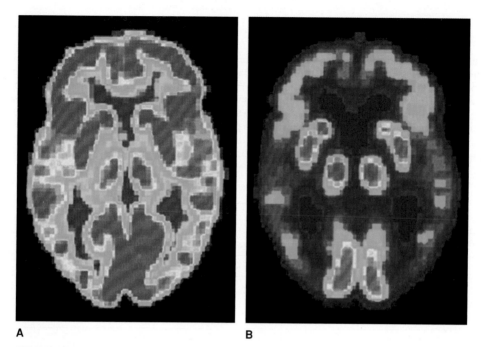

A   B

FIGURE 19.1

A: PET scan of brain of a healthy person. **B:** PET scan of a brain of a person with Alzheimer's disease. The blue areas indicate reduced brain activity. (Images courtesy of the Alzheimer's Disease Education and Referral Center, a service of the National Institute on Aging.)

Alzheimer's disease (AD) primarily affects the cerebral cortex, which is involved in conscious thought and language, the production of acetylcholine (a neurotransmitter involved in memory and learning), and the hippocampus, essential to memory storage. In the regions attacked by this disease, the neurons degenerate and lose their synaptic connections to other neurons. The positron emission tomography (PET) scan in Figure 19.1 shows the reduced brain activity in the brain of a person with AD versus a healthy brain.

Signs and Symptoms

As the neurons of the hippocampus degenerate, short-term memory fails. The ability to perform routine tasks begins to diminish. Once the disease progresses to the cerebral cortex, it begins to take away language and impairs judgment, leading to impulsive emotional outbursts and disturbing behaviors such as the wandering and agitation that are commonly seen in this disorder. The progression to remote memory loss leaves the person with the inability to recognize even close family members or to communicate in any meaningful way. In addition, there is a progressive, irreversible loss of memory that affects temporal and spatial orientation, abstract thinking, ability to carry out

mathematical calculations, and capacity to learn new things or concepts. Personality changes lead to a diminished and lost sense of self as memory fades and with it the mental pictures that give meaning to one's life. Memories erode into small pieces that gradually disappear and are lost beyond recall.

Initially, the person may write down what they want to remember, and then forget to check the written reminder. There is difficulty encoding material to be recalled or an inability to make a connection between the meaning of the spoken word and words to be remembered. Early in the course of the disease, clients are usually aware of their memory deficit and try to compensate for their losses by using **confabulation** (filling in the gaps with fictitious statements), but increasingly they become frightened and anxious about the memory deficits and get discouraged. As the disease progresses, they lose insight into their memory loss and are no longer aware of it.

> **Just the Facts**
>
> Short-term (recent) memory: Remembering for a few minutes or hours
> Long-term (remote) memory: Remembering for a few years; memory is preserved

BOX 19.5

Language Deterioration in Dementia Due to Alzheimer's Disease

- Conversational speech to sentence fragments
- Tends to repeat words and questions (echolalia)
- Repeating one word (paralalia)
- Repeating one syllable (logoconia)
- Unintelligible and repetitive babbling
- Mutism

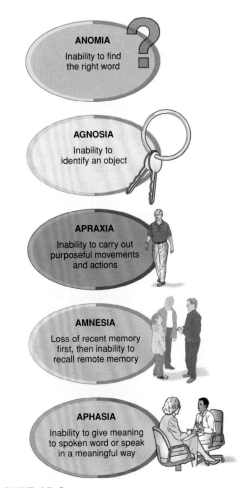

FIGURE 19.2
The Five As of Alzheimer's disease.

There is an inability to acquire and process new information—for example, a new house or address may not be recognized and the person shows up at a previous address. Language difficulties become more marked as the disease progresses (Box 19.5).

The problems related to language include the following:

- **Anomia**—inability to find the right word (e.g., when shown a watch, the client may refer to it as a "timepiece," or referring to someone who has died, may say that the person is at the "resting place" or "sleeping place" instead of the cemetery).
- **Agnosia**—inability to identify an object (e.g., the client may try to eat soup with a knife, eat the paper wrapper on a piece of candy, or attempt to shave with a toothbrush and toothpaste). This can also be sensory (e.g., unable to identify hot temperature [i.e., bath water], recognize the meaning of traffic lights, or recognize themselves in the mirror, thinking there is an intruder in the room).
- **Aphasia**—impairment in the significance or meaning of language that prevents the person from understanding what is heard, following instructions, and communicating needs (e.g., the need to go to the bathroom or to communicate pain).

Visual and spatial skills deteriorate, and the person may get lost while driving a car or walking. The person develops **apraxia**, or an inability to carry out purposeful movements and actions despite intact motor and sensory functioning. The person may try to water plants with a hose but is unable to connect the hose to the water faucet or is unable to transfer food from plate to mouth with silverware when trying to eat. The ability to use correct judgment or to make logical decisions is lost. Usually the first noticeable sign of this is a difficulty in managing finances and is often the deficit that leads families to seek medical attention.

The person may pay bills twice or not pay bills, buy unnecessary items, make large charitable donations, or be unable to balance a checkbook. See Figure 19.2.

In addition, there is evidence of self-neglect as the person shows carelessness and a lack of attention to appearance and dress. Layering of clothing and an unkempt appearance in one who was previously neat and well groomed is typical. Personality and mood changes are noticeable as the person loses interest and energy for doing previously enjoyed activities. Depression is common, with decreasing interaction and social withdrawal. As the disease progresses, agitation and responses of fear and panic (both verbal and physical) may occur with a potential of harm to self and others, referred to as **catastrophic events**. These occurrences are often precipitated by frustration and a perceived threat or fear, often trivial in nature such as a change in routine or environment.

Behavior problems such as stubbornness, resistance to care, abusive language, acting out in response to hallucinations or delusions, or urinating in inappropriate places may occur. Older adults with AD tend to hide articles and develop a suspicion of others, thinking misplaced things have been stolen when the items cannot be found. There may also be increased restlessness that leads to rummaging, wandering, aimless walking (pacing), and interruption of the sleep–wake cycle. This behavior puts the person at risk for injury. Some people exhibit a peak period of agitation and acting-out behavior during the evening hours, which is sometimes referred to as **sundowning syndrome** (Box 19.6).

In advanced AD, the person may be totally unaware of his or her surroundings and require total and constant supervision and care. The people with this degree of impairment are at risk for accidents and infectious diseases that often lead to death. The three most common causes of death in the person with AD are pneumonia, urinary tract infections, and infected decubitus ulcers. Clients live an average of 4 to 10 years, although in some people, the duration from time of diagnosis to death may be as many as 20 years or more. The final phase of the disease may last from a few months to several years, during which time the individual becomes totally disabled. The clinical stages of AD are identified in Table 19.2.

BOX 19.6

Signs and Symptoms of Dementia Due to Alzheimer's Disease

- Confabulation
- Short-term memory loss first—then remote
- Decreasing ability to perform routine tasks
- Hiding articles with inability to relocate them
- Suspiciousness
- Restlessness, rummaging, wandering, and pacing
- Interruption of sleep–wake cycle
- Language deterioration (anomia, aphasia)
- Impaired judgment
- Inability to cognitively be independent in daily activities (money management, paying bills, taking medications)
- Impulsive emotional outbursts (catastrophic events)
- Inability to recognize family or friends
- Inability to recognize familiar objects (agnosia)
- Loss of spatial and temporal orientation
- Loss of abstract thinking and mathematical concepts
- Inability to learn anything new or encode incoming information
- Personality changes
- Inability to carry out purposeful movements (apraxia)
- Stubbornness
- Abusive language
- Hallucinations and delusions
- Eliminating in inappropriate places
- Sundowning

TABLE 19.2 Clinical Stages of Alzheimer's Disease

STAGE	DURATION	CHARACTERISTICS
Mild	1–4 y	Poor short-term memory Unable to acquire new information (may have difficulty balancing a checkbook, preparing a complex meal, or remembering medication schedules) Mild anomia Personality changes Disorientation—may get lost Some decrease in judgment
Moderate	2–10 y	Significant memory loss Impaired judgment (difficulty with simple food preparation, housework or yard work, may require assistance with ADLs) Increased cognitive loss Anxiety, suspiciousness Agitation, depression Problems with sleeping Wandering or pacing Difficulty recognizing family or friends
Severe	8–12 y	Severe cognitive impairment Physical unsteadiness and loss of mobility (requires considerable assistance with personal care and ADLs; often chair or bed bound and dependent on others for care; may be mute) Total loss of speech Loss of appetite, weight loss Incontinence

"Annie's Decline"

Lately, Annie has been coming to the senior citizen center with unmatched earrings and shoes without hose. The supervisor of the center has been concerned about the obvious change in Annie's appearance. One day when Annie is delivering her assigned meals, she walks into the school where she taught for 30 years and tells the secretary, "I don't know where I need to go with this food." When the center is advised of the situation, the supervisor remembers that several people on Annie's route have reported that they have not been receiving their meals. However, when she asks Annie about this, Annie states she must "have left them at another house by mistake." Realizing that there is a problem, the supervisor notifies Annie's daughter, Katy, of the situation. She arranges a visit to her mother's house the next day. She finds piles of unopened mail and bills with notices of nonpayment. There are spoiled food items in the refrigerator and soiled laundry is piled in a corner of the bathroom. Katy realizes something is very wrong with her mother and brings her to the clinic for evaluation. After a diagnostic workup, Annie is given a diagnosis of probable dementia, Alzheimer's type.

What assessment data would the nurse use to support a nursing diagnosis of risk for injury?

_____

_____

Katy feels that her mother can no longer continue to live independently and chooses to admit Annie to a nursing home. Annie does not understand why she has to be there, crying and saying she needs to go—"I have to feed the hungry children." What would be the best nursing approach to Annie at this time?

_____

_____

Annie begins to take food items from the plates of other clients, stating they have stolen "her food." She becomes physically aggressive if they are taken away from her. What nursing approach would be most appropriate when Annie is removing the food?

_____

_____

How can distraction and redirection be used when Annie becomes agitated?

_____

_____

Mind Jogger

What environmental stimuli might cause behaviors to accelerate with evening hours?

Incidence and Etiology

There is clearly a familial pattern with some forms of Alzheimer's disease. Some families exhibit an inherited pattern that suggests possible genetic transmission. There are studies that indicate that early-onset cases (those diagnosed before the age of 65 years) are more likely to be familial than late-onset cases. Estimates of the prevalence of dementia depend on how it is defined, but the incidence increases dramatically after the age of 75, with the risk doubling approximately every 5 years after age 65. More than half of the diagnosed cases of dementia can be attributed to AD. According to a facts and figures report by the Alzheimer's Association in 2014, there are currently as many as 5 million Americans living with Alzheimer's disease, with that number expected to exceed 15 million by 2050. Approximately two thirds of the Americans with Alzheimer's disease are women. Alzheimer's disease is listed as the sixth leading cause of death in the United States.

Mind Jogger

How will this increase in the incidence of Alzheimer's dementia impact nursing as the over-65 segment of the population increases?

Dementia Due to Vascular Disorder

Dementia due to vascular disease is caused by the effects of one or more strokes (cerebrovascular accident [CVA]) on cognitive functioning that is characterized by an abrupt onset and follows a step-like pattern of cerebrovascular disease and symptoms. The pattern of deficit is related to the portion of the brain that has been destroyed by the stroke. Some functions are affected while others may remain intact. Each step is accompanied by a decrease in cognitive functioning.

Signs and Symptoms

In the early stages, personality and insight tend to be better preserved than in the client with AD. Depression is common as the condition advances. Neurological symptoms such as hemiplegia, abnormal reflexes, gait disturbances, and uncontrollable emotional responses may develop as a result of the cerebral infarcts. The person may laugh or cry without a stimulus that would cause the response. There are multiple cognitive deficits such as aphasia, apraxia, agnosia, and the inability to organize thought processes (Box 19.7).

> **Just the Facts**
>
> Vascular changes that start with a decreased blood supply to certain brain areas important in storing and retrieving information may cause memory loss very similar to AD.

Incidence and Etiology

The onset of vascular dementia may occur any time in the older adult but is less common after age 75. The initial onset is typically earlier than the onset of AD. The two types of dementia can coexist in the same person. Vascular dementia tends to be more common in men than in women. The incidence of this form of dementia is much lower than that of the Alzheimer's type, accounting for approximately 20% of all dementias.

Dementia Due to Lewy Body Disease

Lewy body disease is now considered the second most common cause of progressive dementia in which abnormal round deposits of protein called Lewy bodies, develop in nerve cells throughout the brain. The protein associated with this disorder is also associated with Parkinson's disease, but the Lewy bodies are only seen in one portion of the brain.

Signs and Symptoms

Symptoms seen in this disorder share a striking resemblance to those of AD, including disorientation, memory loss, communication and processing decline, and behavior changes. One of the striking variances of Lewy body dementia is the incidence of visual hallucinations of colors, people or animals, paranoia, and delusional thinking. Mental alertness is intermittent with the person seemingly okay one day, and confused, lethargic, distracted, and semi-responsive to the environment the next. Parkinson-like symptoms of slow, rigid movements and shuffling gait are also seen (Box 19.8).

Incidence and Etiology

Lewy body dementia is usually seen in those over 65 years of age, and is more common in men than in women. The average life span from the time of

---

BOX 19.7

Signs and Symptoms of Dementia Due to Vascular Disease

- Series of strokes (CVAs)
- History of hypertension or cerebrovascular disease
- Hemiplegia or weakness of extremities
- Gait disturbances
- Step-like cognitive decline
- Exaggerated reflexes
- Foot drop
- Inability to control emotions
- Aphasia
- Apraxia
- Agnosia
- Decreased thought processing
- Hallucinations and delusions

BOX 19.8

Signs and Symptoms of Dementia Due to Lewy Body Disease

- Cognitive deficits that interfere independence in activities of daily living
- Recurring detailed visual hallucinations
- Fluctuating mental alertness and cognition
- Shuffling gait, stiff or rigid movements
- Depression
- Mild tremors
- Cognitive deficits interfere with independence in daily activities (e.g., paying bills, managing medications)
- Cognitive deficits are not better explained by delirium or another mental disorder.
- Disorder has insidious onset and gradual progression

diagnosis is about 6 to 8 years. Because of its similarity to AD and Parkinson's disease, it is difficult for physicians to give a definitive diagnosis. Findings suggest that one or more of these disorders may coexist in the same individual. Research continues to explore the cause and course of this disease, and its relationship to the other dementias.

Depression and Dementia

Although not categorized as a cognitive disorder, studies show that depression is the most common mental disorder in the older adult population. Depression is categorized as a mood disorder (see Chapter 10) that can occur in any age group. In the older adult, the cognitive deficits of depression tend to be nonprogressive and inconsistent with the degree of those found in dementia. Depression often accompanies the early stages of dementia, particularly in AD. The person still has the mental ability to understand that something is happening, that memory lapses are occurring, and that they are unable to do things that previously were easily accomplished. These disturbing changes naturally lead the person to feelings of loss, decreased self-worth, hopelessness, and depression. These feelings can lead the person to thoughts that life is not worth living. The depression can actually intensify the effects of the disease. It is important to recognize these feelings in the early stages of dementia when the person still may have the ability to carry out a plan for suicide.

As many of the symptoms found in depression are also characteristic of dementia, it may easily go unrecognized. Changes in appetite, changes in sleep patterns, and loss of energy and initiative are common to both disorders. The person may demonstrate other symptoms such as withdrawal from others, self-neglect, and feelings of failure, inadequacy, helplessness, and powerlessness. The diagnostic work-up for all dementia of the AD type includes testing for depression. Usually when asked questions, the depressed person will answer with, "I don't know," indicating a lack of energy to formulate an answer, whereas the demented person will attempt to answer, demonstrating the existing mental deficits.

Risk factors for the development of depression in the early stages of dementia include a previous depressive episode or a very achievement-oriented lifestyle. Difficult family situations or financial strain may also precipitate depressive symptoms such as sadness and emptiness, which may be reinforced by a coexisting dementia. If the existence

> **CLIENT TEACHING NOTE 19.1**
>
> ### Resources for More Information
>
> - Alzheimer's Association
>   225 North Michigan Ave–17th Floor
>   Chicago, IL 60601-7633
>   312-335-8700
>   1-800-272-3900 (24-hour helpline)
>   http://www.alz.org
> - National Institute on Aging—Alzheimer's Disease Education and Referral Center
>   (800)438-4380
>   http://www.nih.gov/nia
> - Lewy Body Dementia Association
>   P.O. Box 451429
>   Atlanta, GA 31145-9429
>   404-935-6444
>   1-800-539–9767 (24-hour helpline)
>   http://www.lewybodydementia.org
> - Family Caregiver Alliance/National Center on Caregiving
>   180 Montgomery Street
>   Suite 1100
>   San Francisco, CA 94104
>   http://www.caregiver.org

of depression is determined, it is important that treatment be initiated, because this can lead to improvement in the person's overall functioning.

In addition to clients with dementia, it is common for caregivers to experience signs of depression. The constant demands of the unpredictable behaviors in the demented person take their toll on the caregiver. The burden increases as an attempt is made to balance this schedule with other family responsibilities. Communication with family and friends may become strained or minimal as the caregiver becomes increasingly protective and isolated. Programs such as support groups can allow the caregiver to express feelings that are shared by others in the group. These groups can also provide information and suggestions for dealing with the problem behaviors and the frustration or fear that may accompany them (Client Teaching Note 19.1).

Treatment of Neurocognitive Disorders in the Older Adult

Currently, there is no cure for dementia due to Alzheimer's or Lewy body disease. This makes treatment difficult and symptomatic in its approach. Management is aimed at controlling the cognitive and behavioral symptoms that result from the progressive decline in the dementias. In Lewy body disease, there is also treatment geared toward controlling the motor movements or Parkinson-like symptoms. Various therapies are combined with medications to reduce the devastating effects of these mental diseases. Much research is being done to determine other approaches to the treatment of AD. Support groups may be of help to spouses and family members who take care of the victims of this disease (Client Teaching Note 19.1).

There are currently several medications available that can sometimes delay the progression of the disease and symptoms. These may differ depending on the type of dementia being treated. The cholinesterase inhibitors are useful in increasing the levels of neurotransmitters or chemical messengers to the portions of the brain affected by AD. They can improve mental alertness and cognition, along with reducing the behavioral problems. The cholinesterase inhibitors can delay worsening of symptoms for 6 to 12 months for some who take them. Another neurotransmitter, glutamate,

is needed for memory and learning processes in the brain. Research shows that an excess of glutamate may lead to destruction of brain cells in the individual with AD. A drug called memantine (Namenda), approved by the FDA in 2003, is a glutamate receptor antagonist that has demonstrated effectiveness in the later stages of the disease. Antipsychotic medications may be useful in decreasing verbal and physical aggressiveness in individuals with AD, and may improve delusional thinking or hallucinations. Persons with Lewy body dementia however, often are very sensitive to these drugs related to the Parkinson-like symptoms and may have an increase in the psychotic symptoms. Parkinson's disease medications may be used to reduce the movement symptoms in the person with Lewy body dementia. Medications used in the treatment of dementia are found in Table 19.3.

The most effective treatment in the older adult with depression is a combination of antidepressant medication and various psychotherapeutic approaches. Nursing observations related to antidepressant therapy should take into consideration the age-related physiological changes that slow the body's response and the elimination

TABLE 19.3 Medications Used in Treatment of Dementia

DRUG CLASSIFICATION	DRUG NAME	COMMON SIDE EFFECTS
Cholinesterase inhibitors	Galantamine (Razadyne—formerly called Reminyl) Donepezil (Aricept) Rivastigmine (Exelon) (Tacrine (Cognex) is rarely prescribed today due to serious side effects and possible liver damage)[a]	Nausea, vomiting, anorexia, diarrhea, abdominal pain, headache, dizziness, rash, urinary frequency, insomnia, blurred vision, muscle cramps
(*N*-methyl-D-aspartate) NMDA receptor antagonist	Memantine (Namenda)[b]	Fatigue, dizziness, headache, insomnia, constipation, nausea, vomiting, anorexia, diarrhea, muscle aches, coughing, rash, frequent urination
Antipsychotics	Risperidone (Risperdal) Haloperidol (Haldol)[c]	Orthostatic hypotension, sedation, drowsiness, headache, insomnia, agitation, anxiety, extrapyramidal symptoms, dry mouth, dyspepsia, nausea, vomiting, diarrhea, constipation, hyperglycemia, cough, photosensitivity, urinary retention, decreased libido
Other alternative therapy methods such as vitamin E, NSAIDs, estrogen are in research-based studies Parkinson's drug	Selegiline (Eldepryl, Carbex)[d]	Can cause increased confusion, hallucinations, and delusions in those with Lewy body disease

[a]Most effective when treatment begun in early stages.
[b]Treatment of moderate to severe Alzheimer's.
[c]May be used to decrease verbal and physical aggressiveness.
[d]May be useful in Lewy body disease.

of drugs in older people. It is also important to monitor for the many side effects caused by these agents and to report and document any adverse effects. Elderly persons may experience negative effects that may worsen other existing conditions.

Application of the Nursing Process for Delirium

Assessment

It is crucial to determine the cause of **disorientation**—the inability to be cognizant of time, direction or location, and person—and mental decline. Sometimes it is a combination of sensory loss (e.g., hearing loss) and an unfamiliar environment (e.g., hospital) for an elderly person, sometimes there is a related mental disorder (e.g., dementia), and other times there is an underlying physical or medical condition. When sensory factors are assessed as an issue, a simple adjustment of lighting or checking the battery in a hearing aid may be all that is needed to resolve the problem. In the case of physical causes, prompt detection and treatment is imperative to restoring mental function.

Assessment will include a complete history and physical examination. Nurses play a major role in obtaining information. If the client is unable to provide information, it may be acquired from family members or others who may be aware of the person's health history and circumstances leading up to the current disorder. Obtain a list of the client's current medications so that the possibility of medication toxicity or interaction can be determined. Treatment and nursing intervention will depend on the precipitating factors. Assessment data should also be considered in comparison to the client's baseline physical condition or previous level of functioning.

Selected Nursing Diagnoses

Although each situation of delirium may differ, some commonalities exist in caring for the client with an acute deteriorating mental state. Nursing diagnoses to address the problems may include the following:

- Risk for Injury
- Risk for Other-Directed Violence
- Altered Thought Processes
- Acute Confusion
- Self-Care Deficit
- Altered Sensory Perception
- Fear
- Disturbed Sleep Pattern
- Imbalanced Nutrition: Less Than Body Requirements
- Deficient Knowledge

Expected Outcomes

Once problems are identified, the planning of realistic outcomes will depend on the individual problems. Outcomes for the client may include the following:

- Remains safe from harm or injury
- Accurately states time, place, person, situation
- Meets basic needs and independently performs ADL
- Responds appropriately to incoming stimuli
- Identifies the fear and focuses on eliminating or reducing the source
- Is free of signs of sleep deprivation
- Regains or maintains ideal body weight for height and age
- Demonstrates understanding of current health problems

Interventions

Most clients with delirium will be cared for in the acute care setting. In providing nursing care for the client, the nurse must carry out all interventions to ensure that permanent brain damage or death is avoided. Because the course of delirium is short and critical, plans of care and goals are short term, and the focus of the medical and nursing teams should be directed toward correcting the underlying problem. Nursing interventions will be directed toward the acute phase of the illness. Those specific for the delirious state may include the following:

- Monitor level of consciousness for further deterioration or improvement.
- Reduce environmental noise.
- Provide regular verbal, visual, or tactile stimulation.
- Provide glasses or hearing aids to facilitate orientation.
- Place family photographs or favorite objects within view.
- Provide a nightlight.
- Reorient client to date, time, and place.

"Hidden Messages"

Frank is a 67-year-old resident of a special dementia unit of a long-term care facility. His family admitted him following an incident in which he drove a neighbor's car to the interstate and proceeded to enter an exit access going the wrong direction. Several vehicles were forced into the median to avoid an accident. He was eventually stopped by police officers who informed his wife, Ruth, that arrangements would have to be made for his safety.

Frank owns a construction business and told the police officers he was "going to work," although he had been unable to work for the past 3 years because of diagnosed early-onset Alzheimer's dementia. Since admission to the nursing home facility, Frank paces the halls, pulling on hand rails, doorknobs, and window casings. He repeatedly runs his hands over all door hinges and latches, kicks the wall and doors, and moves furniture around in the rooms. Frank wears a sock on his left foot, but refuses to wear shoes. He becomes agitated and strikes out with a fisted hand if any attempt is made to put a sock or shoe on the right foot. Frank will only take a bath if Ruth is present. He becomes physically aggressive when nursing personnel try to attend to his hygiene needs unless she is talking to him. The staff has placed pictures of Ruth on several doors in his room and in the shower room hoping to give him a feeling of security with her perceived presence. Ruth comes to the facility several times each day to help with her husband's care.

What may be the precipitating factor in Frank's aggressive behavior?

_____

_____

What methods can the nurse use to deal with the behavior?

_____

_____

What purpose do the pictures serve for Frank?

_____

_____

It is noted that Frank is limping with limited weight bearing on his right foot. An order is received for an x-ray that reveals a comminuted fracture of the third metatarsal. Calcification surrounding the fracture indicates the injury occurred several weeks ago, and it is decided to allow calcification to continue and not to intervene surgically at this point. How is this injury affecting Frank's behavior?

_____

_____

What approach can the nurse use to help Frank with the pain he does not understand?

_____

_____

What nursing approaches may be used to relieve some of the caregiver strain for Ruth?

_____

_____

"Confusion in Motion"

Patty is a 74-year-old woman who worked as a hotel custodian. She is constantly pacing the hallway with a broom, sweeping the floor as she goes. Patty has lost 14 pounds in the 3 months since her admission to the nursing home. She is unable to sit at the table long enough to eat her meals and resumes her constant walking after eating only a few bites.

What nursing diagnosis would the nurse assign to Patty's situation?

_____

_____

What nursing interventions could be used to address the problem?

_____

_____

- Explain all procedures and what is happening to the client.
- Initiate safety precautions.

Evaluation

Evaluation of the effectiveness of the care plan will be based on the degree to which successful reversal of the underlying problem is accomplished. Although most people with delirium will have a full recovery, this likelihood decreases in older people. Many older clients will develop delirium during a hospital stay because of existing medical conditions that increase their risk of complications. There is an increase in the morbidity rate associated with this risk.

Application of the Nursing Process for Dementia

Assessment

Assessment data for the client with dementia should include a past health and medication history. Asking the client questions or reviewing the current level of functioning with family members may help the nurse to obtain data concerning recent and remote memory loss. Other assessment information to obtain includes the following:

- Disorientation
- Mood changes, feelings of hopelessness
- Fear and frustration level—develops as the person is unable to give meaning to incoming sensory messages and leads to agitation and catastrophic reactions
- Inability to concentrate—leads to pacing behaviors
- Suspiciousness, agitation, or aggressive behaviors
- Self-care deficit
- Inappropriate social behavior—public disrobing or sexual behaviors such as masturbation
- Level of mobility, wandering or pacing behaviors
- Judgment ability—safety becomes a major concern
- Sleep disturbance—sleep more often for shorter periods of time
- Speech or language impairment
- Hallucinations, illusions, or delusions
- Bowel and bladder incontinence

- Apathy (flatness of gestures, tone of voice, facial expression)
- Recognition of family members, child, or spouse (may have difficulty deciding to whom feelings should be directed)
- Any decline in nutritional status
- Sensory needs and limitations

Identify the primary caregiver, support systems, and the knowledge base of the family members. The role of caregiver to the demented person is a difficult, stressful, and time-consuming task. A spouse or adult children most often assume this role. It is important for the nurse to actively listen to the feelings and concerns of the family members. The demented person is dependent on the caregiver and often will be reassured and calmed by his or her presence. However, caregivers often feel overwhelmed by the responsibility imposed by the disease as it progresses and may be increasingly isolated as the demented person continues to decline. Words cannot describe the emotional devastation of this disease on the caregiver and family as the one they love vanishes one day at a time. The nurse can assist in locating support groups and respite care (programs to temporarily relieve the burden of primary care giving) alternatives for the family.

Selected Nursing Diagnoses

The problems of caring for the client with dementia are many. Each person must be viewed from the perspective of his or her own particular situation and the losses that are evident and continuous in the person's decline. Nursing diagnoses that may be applicable to the situation may include the following:

- Anxiety, related to accumulative losses
- Ineffective Coping, related to frustration and fear
- Risk for Injury, related to wandering behaviors and disorientation
- Risk for Other-Directed or Self-Directed Violence, related to agitation
- Altered Thought Processes, related to hallucinations or delusions
- Self-Care Deficit, related to cognitive loss
- Altered Sensory Perception, related to agnosia
- Situational Low Self-Esteem, related to hopelessness and losses
- Imbalanced Nutrition: Less Than Body Requirements, related to decreased appetite

- Acute or Chronic Confusion, related to cognitive losses
- Social Isolation, related to anomia and agnosia
- Impaired Verbal Communication, related to anomia and aphasia
- Disturbed Sleep Pattern, related to loss of time orientation
- Caregiver Role Strain, related to dependent state of the victim
- Interrupted Family Processes, related to caregiving roles

> **Mind Jogger**
>
> What symptoms or behaviors might support each of these nursing diagnoses?

Expected Outcomes

Once problems are identified, the planning of realistic outcomes will depend on the individual problems. Outcomes for the client may include the following:

- Demonstrates decreased anxiety levels
- Remains safe and free from injury
- Does not harm self or others
- Experiences minimal catastrophic reactions
- Maintains participation in self-care activities
- Remains oriented at level of ability
- Follows scheduled routine of activity and rest
- Feels valued and accepted

An additional outcome is that the caregiver and family will identify and utilize community support systems.

Interventions

Perhaps one of the most important aspects of caring for the person with dementia is communication. Both verbal and nonverbal approaches must be adapted to the limited ability the demented person has to understand what is being said or the intended meaning. Interventions specific to the client with dementia may include the following:

- Use touch, eye contact, unhurried movements, a smile, or a pleasant affect.
- Speak clearly, softly, and slowly using short, simple words and sentences—a raised voice will trigger agitation.
- Identify yourself and call the person by name at each meeting.
- Avoid questions that challenge memory—instead of asking the person who a relative is, tell them the relative's name.

- Focus on one piece of information at a time.
- Use gestures or cues to accompany speech or commands.
- Use face-to-face contact.
- Repeat questions or commands exactly as they were first stated—saying them another way adds another challenge.
- Validate at the client's level of functioning—this helps the client to cope with feelings of loss.
- Ask questions and comments that allow the client to remember or reminisce on subjects that have emotional meaning for the client. Do not argue or disagree with what the client is saying. When the client is delusional, acknowledge his or her feelings and reinforce reality or divert attention to another issue.
- Recognize the client's feelings and redirect attention to another subject that is pleasant if a client becomes verbally aggressive.
- Keep clocks, pictures, calendars in view to help the client identify with reality.
- Play soft music, which has a soothing effect, or the television can be turned on without sound. Misleading stimuli such as excess noise or television can produce agitation—programs are often too confusing or move too fast.
- Cover mirrors to minimize the illusion that an intruder is in the room, because the client may no longer recognize self in a mirror.

As dementia advances, the ability to independently carry out the steps of self-care is diminished. Nursing interventions that may support the client's self-care deficit may include the following:

- Allow client time to perform those tasks he or she is able to do.
- Assist with dressing—minimize the choices by selecting items of clothing. Different color items help the client to separate socks from pants, for example. Avoid tight clothing or complicated zippers and fasteners—Velcro fasteners decrease frustration with laces and buttons.
- Use step-by-step instructions, cueing as necessary.
- Try again later if client resists care—he or she may forget the issue in a few minutes.
- Maintain a consistent routine or schedule with the same caregivers as much as possible. This will promote calmness and decrease agitation.
- Use tub baths—many clients with dementia are frightened by the falling water of a shower on their skin.

- Use a same-sex person to bathe the client, which is sometimes accepted better by the client.
- Bathe the client at the time the client is accustomed to bathing (day vs. evening).
- Provide rest periods between activities—fatigue produces negative behaviors.
- Use a bed closer to the floor to prevent serious injury when ataxia is present.

Most clients with dementia will have weight loss. Nursing interventions related to maintaining adequate nutritional intake may include the following:

- Monitor intake of food and fluids.
- Provide finger foods that can be eaten while pacing—make sandwiches out of meat, vegetables, or fruit.
- Set one item or bowl of food in front of the client at a time—too many choices may be overwhelming and result in refusal to eat.
- Face the person if feeding—Alzheimer's tends to decrease peripheral vision and a side approach may frighten the client.
- Prevent the client from eating nonfood items such as napkins, food wrappers, or plants.
- Offer between-meal snacks.
- Consider a mechanical alteration in food consistency as the disease progresses, because swallowing may be impaired.

As dementia progresses, the ability to locate the bathroom and follow through with the steps of toileting is lost. The person may become incontinent with little recognition that urination or defecation has occurred. The nurse can best assist the demented client by doing the following:

- Label the bathroom door with a picture or large-print wording.
- Assist with clothing fasteners—simplify clothing (e.g., using pants with an elastic waist).
- Use toileting schedules.
- Watch the client for nonverbal messages such as fidgeting with pants, increased pacing, or going in and out of doors.

When a catastrophic reaction is occurring, distraction and redirection are the most useful interventions. It is important for the nurse not to overreact, as this may increase the intensity of the situation. Remember, the demented person is unable to control the behavior but will quickly forget the incident if allowed time to do so. It is important to intervene to prevent injury to the person or others. Nursing observations should be made as to *who* is involved in the incident (do certain persons tend to trigger the behavior?), *what* is going on in the environment at the time of the incident, *where* the incidents tend to occur (does one location precipitate the behavior more than others), *when* the person tends to become more agitated (is there a particular time of day when the incidents reoccur), and *why* the person might be responding with agitation (e.g., pain, infection, uncomfortable clothing, incontinence).

Mind Jogger

What type of situation might cause a catastrophic response?

Just the Facts

Key areas of concern in the care of the person with dementia include communication, self-care deficit, nutrition, safety, fatigue, and confusion.

Evaluation

Outcomes for persons with dementia must be considered on a day-to-day and moment-to-moment basis, because their behavior is a response to the immediate world around them. The most important thing that caregivers can do is provide a safe environment and protection from injury. The nursing interventions suggested here allow clients to participate in self-care to the extent of their ability. With the assistance of caregivers and nursing personnel in controlling the environment, the person is helped to control the impulsive aggressive actions precipitated by frustration and confusion. Reassurance and calm are encouraged by consistency and simple, routine day-to-day activities. The nurse's reflection and evaluation of what works and what does not work with each client will promote a more positive outcome to a very devastating situation. In addition, it is anticipated that the caregiver will understand the disease process and demonstrate adaptive coping strategies in dealing with the stress of the caregiver role.

Summary

- Aging is an inevitable part of life in which changes occur that may have natural causes or be imposed by environmental and societal factors. Many older adults continue to live active and viable lives beyond the retirement age, whereas others are restricted by decreased income and limitations imposed by chronic illness.
- With age comes the reality of loss in ways that may present the elderly person with emotional hurdles that are difficult to confront. Although some older persons may have conditioned coping adaptability, others may encounter difficulty in meeting these mental challenges.
- The aging person is often unaware of the signs that indicate a need for professional help in dealing with the psychological issues. The lack of resources available to allow treatment of mental disorders in this segment of the population further discourages older adults from seeking help.
- Although some cognitive decline is probable as one ages, it is subtle and causes few complications for the person. In contrast, cognitive impairment leads to a significant memory loss and a decline in the ability to perform activities of daily living.

- The two most common causes of cognitive impairment are delirium and dementia.
- Delirium is marked by a sudden onset of a disturbance of consciousness and follows a short and critical course. In most cases, with treatment of the underlying cause, this disorder is reversible. Treatment is dependent on the cause, with the goal being to restore a previous level of functioning. Many older adults develop delirium as a complication of an existing medical problem, which leads to a decrease in the likelihood of a full recovery.
- In contrast, dementia is characterized by a deterioration in cognitive functioning that is irreversible and progressive, leaving the person with only a shadow of past experiences.
- The most common types of progressive dementias are AD (most common), vascular disorder, and Lewy body disease.
- AD develops slowly; its destructive process leaves the person with an inability to recognize what once were familiar objects, functions, and people.
- Personality and mood changes accompany a loss of interest and energy in previously enjoyed activities. Behavior problems arise out of the fear and confusion

the person is faced with as he or she attempts to cope with stimuli that are not understood.

- In advanced dementia, the person may be totally unaware of the environment and require constant care.
- Nursing interventions should be directed at providing for the safety and basic needs of the person. Use of simple one-step commands in a stable and consistent environment provides a milieu that offers security and comfort to the demented person and promotes an optimal response.
- Excessive or misunderstood stimuli lead to fear, which in turn may result in outbursts or catastrophic events. These are best managed by a calm approach, using redirection and refocusing of the person's attention.
- The symptoms of depression are often seen in the person with dementia. However, it is important to recognize the existence of depression in many older adults who are not demented.

- Because these two disorders have similar symptoms, a diagnostic work-up is essential to distinguish between the two conditions. Treatment usually leads to improvement in the cognitive level and overall functioning of the person.
- It is important for the nurse to make assessments that provide a database from which applicable nursing diagnoses can be formulated. Plans of care should focus on providing a reasonable and measurable outcome.
- Nursing interventions are directed at maximizing the functional ability of the person with cognitive impairment. Whether the impairment be delirium or dementia, it is the responsibility of the nurse to initiate actions that, to whatever degree possible, improve the quality of the person's life and that of family members.

Bibliography

Alzheimer's Association. (2014). Latest medication for memory loss. Retrieved April 11, 2014, from http://www.alz.org/alzheimers_disease_standard_prescriptions.asp

American Psychiatric Association. (2013). *Diagnostic and statistical manual of mental disorders* (5th ed.). Washington, DC: American Psychiatric Association.

Ballard, C., Aarsland, D., Francis, P., & Corbett, A. (2013). Neuropsychiatric symptoms in patients with dementias associated with cortical Lewy Bodies: Pathophysiology, clinical features, and pharmacological management. *Drugs and Aging, 30*(8), 603–611. Retrieved April 11, 2014.

Castel, A. D., Balota, D. A., & McCabe, D. P. (2009). Memory efficiency and the strategic control of attention at encoding: Impairments of value-directed remembering in Alzheimer's Disease. *Neuropsychology, 23*(3), 297–306. Retrieved April 11, 2014, from http://www.apa.org/journals/releases/neu233297.pdf.

Fox, C., Maidment, I., Moniz-Cook, E., White, J., Rene Thyrian, J., Young J., Katona, C., Chew-Graham, C. A. (2013). Optimising primary care for people with dementia. *Mental Health in Family Medicine, 10*(3), 143–151. Retrieved April 11, 2014.

Glass, R. M. (2001). JAMA patient page: Alzheimer's disease. *JAMA, 286*(17), 2194.

Henry, J. D., Rendell, P. G., Scicluna, A., Jackson, M., & Phillips, L. H. (2009). Emotion experience, expression, and regulation in Alzheimer's disease. *Psychology and Aging, 24*(1), 252–257. Retrieved April 11, 2014.

Laurenhue, K. (2006). *Activities of Daily Living: An ADL Guide for Alzheimer's Care.* Bradenton, FL: Wiser Now, Inc.

Mace, N. L., & Rabins, P. V. (2011). *The 36-hour day: A family guide to caring for people with Alzheimer's disease, related dementias, and memory loss in later life,* 5th ed. Baltimore, MD: The Johns Hopkins University Press.

National Institute on Aging. (2014). Alzheimer's disease medications fact sheet. Retrieved April 11, 2014, from, http://www.nia.nih.gov/alzheimers/publication/alzheimers-disease-medications-fact-sheet

National Institute on Aging, National Institute of Health. (2011). Alzheimer's disease, unraveling the mystery. NIH Publication Number 03-3782. Retrieved April 11, 2014, from, http://www.nia.nih.gov/Alzheimers/Publications/Unraveling/.

Nicholson, L. (2013). Risk of suicide in patients with dementia: a case study. *Nursing Standard, 28*(11), 43–49. Retrieved April 11, 2014.

Nordgren, L., & Engstrom, G. (2014). Effects of dog-assisted intervention on behavioral and psychological symptoms of dementia. *Nursing Older People, 26*(3), 31–38. Retrieved April 11, 2014.

Radin, L., & Radin, G. (2008). *What If It's Not Alzheimer's? A Caregiver's Guide to Dementia,* 2nd ed. New York, NY: Prometheus Books.

Smyer, M. A., & Qualls, S. H. (1999). *Aging and mental health.* London: Blackwell Publishers, Inc.

Student Worksheet

Fill in the Blank

Fill in the blank with the correct answer.

1. The most common causes of cognitive impairment are _____, _____, and _____.

2. Delirium is characterized by a change in _____ and a change in cognition that occur in a _____ period of time.

3. An altered response to the effects of medication is seen in older people because of the decreased ability of the body to _____.

4. Dementia is characterized by mental decline that is _____ and _____.

5. The three most common causes of death in the person with Alzheimer's dementia are _____, _____, and _____.

6. Periods of agitation in the client with Alzheimer's disease are referred to as _____.

Matching

Match the following terms to the most appropriate phrase.

1. _____ Confabulation
2. _____ Paralalia
3. _____ Anomia
4. _____ Echolalia
5. _____ Apraxia
6. _____ Logoconia
7. _____ Agnosia
8. _____ Aphasia

a. Inability to carry out purposeful movement
b. Repetitive verbalization of one word
c. Inability to understand what is heard
d. Filling in the gaps with fictitious statements
e. Inability to find the right word
f. Repeating words or questions
g. Inability to identify an object
h. Repeating one syllable

Multiple Choice

Select the best answer from the multiple-choice items.

1. Hosea, a client diagnosed with Alzheimer's dementia, goes into the bathroom. As he glances in the mirror, he pulls up his pants and wanders back into the dayroom where he urinates in the trash can. This is an example of:
   a. Amnesia
   b. Anomia
   c. Agnosia
   d. Apraxia

2. Hosea's behavior is most likely related to:
   a. Anxiety created by an illusion that someone else is in the bathroom.
   b. Inability to remember why he is in the bathroom.
   c. Failure to recognize the purpose of the commode.
   d. Difficulty in managing his clothing to facilitate using the bathroom.

3. The nurse is caring for a client who is diagnosed with delirium related to urosepsis. Which of the following would correctly describe the course of this cognitive disorder?
   a. Progressive
   b. Insidious onset
   c. Reversible
   d. Long term

4. Lilly is telling her family about her trip to the doctor yesterday afternoon. Although she is ill, she is unable to recall the reason for the visit and states she just needed some papers filled out. Which of the following describes Lilly's behavior?
   a. Anomia
   b. Confabulation
   c. Sundowning
   d. Logoconia

5. The nurse is feeding a nursing home resident who is diagnosed with Alzheimer's dementia. As the nurse attempts to place a spoonful of food in the resident's mouth, the resident says, "I don't want it, I don't want it, I don't want it." The term referring to this level of spoken language is:
   a. Babbling
   b. Paralalia
   c. Logoconia
   d. Echolalia

6. The nurse prepares to administer oral medication to Max, an elderly client with Alzheimer's disease. As the nurse attempts to put the tablets in his mouth, Max curses and strikes the nurse's hand. The nurse's best choice of action at this time would be to
   a. Explain to Max that the medications are to help him get better.
   b. Leave Max alone and give the medication at a later time.
   c. Omit the dose and document the medication as refused.
   d. Call the physician and report the incident.

7. The nurse asks Mary, a client with dementia, to sit down so her shoestrings can be retied. Mary looks blankly at the nurse and continues to pace. How can the nurse best help Mary to understand this command?
   a. Repeat the command using different words to explain what is meant.
   b. Explain why it is important to keep her shoestrings tied.
   c. Guide her to a chair and point to the chair seat while telling her to sit.
   d. Allow her to pace and retie the shoestring when she sits down on her own.

8. Daisy has sustained several lacerations and bruises from falling as she gets out of bed and attempts to ambulate to the bathroom. With a memory deficit, Daisy does not remember verbal reminders to call for help when she needs to go to the bathroom. Which of the following nursing interventions would be the best approach to provide for her safety?
   a. Provide a bed closer to the floor.
   b. Provide a bedside commode.
   c. Place full side rails on the bed.
   d. Ask the doctor for a sedative at bedtime.

9. A client with AD is given a breakfast tray of eggs, bacon, canteloupe, oatmeal, toast, milk, juice, and coffee. The client proceeds to get up and wander away from the table. The appropriate nursing action is to:
   a. Save the tray and allow the client to eat at a later time.
   b. Redirect client back to table and provide one food item at a time.
   c. Accept actions to indicate client is not hungry.
   d. Verbally tell the client their breakfast is ready.

10. The family member of a client with AD approaches the nurse and says, "Mom doesn't recognize me. She thinks her son is a little boy. How can I make her understand who I am?" The nurse's best response would be:
    a. "Remind her you are grown and that she does not have a little boy anymore."
    b. "Give her current pictures of you to remind her you are grown."
    c. "Ask her each time if she knows who you are before you tell her."
    d. "Tell her who you are each time and let her reminisce about your childhood."

Appendix A
DSM-5 *Classification of Mental Disorders*

Neurodevelopmental Disorders

Intellectual Disabilities (Intellectual Developmental Disorder)

317	Mild
318.0	Moderate
318.1	Severe
318.2	Profound
315.8	Global Developmental Delay
319	Unspecified Intellectual Disability (Intellectual Developmental Disorder)

Communication Disorder

315.39	Language Disorder
315.39	Speech Sound Disorder
315.35	Childhood-Onset Fluency Disorder (Stuttering)
315.39	Social (Pragmatic) Communication Disorder
307.9	Unspecified Communication Disorder

Autism Spectrum Disorder

299.00	Autism Spectrum Disorder

Attention Deficit/Hyperactivity Disorder

_._ (_._)	Attention Deficit/Hyperactivity Disorder
314.01	Combined Presentation
314.00	Predominantly Inattentive Presentation
314.01	Predominantly Hyperactive/Impulsive Presentation

Specific Learning Disorder

_._ (_._)	Specific Learning Disorder
315.00	With Impairment in Reading
315.2	With Impairment in Written Expression
315.1	With Impairment in Mathematics

Motor Disorders

315.4	Developmental Coordination Disorder
307.3	Stereotypic Movement Disorder

Tic Disorders

307.23	Tourette's Disorder
307.22	Persistent (Chronic) Motor or Vocal Tic Disorder
307.21	Provisional Tic Disorder
307.20	Other Specified Tic Disorder
307.20	Unspecified Tic Disorder

Other Neurodevelopmental Disorders

315.8	Other Specified Neurodevelopmental Disorder
315.9	Unspecified Neurodevelopmental Disorder

Schizophrenia Spectrum and Other Psychotic Disorders

301.22	Schizotypal (Personality) Disorder
297.1	Delusional Disorder
298.8	Brief Psychotic Disorder
295.40	Schizophreniform Disorder
295.90	Schizophrenia
_._ (_._)	Schizoaffective Disorder
295.70	Bipolar Type
295.70	Depressive Type
_._ (_._)	Substance/Medication-Induced Psychotic Disorder
_._ (_._)	Psychotic Disorder Due to Another Medical Condition
293.81	With Delusions
293.82	With Hallucinations
293.89	Catatonia Associated With Another Mental Disorder (Catatonia Specific)
293.89	Catatonic Disorder Due to Another Medical Condition
293.89	Unspecified Catatonia
298.8	Other Specified Schizophrenia Spectrum and Other Psychotic Disorder
298.9	Unspecified Schizophrenia Spectrum and Other Psychotic Disorder

Bipolar and Related Disorders

_._ (_._)	Bipolar I Disorder
_._ (_._)	Current or Most Recent Episode Manic
296.41	Mild
296.42	Moderate
296.43	Severe
296.44	With Psychotic Features
296.45	In Partial Remission
296.46	In Full Remission
296.40	Unspecified
296.40	Current or Most Recent Episode Hypomanic
296.45	In Partial Remission
296.46	In Full Remission
296.40	Unspecified
_._ (_._)	Current or Most Recent Episode Depressed
296.51	Mild
296.52	Moderate
296.53	Severe
296.54	With Psychotic Features
296.55	In Partial Remission
296.56	In Full Remission
296.50	Unspecified
296.7	Current or Most Recent Episode Unspecified
296.89	Bipolar II Disorder
301.13	Cyclothymic Disorder
_._ (_._)	Substance/Medication-Induced Bipolar and Related Disorder
293.83	Bipolar and Related Disorder Due to Another Medical Condition
	With Manic Features
	With Manic- or Hypomanic-Like Episode
	With Mixed Features
296.89	Other Specified Bipolar and Related Disorder
296.80	Unspecified Bipolar and Related Disorder

Depressive Disorders

296.99	Disruptive Mood Dysregulation Disorder
_._ (_._)	Major Depressive Disorder
_._ (_._)	Single Episode
296.21	Mild
296.22	Moderate
296.23	Severe
296.24	With Psychotic Features
296.25	In Partial Remission
296.26	In Full Remission
296.20	Unspecified
_._ (_._)	Recurrent Episode
296.31	Mild
296.32	Moderate
296.33	Severe
296.34	With Psychotic Features
296.35	In Partial Remission
296.36	In Full Remission
296.30	Unspecified
300.4	Persistent Depressive Disorder (Dysthymia)
625.4	Premenstrual Dysphoric Disorder
_._ (_._)	Substance/Medication-Induced Depressive Disorder
293.83	Depressive Disorder Due to Another Medical Condition
	With Depressive Features
	With Major Depressive-Like Episode
	With Mixed Features
311.	Other Specified Depressive Disorder
311.	Unspecified Depressive Disorder

Anxiety Disorders

309.21	Separation Anxiety Disorder
312.23	Selective Mutism
300.29	Specific Phobia
	Animal
	Natural Environment
	Blood-Injection-Injury
	Fear of Blood
	Fear of Injections and Transfusions
	Fear of Other Medical Care
	Fear of Injury
	Situational
	Other
300.23	Social Anxiety Disorder (Social Phobia)
300.01	Panic Disorder
_._ (_._)	Panic Attack Specifier
300.22	Agoraphobia
300.02	Generalized Anxiety Disorder
_._ (_._)	Substance/Medication-Induced Anxiety Disorder
293.84	Anxiety Disorder Due to Another Medical Condition
300.09	Other Specified Anxiety Disorder
300.00	Unspecified Anxiety Disorder

Obsessive-Compulsive and Related Disorders

300.3	Obsessive-Compulsive Disorder
300.7	Body Dysmorphic Disorder
300.3	Hoarding Disorder
312.39	Trichotillomania (Hair-Pulling Disorder)
698.4	Excoriation (Skin-Picking) Disorder

_._ (_._)	Substance/Medication-Induced Obsessive-Compulsive and Related Disorder
294.8	Obsessive-Compulsive and Related Disorder Due to Another Medical Condition
300.3	Other Specified Obsessive-Compulsive and Related Disorder
300.3	Unspecified Obsessive-Compulsive and Related Disorder

Trauma- and Stressor-Related Disorder

313.89	Reactive Attachment Disorder
313.89	Disinhibited Social Engagement Disorder
309.81	Posttraumatic Stress Disorder (Includes Posttraumatic Stress Disorder for Children 6 Years and Younger)
308.3	Acute Stress Disorder
_._ (_._)	Adjustment Disorders
309.0	With Depressed Mood
309.24	With Anxiety
309.24	With Mixed Anxiety and Depressed Mood
309.28	With Disturbance of Conduct
309.4	With Mixed Disturbance of Emotions and Conduct
309.4	Unspecified
309.89	Other Specified Trauma- and Stressor-Related Disorder
309.9	Unspecified Trauma- and Stressor-Related Disorder

Dissociative Disorders

300.14	Dissociative Identity Disorder
300.12	Dissociative Amnesia
300.13	With Dissociative Fugue
300.6	Depersonalization/Derealization Disorder
300.15	Other Specified Dissociative Disorder
300.15	Unspecified Dissociative Disorder

Somatic Symptom and Related Disorders

300.82	Somatic Symptom Disorder
	Specify if: With Predominant Pain
	Persistent
	Specify Current Severity: Mild, Moderate, Severe
300.7	Illness Anxiety Disorder (Care-Seeking Type, Care Avoidant Type)
300.11	Conversion Disorder (Functional Neurological Symptom Disorder)
	With Weakness or Paralysis
	With Abnormal Movement
	With Swallowing Symptoms
	With Speech Symptom
	With Attacks or Seizures
	With Anesthesia or Sensory Loss
	With Special Sensory Symptom
	With Mixed Symptoms
316	Psychological Factors Affecting Other Medical Conditions
300.19	Factitious Disorder (Imposed on Self, Imposed on Another)
300.89	Other Specified Somatic Symptom and Related Disorder
300.82	Unspecified Somatic Symptom and Related Disorder

Feeding and Eating Disorders

307.52	Pica
	In Children
	In Adults
307.53	Rumination Disorder
307.59	Avoidant/Restrictive Food Intake Disorder
307.1	Anorexia Nervosa (Restricting Type, Binge-Eating/Purging Type)
307.51	Bulimia Nervosa
307.51	Binge-Eating Disorder
307.59	Other Specified Feeding or Eating Disorder
307.50	Unspecified Feeding or Eating Disorder

Elimination Disorders

307.6	Enuresis
307.7	Encopresis
_._ (_._)	Other Specified Elimination Disorder
788.39	With Urinary Symptoms
787.60	With Fecal Symptoms
_._ (_._)	Unspecified Elimination Disorder
788.30	With Urinary Symptoms
787.60	With Fecal Symptoms

Sleep–Wake Disorders

780.52	Insomnia Disorder
780.54	Hypersomnolence Disorder
_._ (_._)	Narcolepsy
347.00	Narcolepsy Without Cataplexy but With Hypocretin Deficiency
347.01	Narcolepsy With Cataplexy but Without Hypocretin Deficiency
347.00	Autosomal Dominant Cerebellar Ataxia, Deafness, and Narcolepsy
347.00	Autosomal Dominant Narcolepsy, Obesity, and Type 2 Diabetes
347.10	Narcolepsy Secondary to Another Medical Condition

Breathing-Related Sleep Disorders

327.21	Obstructive Sleep Apnea
_._ (_._)	Central Sleep Apnea
327.21	Idiopathic Central Sleep Apnea
786.04	Cheyne-Stokes Breathing
780.57	Central Sleep Apnea Comorbid With Opioid Use
_._ (_._)	Sleep-Related Hypoventilation
327.24	Idiopathic Hypoventilation
327.25	Congenital Central Alveolar Hypoventilation
327.26	Comorbid Sleep-Related Hypoventilation
_._ (_._)	Circadian Rhythm Sleep-Wake Disorders
307.45	Delayed Sleep Phase Type
307.45	Advanced Sleep Phase Type
307.45	Irregular Sleep-Wake Type
307.45	Non-24-Hour Sleep-Wake Type
307.45	Shift Work Type
307.45	Unspecified Type

Parasomnias

_._ (_._)	Non-Rapid Eye Movement Sleep Arousal Disorders
307.46	Sleepwalking Type
307.46	Sleep Terror Type
307.47	Nightmare Disorder

327.42	Rapid Eye Movement Sleep Behavior Disorder
333.94	Restless Legs Syndrome
_._ (_._)	Substance/Medication-Induced Sleep Disorder
780.52	Other Specified Insomnia Disorder
780.52	Unspecified Insomnia Disorder
780.54	Other Specified Hypersomnolence Disorder
780.54	Unspecified Hypersomnolence Disorder
780.59	Other Specified Sleep-Wake Disorder
780.59	Unspecified Sleep-Wake Disorder

Sexual Dysfunctions

302.74	Delayed Ejaculation
302.72	Erectile Disorder
302.73	Female Orgasmic Disorder
302.72	Female Sexual Interest/Arousal Disorder
302.76	Genito-Pelvic Pain/Penetration Disorder
302.71	Male Hypoactive Sexual Desire Disorder
302.75	Premature Ejaculation
_._ (_._)	Substance/Medication-Induced Sexual Dysfunction
302.79	Other Specified Sexual Dysfunction
302.70	Unspecified Sexual Dysfunction

Gender Dysphoria

_._ (_._)	Gender Dysphoria
302.6	Gender Dysphoria in Children
302.85	Gender Dysphoria in Adolescents and Adults
302.6	Other Specified Gender Dysphoria
302.6	Unspecified Gender Dysphoria

Disruptive, Impulse-Control, and Conduct Disorders

313.81	Oppositional Defiant Disorder
312.34	Intermittent Explosive Disorder
_._ (_._)	Conduct Disorder
312.81	Childhood-Onset Type
312.82	Adolescent-Onset Type
312.89	Unspecified Onset
301.7	Antisocial Personality Disorder
312.33	Pyromania
312.32	Kleptomania
312.89	Other Specified Disruptive, Impulse-Control, and Conduct Disorder
312.9	Unspecified Disruptive, Impulse-Control, and Conduct Disorder

Substance-Related and Addictive Disorders

Substance-Related Disorders

Alcohol-Related Disorders

_._ (_._)	Alcohol Use Disorder
305.00	Mild
303.90	Moderate
303.90	Severe
303.00	Alcohol Intoxication
291.81	Alcohol Withdrawal
_._ (_._)	Other Alcohol-Induced Disorders
291.9	Unspecified Alcohol-Related Disorder

Caffeine-Related Disorders

305.90	Caffeine Intoxication
292.0	Caffeine Withdrawal
_._ (_._)	Other Caffeine-Induced Disorders
292.9	Unspecified Caffeine-Related Disorder

Cannabis-Related Disorders

_._ (_._)	Cannabis Use Disorder
305.20	Mild
304.30	Moderate
304.30	Severe
292.89	Cannabis Intoxication
292.0	Cannabis Withdrawal
_._ (_._)	Other Cannabis-Induced Disorders
292.9	Unspecified Cannabis-Related Disorders

Hallucinogen-Related Disorders

_._ (_._)	Phencyclidine Use Disorder
305.90	Mild
304.60	Moderate
304.60	Severe
_._ (_._)	Other Hallucinogen Use Disorder
305.30	Mild
304.50	Moderate
304.50	Severe
292.89	Phencyclidine Intoxication
292.89	Other Hallucinogen Intoxication
292.89	Hallucinogen Persisting Perception Disorder
_._ (_._)	Other Phencyclidine-Induced Disorders
_._ (_._)	Other Hallucinogen-Induced Disorders
292.9	Unspecified Phencyclidine-Related Disorder
292.9	Unspecified Hallucinogen-Related Disorder

Inhalant-Related Disorders

_._ (_._)	Inhalant Use Disorder
305.90	Mild
304.60	Moderate
304.60	Severe
292.89	Inhalant Intoxication
_._ (_._)	Other Inhalant-Induced Disorders
292.9	Unspecified Inhalant-Related Disorder

Opioid-Related Disorders

_._ (_._)	Opioid Use Disorder
305.50	Mild
304.00	Moderate
304.00	Severe
292.89	Opioid Intoxication
292.0	Opioid Withdrawal
_._ (_._)	Other Opioid-Induced Disorders
292.9	Unspecified Opioid-Related Disorder

Sedative, Hypnotic, or Anxiolytic-Related Disorders

_._ (_._)	Sedative, Hypnotic, or Anxiolytic Use Disorder
305.40	Mild
304.10	Moderate
304.10	Severe
292.89	Sedative, Hypnotic, or Anxiolytic Intoxication
292.0	Sedative, Hypnotic, or Anxiolytic Withdrawal
_._ (_._)	Other Sedative-, Hypnotic-, or Anxiolytic-Induced Disorders
292.9	Unspecified Sedative-, Hypnotic-, or Anxiolytic-Related Disorder

Stimulant-Related Disorders

_._ (_._)	Stimulant Use Disorder
	Mild
305.70	Amphetamine-Type Substance
305.60	Cocaine
305.70	Other or Unspecified Stimulant
	Moderate
304.40	Amphetamine-Type Substance
304.20	Cocaine
304.40	Other or Unspecified Stimulant
	Severe
304.40	Amphetamine-Type Substance
304.20	Cocaine
304.40	Other or Unspecified Stimulant
292.89	Stimulant Intoxication
292.89	Amphetamine or Other Stimulant, Without Perceptual Disturbances
292.89	Cocaine, Without Perceptual Disturbances
292.89	Amphetamine or Other Stimulant, With Perceptual Disturbances
292.89	Cocaine, With Perceptual Disturbances
292.0	Stimulant Withdrawal
_._ (_._)	Other Stimulant-Induced Disorders
292.9	Unspecified Stimulant-Related Disorder

Tobacco-Related Disorders

_._ (_._)	Tobacco Use Disorder
305.1	Mild
305.1	Moderate
305.1	Severe
292.0	Tobacco Withdrawal
_._ (_._)	Other Tobacco-Induced Disorders
292.9	Unspecified Tobacco-Related Disorder

Other (or Unknown) Substance Intoxication

_._ (_._)	Other (or Unknown) Substance Use Disorder
305.90	Mild
304.90	Moderate
304.90	Severe
292.89	Other (or Unknown) Substance Intoxication
292.0	Other (or Unknown) Substance Withdrawal
_._ (_._)	Other (or Unknown) Substance-Induced Disorders
292.9	Unspecified Other (or Unknown) Substance-Related Disorder

Non-Substance-Related Disorders

312.31	Gambling Disorder

Neurocognitive Disorders

_._ (_._)	Delirium
_._ (_._)	Substance Intoxication Delirium
_._ (_._)	Substance Withdrawal Delirium
292.81	Medication-Induced Delirium
293.0	Delirium Due to Another Medical Condition
293.0	Delirium Due to Multiple Etiologies
780.09	Other Specified/Unspecified Delirium
293.0	Delirium Due to Multiple Etiologies
780.09	Other Specified Delirium
780.09	Unspecified Delirium

Major and Mild Neurocognitive Disorders

Major or Mild Neurocognitive Disorder Due to Alzheimer's Disease

_._ (_._)	Probable Major Neurocognitive Disorder Due to Alzheimer's Disease
294.11	With Behavioral Disturbance
294.10	Without Behavioral Disturbance
331.9	Possible Major Neurocognitive Disorder Due to Alzheimer's Disease
331.83	Mild Neurocognitive Disorder Due to Alzheimer's Disease

Major or Mild Frontotemporal Neurocognitive Disorder

_._ (_._)	Probable Major Frontotemporal Neurocognitive Disorder
294.11	With Behavioral Disturbance
294.10	Without Behavioral Disturbance
331.9	Possible Major Neurocognitive Disorder Due to Frontotemporal Lobar Degeneration
331.83	Mild Neurocognitive Disorder Due to Frontotemporal Lobar Degeneration

Major or Mild Neurocognitive Disorder With Lewy Bodies

	Probable Major Neurocognitive Disorder with Lewy Bodies
294.11	With Behavioral Disturbance
294.10	Without Behavioral Disturbance
331.9	Possible Major Neurocognitive Disorder With Lewy Bodies
331.83	Mild Neurocognitive Disorder With Lewy Bodies

Major or Mild Vascular Neurocognitive Disorder

_._ (_._)	Probable Major Vascular Neurocognitive Disorder
290.40	With Behavioral Disturbance
290.40	Without Behavioral Disturbance
331.9	Possible Major Vascular Neurocognitive Disorder
331.83	Mild Neurocognitive Disorder

Major or Mild Neurocognitive Disorder Due to Traumatic Brain Injury

_._ (_._)	Major Neurocognitive Disorder Due to Traumatic Brain Injury
294.11	With Behavioral Disturbance
294.10	Without Behavioral Disturbance
331.83	Mild Neurocognitive Disorder Due to Traumatic Brain Injury

Major or Mild Neurocognitive Disorder Due to HIV Infection

_._ (_._)	Major Neurocognitive Disorder Due to HIV Infection
294.11	With Behavioral Disturbance
294.10	Without Behavioral Disturbance
331.83	Mild Neurocognitive Disorder Due to HIV Infection

Major or Mild Neurocognitive Disorder Due to Prion Disease

_._ (_._)	Major Neurocognitive Disorder Due to Prion Disease
294.11	With Behavioral Disturbance
294.10	Without Behavioral Disturbance
331.83	Mild Neurocognitive Disorder Due to Prion Disease

Major or Mild Neurocognitive Disorder Due to Parkinson's Disease

_._ (_._)	Major Neurocognitive Disorder Due to Parkinson's Disease
294.11	With Behavioral Disturbance
294.10	Without Behavioral Disturbance
331.9	Major Neurocognitive Disorder Possibly Due to Parkinson's Disease
331.83	Mild Neurocognitive Disorder Due to Parkinson's Disease

Major or Mild Neurocognitive Disorder Due to Huntington's Disease

_._ (_._)	Major Neurocognitive Disorder Due to Huntington's Disease
294.11	With Behavioral Disturbance
294.10	Without Behavioral Disturbance
331.83	Mild Neurocognitive Disorder Due to Huntington's Disease

Major or Mild Neurocognitive Disorder Due to Another Medical Condition

_._ (_._)	Major Neurocognitive Disorder Due to Another Medical Condition
294.11	With Behavioral Disturbance
294.10	Without Behavioral Disturbance
331.83	Mild Neurocognitive Disorder Due to Another Medical Condition

Major or Mild Neurocognitive Disorder Due to Multiple Etiologies

_._ (_._)	Major Neurocognitive Disorder Due to Multiple Etiologies
294.11	With Behavioral Disturbance
294.10	Without Behavioral Disturbance
331.83	Mild Neurocognitive Disorder Due to Multiple Etiologies

Unspecified Neurocognitive Disorder

799.59	Unspecified Neurocognitive Disorder

Personality Disorders

Cluster A Personality Disorders

301.0	Paranoid Personality Disorder
301.20	Schizoid Personality Disorder
301.22	Schizotypal Personality Disorder

Cluster B Personality Disorders

301.7	Antisocial Personality Disorder
301.83	Borderline Personality Disorder
301.50	Histrionic Personality Disorder
301.80	Narcissistic Personality Disorder

Cluster C Personality Disorders

301.82	Avoidant Personality Disorder
301.6	Dependent Personality Disorder
301.4	Obsessive-Compulsive Personality Disorder

Other Personality Disorders

310.1	Personality Change Due to Another Medical Condition
301.89	Other Specified Personality Disorder
301.9	Unspecified Personality Disorder

Paraphilic Disorders

302.82	Voyeuristic Disorder
302.4	Exhibitionistic Disorder
302.89	Frotteuristic Disorder
302.83	Sexual Masochism Disorder
302.84	Sexual Sadism Disorder
302.2	Pedophilic Disorder
302.81	Fetishistic Disorder
302.3	Transvestic Disorder
302.89	Other Specified Paraphilic Disorder
302.9	Unspecified Paraphilic Disorder

Other Mental Disorders

294.8	Other Specified Mental Disorder Due to Another Medical Condition
294.9	Unspecified Mental Disorder Due to Another Medical Condition
300.9	Other Specified Mental Disorder
300.9	Unspecified Mental Disorder

Medication-Induced Movement Disorders and Other Adverse Effects of Medication

332.1	Neuroleptic-Induced Parkinsonism
332.1	Other Medication-Induced Parkinsonism
333.92	Neuroleptic Malignant Syndrome
333.72	Medication-Induced Acute Dystonia
333.99	Medication-Induced Acute Akathisia
333.85	Tardive Dyskinesia
333.72	Tardive Dystonia
333.99	Tardive Akathisia
333.1	Medication-Induced Postural Tremor
333.99	Other Medication-Induced Movement Disorder
_._ (_._)	Antidepressant Discontinuation Syndrome
995.29	Initial Encounter
995.29	Subsequent Encounter
995.29	Sequelae
_._ (_._)	Other Adverse Effect of Medication
995.20	Initial Encounter
995.20	Subsequent Encounter
995.20	Sequelae

Other Conditions that May Be a Focus of Clinical Attention

Relationship Problems
Problems Related to Family Upbringing

V61.20	Parent-Child Relational Problem
V61.8	Sibling Relational Problem
V61.8	Upbringing Away From Parents
V61.29	Child Affected by Parental Relationship Distress

Other Problems Related to Primary Support Group

V61.10	Relationship Distress With Spouse or Intimate Partner
V61.03	Disruption of Family by Separation or Divorce
V61.8	High Expressed Emotion Level Within Family
V62.82	Uncomplicated Bereavement

Abuse and Neglect

Child Maltreatment and Neglect Problems

Child Physical Abuse

Child Physical Abuse, Confirmed

995.54	Initial Encounter
995.54	Subsequent Encounter

Child Physical Abuse, Suspected

995.54	Initial Encounter
995.54	Subsequent Encounter

Other Circumstances Related to Child Physical Abuse

Child Sexual Abuse

Child Sexual Abuse, Confirmed

995.53	Initial Encounter
995.53	Subsequent Encounter

Child Sexual Abuse, Suspected

995.53	Initial Encounter
995.53	Subsequent Encounter

Other Circumstances Related to Child Sexual Abuse

Child Neglect

Child Neglect, Confirmed

995.52	Initial Encounter
995.52	Subsequent Encounter

Child Neglect, Suspected

995.21	Initial Encounter
995.21	Subsequent Encounter

Other Circumstances Related to Child Psychological Abuse

Adult Maltreatment and Neglect Problems

Spouse or Partner Violence, Physical
Spouse or Partner Violence, Physical, Confirmed

995.81	Initial Encounter
995.81	Subsequent Encounter

Spouse or Partner Violence, Physical, Suspected

995.81	Initial Encounter
995.81	Subsequent Encounter

Other Circumstances Related to Spouse or Partner Violence, Physical
Spouse or Partner Violence, Sexual
Spouse or Partner Violence, Sexual, Confirmed

995.83	Initial Encounter
995.83	Subsequent Encounter

Spouse or Partner Violence, Suspected

995.83	Initial Encounter
995.83	Subsequent Encounter

Other Circumstances Related to Spouse or Partner Violence, Sexual
Spouse or Partner, Neglect
Spouse or Partner Neglect, Confirmed

995.85	Initial Encounter
995.85	Subsequent Encounter

Spouse or Partner Neglect, Suspected

995.85	Initial Encounter
995.85	Subsequent Encounter

Other Circumstances Related to Spouse or Partner Neglect

Spouse or Partner Abuse, Psychological

Spouse or Partner Abuse, Psychological, Confirmed

995.82	Initial Encounter
995.82	Subsequent Encounter

Spouse or Partner Abuse, Psychological, Suspected

995.82	Initial Encounter
995.82	Subsequent Encounter

Other Circumstances Related to Spouse or Partner Abuse, Psychological

Adult Abuse by Nonspouse or Nonpartner

995.81	Adult Physical Abuse by Nonspouse or Nonpartner, Confirmed
995.81	Adult Physical Abuse by Nonspouse or Nonpartner, Suspected
995.83	Adult Sexual Abuse by Nonspouse or Nonpartner, Confirmed

995.83	Adult Sexual Abuse by Nonspouse or Nonpartner, Suspected
995.82	Adult Psychological Abuse by Nonspouse or Nonpartner, Confirmed
995.82	Adult Psychological Abuse by Nonspouse or Nonpartner, Suspected

Other Circumstances Related to Adult Abuse by Nonspouse or Nonpartner

Educational and Occupational Problems

Educational Problems
| V62.3 | Academic or Educational Problems |

Occupational Problems
| V62.21 | Problem Related to Current Military Deployment Status |
| V62.29 | Other Problem Related to Employment |

Housing and Economic Problems
Housing Problems
V60.0	Homelessness
V60.1	Inadequate Housing
V60.89	Discord with Neighbor, Lodger, or Landlord
V60.6	Problem Related to Living in a Residential Institution

Economic Problems
V60.2	Lack of Adequate Food or Safe Drinking Water
V60.2	Extreme Poverty
V60.2	Low Income
V60.2	Insufficient Social Insurance or Welfare Support
V60.2	Unspecified Problem Related to Social Environment

Other Problems Related to the Social Environment
V62.89	Phase of Life Problem
V60.3	Problem Related to Living Alone
V62.4	Acculturation Difficulty
V62.4	Social Exclusion or Rejection
V62.4	Target of (Perceived) Adverse Discrimination or Persecution
V62.9	Unspecified Problem Related to Social Environment

Problems Related to Crime or Interaction With the Legal System
| V62.89 | Victim of Crime |
| V62.5 | Conviction in Civil or Criminal Proceedings Without Imprisonment |

V62.5	Imprisonment or Other Incarceration
V62.5	Problems Related to Release From Prison
V62.5	Problems Related to Other Legal Circumstances

Other Health Service Encounters for Counseling and Medical Advice
| V65.49 | Sex Counseling |
| V65.40 | Other Counseling or Consultation |

Problems Related to Other Psychosocial, Personal, and Environmental Circumstances
V62.89	Religious or Spiritual Problem
V61.7	Problems Related to Unwanted Pregnancy
V61.5	Problems Related to Multiparity
V62.89	Discord With Social Service Provider (Probation Officer, Case Manager, or Social Services Worker)
V62.89	Victim of Terrorism or Torture
V62.22	Exposure to Disaster, War, or Other Hostilities
V62.89	Other Problem Related to Psychosocial Circumstances
V62.9	Unspecified Problem Related to Unspecified Psychosocial Circumstances

Other Circumstances of Personal History
V15.49	Other Personal History of Psychological Trauma
V15.59	Personal History of Self-Harm
V62.22	Personal History of Military Deployment
V15.89	Other Personal Risk Factors
V69.9	Problem Related to Lifestyle
V71.01	Adult Antisocial Behavior
V71.02	Child or Adolescent Antisocial Behavior

Problems Related to Access to Medical and Other Health Care
| V63.9 | Unavailability or Inaccessibility of Health Care Facilities |
| V63.8 | Unavailability or Inaccessibility of Other Helping Agencies |

Nonadherence to Medical Treatment
V15.81	Nonadherence to Medical Treatment
278.00	Overweight or Obesity
V65.2	Malingering
V40.31	Wandering Associated With a Mental Disorder
V62.89	Borderline Intellectual Functioning

Appendix B
Mini-Mental Status Exam

Orientation	Ask the year, season, date, day, month, state, county, town, hospital, floor	5 _____ 5 _____
Concentration	Repeat and ask person to remember three words	3 _____
Attention and Processing	Ask person to do serial 7s (five times) or spell WORLD backward	5 _____
Recall	Ask person to recall the above three items	3 _____
Language	Ask person to name two common objects when shown (i.e., watch, clock, glasses)	2 _____
	Ask person to repeat "no ifs and no buts"	1 _____
Command	Give person a plain piece of paper with a three-step command—"take this paper, fold it, place it on table"	3 _____
Read and Do	Show person **Close Your Eyes** in big letters Observe if person does what is asked	1 _____
Write a Sentence	Ask person to write a sentence with proper grammar	1 _____
Copy	Ask person to copy the overlapping pentagons below	1 _____ **TOTAL** ____/30

Folstein, M. F., Folstein, S. E., & McHugh, P. R. (1975). "Mini-Mental State": A practical method for grading the cognitive state of patients for the clinician. *Journal of Psychiatric Research, 12,* 189–198.

Appendix C

North American Nursing Diagnosis Association (NANDA) Nursing Diagnoses Most Frequently Used in Mental Health and Psychiatric Settings

- Acute Confusion
- Acute Pain
- Activity Intolerance (Actual or Risk for)
- Adult Failure to Thrive
- Altered Thought Processes
- Anxiety
- Bowel Incontinence
- Caregiver Role Strain
- Caregiver Role Strain (Risk for)
- Chronic Confusion
- Chronic Low Self-Esteem
- Chronic Pain
- Chronic Sorrow
- Complicated Grieving (Actual or Risk for)
- Compromised Family Coping
- Conflict, Decisional
- Conflict, Parental role
- Constipation
- Decisional Conflict
- Decreased Cardiac Output
- Defensive Coping
- Deficient Fluid Volume (Actual or Risk for)
- Delayed Growth and Development (Actual or Risk for)
- Delayed Surgical Recovery
- Diarrhea
- Disabled Family Coping
- Disturbed Body Image
- Disturbed Personal Identity (Actual or Risk for)
- Disturbed Sleep Pattern
- Dysfunctional Family Processes
- Excess Fluid Volume (Actual or Risk For)
- Fatigue
- Fear
- Functional Urinary Incontinence
- Grieving
- Hopelessness
- Hyperthermia
- Hypothermia

- Impaired Adjustment
- Impaired Comfort
- Impaired Dentition
- Impaired Gas Exchange
- Impaired Home Maintenance
- Impaired Memory
- Impaired Oral Mucous Membrane
- Impaired Parenting
- Impaired Physical Mobility
- Impaired Skin Integrity
- Impaired Social Interaction
- Impaired Transfer Ability
- Impaired Urinary Incontinence
- Impaired Walking
- Impaired Wheelchair Mobility
- Impaired Verbal Communication
- Ineffective Airway Clearance
- Ineffective Breathing Pattern
- Ineffective Coping
- Ineffective Community Coping
- Ineffective Denial
- Ineffective Infant Feeding Pattern
- Ineffective Peripheral Tissue Perfusion (Actual or Risk For)
- Ineffective Relationship (Actual or Risk for)
- Ineffective Role Performance
- Ineffective Self-Health Maintenance
- Ineffective Thermoregulation
- Interrupted Family Processes
- Insomnia
- Moral Distress
- Nausea
- Noncompliance
- Imbalanced Nutrition: Less Than Body Requirements
- Imbalanced Nutrition: More Than Body Requirements
- Impaired Environmental Interpretation Syndrome
- Impaired Individual Resilience

- Impaired Spontaneous Ventilation
- Impaired Swallowing
- Impaired Tissue Integrity
- Impaired Urinary Elimination
- Latex Allergy Response
- Pain
- Parental Role Conflict
- Post-Trauma Syndrome
- Powerlessness (Actual or Risk for)
- Rape-Trauma Syndrome
- Readiness for Enhanced Decision-Making
- Readiness for Enhanced Hope
- Relocation Stress Syndrome (Actual or Risk for)
- Risk for Activity Intolerance
- Risk for Aspiration
- Risk for Bleeding
- Risk for Chronic Low Self-Esteem
- Risk for Contamination
- Risk for Decreased Cardiac Tissue Perfusion
- Risk for Electrolyte Imbalance
- Risk for Falls
- Risk for Impaired Attachment
- Risk for Impaired Religiosity
- Risk for Ineffective Cerebral Tissue Perfusion
- Risk for Infection
- Risk for Injury
- Risk for Loneliness
- Risk for Other-Directed Violence
- Risk for Chronic Low Self-Esteem
- Risk for Ineffective Renal Perfusion
- Risk for Peripheral Neurovascular Dysfunction
- Risk for Poisoning
- Risk for Self-Directed Violence
- Risk for Situational Low Self-Esteem
- Risk for Suicide
- Risk for Thermal Injury
- Risk for Trauma
- Risk for Vascular Trauma
- Risk-Prone Health Behavior
- Self-Care Deficit (Bathing, Hygiene, Feeding, Dressing, Grooming, Toileting)
- Self-Mutilation (Actual or Risk for)
- Sensory/Perceptual Alteration (Specify Visual, Auditory, Tactile, Kinesthetic, Gustatory, Olfactory)
- Sexuality Pattern (Ineffective)
- Situational Low Self-Esteem
- Social Isolation
- Spiritual Distress
- Spiritual Well-Being, Potential for Enhancement
- Spontaneous Ventilation, Inability to Sustain
- Stress Overload
- Stress Urinary Incontinence
- Suffocation, Risk for
- Suicide, Risk for
- Urinary Retention
- Wandering

Adapted from North American Nursing Diagnosis Association (NANDA) (2012). *NANDA nursing diagnoses: Definitions and classification 2012–2014*. Oxford, UK: Wiley-Blackwell Publishers.

Appendix D
Anxiety Scale (Sample)

Anxiety scales are rating scales developed to quantify the severity of anxiety symptoms a person is feeling at the present time. There is no right or wrong answer to the questions. A 5-point scale is used for rating each item:

0 = Not present
1 = Rarely
2 = Some of the time
3 = Much of the time
4 = All or most of the time

1. **Anxious feelings**
   Worry   _____
   Anticipate the worst   _____
   Sudden panic   _____

2. **Tension**
   Startle easily   _____
   Cry easily   _____
   Restless   _____
   Tremors   _____

3. **Fears**
   Fear of dark   _____
   Fear of strangers   _____
   Fear of being alone   _____
   Fear of animals   _____
   Fear of closed spaces   _____
   Fear of public places   _____
   Fear of crowds   _____
   Fear with no real cause   _____

4. **Insomnia**
   Difficulty falling asleep   _____
   Difficulty staying asleep   _____
   Uncomfortable dreams   _____

5. **Thinking**
   Problems concentrating   _____
   Memory blanks   _____
   Lose train of thought   _____

6. **Depressed mood**
   Decreased interest in
       previously enjoyed activities   _____
   Reduced contact with
       friends and family   _____

7. **Somatic complaints**
   Dizziness   _____
   Nausea   _____
   Constipation   _____
   Chest pain   _____
   Choking sensation   _____
   Palpitations   _____
   Shortness of breath   _____

Appendix E

Beck's Depression Scale

The questionnaire is completed by the individual or with the help of an examiner.

Directions:

Please read each group of statements carefully. Then pick out one statement in each group, which best accounts for the way you have been feeling the PAST WEEK, INCLUDING TODAY! Circle the letter of the statement that best describes this feeling. If several statements in the group seem to apply equally well, choose only one answer and circle the appropriate response.

(a) I do not feel sad
(b) I feel sad
(c) I am sad all the time and I can't snap out of it
(d) I am so sad or unhappy that I can't stand it

(a) I am not particularly discouraged about the future
(b) I feel discouraged about the future
(c) I feel I have nothing to look forward to
(d) I feel that the future is hopeless and that things cannot improve

(a) I don't have thoughts of killing myself
(b) I have thoughts of killing myself, but I would not carry it out
(c) I would like to kill myself
(d) I would kill myself if I had the chance

(a) I get as much satisfaction out of things as I used to
(b) I don't enjoy things the way I used to
(c) I don't get real satisfaction out of anything anymore
(d) I am dissatisfied or bored with everything

(a) I don't feel particularly guilty
(b) I feel guilty a good part of the time
(c) I feel quite guilty most of the time
(d) I feel guilty all of the time

(a) I make decisions about as well as I ever could
(b) I put off making decisions more than I used to
(c) I have lost most of my interest in other people
(d) I have lost all of my interest in other people

(a) I can work about as well as before
(b) It takes an extra effort to get started at doing something
(c) I have to push myself very hard to do anything
(d) I can't do any work at all

(a) I don't feel I am any worse than anybody else
(b) I am critical of myself for my weakness or mistake
(c) I blame myself all the time for my faults
(d) I blame myself for everything bad that happens

(a) My appetite is no worse than usual
(b) My appetite is not as good as it used to be
(c) My appetite is much worse now
(d) I have no appetite at all anymore

(a) I don't feel disappointed in myself
(b) I am disappointed in myself
(c) I am disgusted with myself
(d) I hate myself

(a) I do not feel like a failure
(b) I feel I have failed more than the average person
(c) As I look back on my life, all I can see is a lot of failures
(d) I feel I am a complete failure as a person

(a) I don't cry any more than usual
(b) I cry more now than I used to
(c) I cry all the time now
(d) I used to be able to cry, but now I can't cry even though I want to

(a) I am no more irritated now than I ever am
(b) I get annoyed or irritated more easily than I used to
(c) I feel irritated all the time now
(d) I don't get irritated at all by the things that used to irritate me

(a) I don't feel I am being punished
(b) I feel I may be punished
(c) I expect to be punished
(d) I feel I am being punished

(a) I don't get more tired than usual
(b) I get tired more easily than I used to
(c) I get tired from doing almost anything
(d) I am too tired to do anything

(a) I don't feel I look any worse than I used to
(b) I am worried that I am looking old/unattractive
(c) I feel that there are permanent changes in my appearance that make me look unattractive
(d) I believe that I look ugly

(a) I have not lost interest in other people
(b) I am less interested in other people than I used to be
(c) I have lost most of my interest in other people
(d) I have lost all of my interest in other people

(a) I haven't lost much weight, if any, lately
(b) I have lost more than 5 pounds
(c) I have lost more than 10 pounds
(d) I have lost more than 15 pounds

(a) I have not noticed any recent change in my interest in sex
(b) I am less interested in sex than I used to be
(c) I am much less interested in sex now
(d) I have lost interest in sex completely

(a) I am no more worried about my health than usual
(b) I am worried about physical problems such as aches and pains, or upset stomach, or constipation
(c) I am very worried about physical problems and it's hard to think of much else
(d) I am so worried about my physical problems that I cannot think about anything else

(a) I can sleep as well as usual
(b) I don't sleep as well as I used to
(c) I wake up 1 to 2 hours earlier than usual and find it hard to get back to sleep
(d) I wake up several hours earlier than I used to and cannot get back to sleep

SCORING: (1) = 1 point
(2) = 2 points
(3) = 3 points
(4) = 4 points
Score is totaled to determine evidence of depression symptoms.

Appendix F
Answers to Student Worksheet

Chapter 1
Fill in the Blank
1. Balance
2. Fight or flight
3. Overreaction
4. Unpredictability
5. Empty clichés

Matching
1. **C**
2. **E**
3. **H**
4. **D**
5. **I**
6. **B**
7. **A**
8. **F**
9. **G**

Multiple Choice
1. **Correct Answer: B,** Indicates feeling of isolation or possible depression. A: Shows active interaction with others. C: Indicates person is comfortable being alone. D: Adaptive coping.
2. **Correct Answer: C,** Criteria for diagnosis of mental disorder include the problem interferes with interpersonal relationships. A, B, D: Indicators of a healthy mental state.
3. **Correct Answer: C,** Indicates overall exhaustion and apathy toward her work. A: A temporary mental get away that replenishes energy. B: Disorganization of mental state not evident. D: Is not specific descriptive of work-related stress.
4. **Correct Answer: A,** Recognizes individual strengths and weaknesses. B: Unrealistic view of one's abilities. C: Indicates negative view of self. D: Self-defeat through negative view of self.
5. **Correct Answer: B,** Temporarily relieves the anxiety but problem still exists. A: With adaptive coping, the problem would be resolved. C: Maladaptive would mean unsuccessful methods are used to reduce anxiety. D: Dysfunctional would indicate no attempt is made to reduce anxiety
6. **Correct Answer: B,** Offers opportunity for client to talk about present feelings. A: Closes the conversation and minimizes client's feelings. C: Belittles client's statement and feelings. D: "Why" puts client on the defensive to respond.
7. **Correct Answer: C,** Avoiding reality of the situation. A: Bargaining cannot occur until reality of inevitable is acknowledged. B: There is no evidence of feelings of bitterness. D: Depression indicates a loss of hope and mourning for that which is gone.
8. **Correct Answer: D,** Seen in person who is facing death in the near future. A: Would indicate the situation has been resolved successfully. B: Grief experienced after the death. C: Adapting to loss.
9. **Correct Answer: B,** Will provide data about the client's view of the present situation. A: Assesses support system. C: Assesses coping skills and strategies. D: Does not invite the client to verbalize feelings.

Chapter 2
Fill in the Blank
1. Concealed hurt
2. Perception
3. Bullying
4. Domestic violence
5. Verbal or physical

Matching
1. **D**
2. **F**
3. **E**
4. **G**
5. **C**
6. **B**
7. **A**

Multiple Choice
1. **Correct Answer: C,** In severe anxiety, the client lacks logical thought processes and presents increasing sympathetic physiologic response. A: Mild anxiety is motivational with good reasoning and logical thought process. B: In moderate anxiety, the autonomic response is less obvious and person is still functional with decreased concentration and problem-solving. D: In panic level, there is disorientation and irrational behavior with hysteria.
2. **Correct Answer: C,** Suicidal gesture indicates the person has defined their plan and may be about ready to carry out the plan. A: Suicidal erosion is the accumulation of negative experiences that may lead to suicidal thoughts. B: Suicidal ideation indicates a verbalized thought or idea that includes the person's desire to do self-harm or destruction. D: A suicidal attempt means the person has actually carried out the suicide plan.
3. **Correct Answer: A,** Situational crisis related to a series of unpredictable events in his life that leave him void of coping skills. B: Maturational crisis refers to a predictable period of development in life stages when the person may be unable to adjust and move to next phase. C: Developmental crisis refers to same as maturational crisis. D: Identity crisis would be applicable to adolescent developmental stage.
4. **Correct Answer: A, B, D,** All factors that are warning signs for violence. C: Action packed movies can be enjoyed without related violent behavior. E: Numerous relationships do not necessarily indicate violence.
5. **Correct Answer: C,** Occurring daily verbally and is frightening to the girl. A: Situational and not necessarily daily. B: Adult is present and not necessarily daily. D: Isolated media incident.

Chapter 3
Fill in the Blank
1. Personality traits
2. Temperament

3. Equilibration
4. Assimilation
5. Accommodation
6. Solid self

Matching
1. **C**
2. **G**
3. **B**
4. **D**
5. **H**
6. **A**
7. **F**
8. **E**

Multiple Choice
1. **Correct Answer: C,** Despair. Demonstrates a lack of fulfillment and satisfaction with life choices in age group over 65 years. A, B, D: All relate to earlier life stages of development.
2. **Correct Answer: A,** Phallic. Period in which child struggles to accept a sexual identity and resolves this conflict by identifying with the parent of the same sex. This child is identifying with his father. B: Child 2 to 4 years is developing an awareness and control of elimination. C: Sexual desires are subdued in the school-age child. D: Puberty and adolescence with heightened sexual feelings and urges.
3. **Correct Answer: B,** Preoperational. Egocentric view and centration in which child is unable to see another point of view except his own. A: Involves growth of abilities related to five senses and motor function. C: Child decenters and recognizes combinations are reversible. D: Abstract thought process and problem solving.
4. **Correct Answer: C,** Postconventional—stage 5. Choice based on the number of people who would be affected and hurt by telling his friend the truth. A: No indication that there is personal gain from the choice. B: Does not show influence either by society or the law. D: There is no law of society that is involved in this decision.
5. **Correct Answer: D,** Reinforcement of early learning experiences. Observed and learned behavior with reinforcement of punishment and aggression. A, B: Behaviorism implies that thinking and feeling are irrelevant. C: Assault does not relate to an environmental threat to survival.
6. **Correct Answer: A,** Social learning theory. Actions based on observation and imitation of others for approval. B: Behaviors are result of conscious choice, not conditioning which is automatic. C: Freudian focus on adolescent sexuality not an issue in this situation. D: Feelings and peer relationships would be irrelevant in behaviorism.
7. **Correct Answer: B,** An internal locus of control. Awareness that behaviors are the result of own choices with option for change. A: Reflects Freudian theory of personality development. C: Does not indicate behavior is influenced by external forces. D: Freudian theory.
8. **Correct Answer: C,** Denial. Ego refuses to see the truth because the trauma of the rape is too painful at this time. A: No blame is being attributed by the client. B: No physical symptoms are present as a result of emotional conflict. D: Client is not offering justification for the behavior.
9. **Correct Answer: A,** Trust versus mistrust. Client is plagued by suspicion and inability to believe in the credibility of company policies. B: Feelings not based on fear of independence. C: Does not indicate a feeling of inadequacy in himself. D: Does not indicate a fear of failure or feeling of unworthiness.

10. **Correct Answer: B,** Conventional, stage 3. Actions to meet the expectations of the peer group. A: Personal gain was not the motive of the young person's actions. C: Actions do not reflect a choice to act for the good of society. D: Actions not prompted by a fear of punishment.

Chapter 4
Fill in the Blank
1. Psychotropic/antipsychotic
2. Linda Richards
3. Ethics
4. Informed consent
5. Confidentiality
6. Thinking

Matching
1. **E**
2. **C**
3. **D**
4. **G**
5. **B**
6. **F**
7. **A**

Multiple Choice
1. **Correct Answer: A,** Dorothea Dix—worked tirelessly to encourage legislation to improve care for the mentally ill. B: Linda Richards was the first American trained nurse who later was involved in training nurses to care for mentally ill. C: Florence Nightingale paved the way for the nursing profession. D: Harriett Bailey wrote the first psychiatric nursing textbook.
2. **Correct Answer: C,** Evidence of mental state posing an immediate threat to self or others is required to have an OPC granted by a court official. A, B, and D: Do not indicate an immediate threat to client safety or that of others and would not be the reason for involuntary commitment.
3. **Correct Answer: A,** Coping abilities both past and present would be included in a psychological assessment. B, C, and D: All would be included in the planning phase of the client care plan for this client.
4. **Correct Answer: C,** An inmate with a history of mental illness will need referral to be further evaluated for any current symptoms and treatment. A, B, D: All are common responses of inmates toward confinement.
5. **Correct Answer: D,** Outpatient care offers client treatment without admission to a mental health inpatient unit. A: Referral indicates the client has already consented to treatment. B: Question specifically asks about the physician action of referral. C: Treatment plan is discussed at the time of admission for treatment.
6. **Correct Answer: B,** Intent to commit a crime is a legal reason for disclosure. A: Information cannot be given to wife unless client has given consent. C: Only personnel directly involved in client care legally have access to the information. D: Disclosure to the media would violate HIPPA policies.
7. **Correct Answer: C,** The initial action should be to try to de-escalate the behavior by a calm and nonthreatening approach. This will allow the client a chance to regain control of their behavior without the use of restraint. A: Sedation may be necessary if behavior becomes unmanageable by nonrestraining methods. B: Threat of seclusion or restraint is inappropriate. D: Nurses have obligation to protect the safety of all clients. To allow the confrontation to continue could pose a threat to all involved.

8. **Correct Answer: A,** Chemical restraint is the least restrictive. B: Seclusion should only be used if behavior cannot be controlled by other means and requires a time frame. C: Seclusion would only be used if sedation was not effective in behavior management. D: Physical restraint is most restrictive and only used in an emergency situation.

9. **Correct Answer: C,** Seclusion is never appropriate when a client is suicidal. A, B, D: All indicate inappropriate social behaviors for which seclusion may be used until client regains control or is determined to be ineffective.

10. **Correct Answer: C,** Since competency of the client may be questionable at the point of admission, it would be advisable to include a family member to verify information was received. A: If present psychological state of the client is irrational, it will not help to go over the information again. B: It is important that information on client rights and unit policies is explained at the time of admission. D: A co-worker cannot legally provide a signed statement of understanding from the client or family.

Chapter 5
Fill in the Blank
1. Social; therapeutic
2. Psychotherapy
3. Caregiver
4. Therapeutic process
5. Psychotropic
6. Lipid solubility
7. Cumulative effects

Matching
1. **F**
2. **E**
3. **D**
4. **C**
5. **A**
6. **B**
7. **G**

Multiple Choice
1. **Correct Answer: C,** Monitoring behavioral responses to therapy. Observation of behavior and response to treatment is the responsibility of the nurse. A: Role of the psychologist. B: Done by psychiatrist or therapist. D: This is the responsibility of the social worker.

2. **Correct Answer: A,** Model an appropriate response to the situation. Modeling is an effective method of reinforcing socially appropriate behavior. B: Assessment data. C: Reprimands are not therapeutic and demean the client. D: Does not involve client interaction.

3. **Correct Answer: D,** Clinical social worker. Social worker works with community agencies to secure continued support and care for the client. A: Works with direct day-to-day care of the client. B: May be involved with psychotherapy. C: Not a nursing function.

4. **Correct Answer: B,** Advocate. As a client advocate, the nurse functions to protect the rights of the client through acceptance, respect, and support of the client's perspective and decisions. A: Providing information about the problem and how treatment works. C: Active listening and therapeutic communication. D: Implementation of nursing interventions.

5. **Correct Answer: A,** Caregiver. Observation of response to treatment and assessment are part of the caregiver role. B: Therapeutic

interaction with the client. C: Patient teaching. D: Protecting patient rights.

6. **Correct Answer: C,** Modeling appropriate ways to communicate feelings. Modeling assists the client with communication skills and social interaction. A: No guidance or supportive intervention has occurred. B: Isolating the client will not support improved social skills. D: Punitive methods are not therapeutic.

7. **Correct Answer: B,** They will reduce symptoms and assist to restore functional levels of living. Psychotropic agents used in combination with therapy will reduce the disabling symptoms and promote a manageable level of living. A: Drugs by themselves cannot help the client with the behaviors imposed by the illness. Therapy helps the client to understand the symptoms and how to manage them. C: These drugs can reduce the symptoms, but there is no guarantee that they will ever be totally free of them. D: Psychotropic agents are not curative.

8. **Correct Answer: A,** Slowed metabolic rate and renal excretion time. Slowed metabolic rate and renal excretion time allow the drug to remain in the body longer. B: There is a higher fat composition of tissue in the older adult. C, D: There is less serum albumin and protein to bind with the drug which allows more of the free drug to circulate in the blood.

9. **Correct Answer: B,** "I take so much medication every day but I just seem to feel worse later." Feeling worse after taking several medications could indicate the client is experiencing side effects from drug interactions. The nurse should ask more questions to clarify the statement. A: Indicates a need for explanation of diagnostic need for medication. C: Information would be noted to alert physician to client request. D: Client is taking medication correctly to assist with difficulty swallowing.

10. **Correct Answer: D,** Dry skin with decreased intake of fluids. Dry skin with decreased fluid intake could indicate dehydration which increases the concentration of the drug in the body. A: Indicates safety issue related to side effects. B: Increased drowsiness is side effect of antidepressant medication. C: Usual symptoms of depressed state.

Chapter 6
Fill in the Blank
1. Problem-solving
2. Subjective
3. Objective
4. Contributing factor
5. Collaboratively

Matching
1. **C**
2. **D**
3. **A**
4. **E**
5. **F**
6. **B**

Multiple Choice
1. **Correct Answer: A,** Subjective data is best documented using exact words as stated by the client to avoid attempts at interpreting the intended meaning. B: This can validate subjective data but cannot provide client perspective. C: Objective data. D: Nurse's perspective may differ from intended meaning.

2. **Correct Answer: D,** Establishes setting in which the client can feel safe, secure, and free to express feelings and thoughts without

reprisal. A: Cooperation of the client is a result of the trusting relationship. B: Provides information but does not establish trust. C: Trusting relationship is initiated by the nurse.

3. **Correct Answer: B,** Mood and affect are components of the mental status assessment. A, C: Do not relate to mental status. D: Established from collected data in next step of process.

4. **Correct Answer: A,** Term referring to a flat or absent emotional expression. B: Refers to memory of the past. C: Used to reference slowed motor activity. D: Attitude of indifference toward environment and others.

5. **Correct Answer: B,** Indicates the client may be having auditory hallucinations. A: Coping mechanism to deal with present threat to self. C: Indicates disturbance in thought processes. D: Short-term memory issue.

6. **Correct Answer: A,** Ability to perceive and understand illness and symptoms is described as insight into the present problem. B: Level of consciousness and processing. C: Alertness to person, place, time. D: Describes decision-making ability.

7. **Correct Answer: D,** Clarification or evaluation of client understanding about the drug. A: Occurs prior to implementation of planned interventions. B: Identifies the problem. C: Question clearly describes phase following nursing intervention.

8. **Correct Answer: D,** Evaluation is a form of reassessment, additional planning, and revamping nursing strategies for effective outcomes. A, B, C: All involved in reevaluation once evaluation has taken place—process is incomplete and cannot be validated until evaluation has occurred.

Chapter 7
Fill in the Blank
1. Congruent
2. Intermittent
3. Blocking
4. Neologism
5. Loose association
6. Kinesics
7. Arm's length

Matching
1. **F**
2. **D**
3. **A**
4. **C**
5. **E**
6. **B**

Multiple Choice
1. **Correct Answer: B,** Reinforces reality while acknowledging and validates the symptoms are real and frightening to the client. A: Minimizes the client's feelings. C: Belittling statement. D: Puts the client on the defensive.

2. **Correct Answer: D,** Clarification to verify perceived meaning of client statement. A: Minimizes the client's feelings. B: False reassurance with superficial attitude. C: Minimizing or belittling and devalues the client's feelings.

3. **Correct Answer: A,** Client behavior indicates anxiety about the topic. Silence will allow the client to continue talking when able. B: Client has not stated feelings about the situation. C: Nonverbal behavior leads the nurse to wait rather than restating at this time. D: Concentrating not an issue at this point.

4. **Correct Answer: B,** Open-ended statement that allows the client to talk freely about the issue. A: Could be used later in the interac-

tion. C: Belittling the client's feelings. D: Could be used later in the interaction.

5. **Correct Answer: A,** Validates nurse's perception of client's feelings and offers the client an opportunity to talk about them. B: Minimizes the client's fears and anxiety. C, D: False reassurance.

6. **Correct Answer: D,** Client's statement indicates a feeling of being controlled by women. A: "Why" puts the client on defensive. B: Belittling comment. C: Block closed-ended statement.

7. **Correct Answer: B,** Open-ended statement allows the client to discuss feelings freely. A: Would allow "yes or no" answer. C: Could be answered in one word. D: "Yes or no" question.

8. **Correct Answer: D,** Focusing helps the client concentrate on a specific issue that may be uncomfortable to talk about. A, C: Allow "yes or no" answer. B: Puts the client on defensive and demands an answer.

Chapter 8
Fill in the Blank
1. Empathy
2. Self-awareness
3. Situation; needs
4. Independence
5. Boundaries
6. Anxiety

Matching
1. **C**
2. **D**
3. **F**
4. **B**
5. **A**
6. **E**

Multiple Choice
1. **Correct Answer: D,** Trust is dependent on consistent honesty and demonstrated genuine concern of the nurse. A: Sympathy allows the nurse to meld into the client's problem and is nontherapeutic. B: Clients are accepted as they come to us for treatment. C: It is not the quantity but the quality of that time spent with the client.

2. **Correct Answer: D,** Client is attempting to manipulate the nurse into a triangle of dependence by complaining about others and showing favoritism. A: Statement does not indicate client is evading discharge. B: Not relevant. C: There are no conflicting statements.

3. **Correct Answer: A,** Changing the topic will remove the immediate threat to the client. B: Threatens the client and is nontherapeutic and unethical. C: Distance should be maintained—touching an aggressive client is unsafe. D: Does not attempt to understand meaning behind the behavior.

4. **Correct Answer: A,** An awareness of our own thinking and behavior allows us to try to elicit this same honesty and openness in the client toward recognition of the problem and opportunity for change. B: Provides information about the client at the present time. C: Key to insight is in "thinking" using knowledge base. D: Used to facilitate interactions between client and nurse.

5. **Correct Answer: A,** Explanations of rules and boundaries are explained at the beginning of the relationship to establish a baseline for the next phase. B: Period of planning and goals to improve client's behavior. C: Client is able to practice learned skills. D: Not a phase of the relationship, but an anticipated outcome.

6. **Correct Answer: B,** Nurse should encourage the client to have increased interaction with others promoting reliance on his or her own ability to deal with problems. This promotes independence in getting along with others toward discharge. A: Time spent with client is continued until discharge. C: The nurse–client relationship must not extend beyond the termination phase. D: This is a focus in the working phase.

7. **Correct Answer: C,** Any contact by phone, mail, e-mail, or socialization with any client following discharge is in clear violation of professional ethics. A, B, D: All within acceptable roles of the nurse.

8. **Correct Answer: D,** Focusing on the client's problem and feelings without responding to the attempted personal reference. A: Encourages further isolated contact and overinvolvement with the client. B: Demeans client without recognizing the feelings behind the statement. C: Focuses on the nurse and is risking overinvolvement.

9. **Correct Answer: A,** Accepting a client's gift is overinvolvement and violates professional limits for behavior. B, C, D: All are acceptable within the nurse–client relationship.

Chapter 9
Fill in the Blank
1. Connect; stimulus
2. Automatic relief behaviors
3. Specific phobia
4. Embarrassment
5. Obsessions
6. Rapid onset

Matching
1. **F**
2. **G**
3. **E**
4. **H**
5. **D**
6. **C**
7. **B**
8. **A**

Multiple Choice
1. **Correct Answer: C,** Reassurance and calm relays a sense of security to client in panic. A: Does not provide the initial reassurance. B: Client in panic is unable to listen to any explanation. D: Touching or approaching can pose additional threat or invade personal space.

2. **Correct Answer: D,** Linking the behavior to a particular situation can help client develop an awareness of feelings that precede anxiety attacks. A: False reassurance that minimizes client's feelings. B: Nurse should remain with client until symptoms abate. C: Every effort should be made to access client feelings behind the anxiety.

3. **Correct Answer: B,** Feelings of suffocation are triggered by sympathetic nervous system that usually accompany a state of panic. A, C: Not typically displayed in panic state. D: Person in panic attack cannot think logically.

4. **Correct Answer: D,** Anticipatory anxiety comes well in advance of a particular situation leading to thoughts of dread and actions to avoid the situation. B, C, D: Do not describe the irrational fear posed by a specific phobic situation.

5. **Correct Answer: D,** With the person experiencing excessive anxiety, it is important to initially take steps to lower the anxiety level. A: Is not established immediately. B: Not an initial outcome. C: Not an initial outcome.

6. **Correct Answer: C,** Demonstrates progress of client in coping with fear of being in public place. A: Relates to person with social phobia. B: Does not relate to agoraphobia. D: Assessment of client with OCD.

7. **Correct Answer: D,** Recognizes client need to perform rituals to deal with acute anxiety created by the obsessive thoughts. B: Inappropriate and punitive. C: Conforming to a schedule would lead to extreme anxiety for the client.

8. **Correct Answer: A,** Smoking decreases the sedative and antianxiety effects of benzodiazepine agents. B, C, D: No additional health teaching indicated.

9. **Correct Answer: C,** Anxiolytic agents are contraindicated during pregnancy and lactation. The client is asking for medication so the fact she is breast-feeding should be reported. A, B, D: Are all common symptoms of panic attack.

10. **Correct Answer: B,** Anxiolytic medications should not be combined with alcohol or other CNS depressants. A: The most common side effect is drowsiness which tends to improve as adjustment to drug occurs. C: Clients may experience some lag time before onset of therapy and reduction of symptoms. D: Most anxiolytics are prescribed for short time frames related to a potential for abuse.

Chapter 10
Fill in the Blank
1. Four
2. Cyclothymic
3. Dysthymia
4. Persecution
5. Lithium carbonate
6. 3
7. Random

Matching
1. **J**
2. **F**
3. **D**
4. **G**
5. **A**
6. **B**
7. **H**
8. **I**
9. **E**
10. **C**

Multiple Choice
1. **Correct Answer: C,** It is important to provide nutrition for the increased energy level when the client is unable to sit long enough to eat. A: Client in manic state will go for long periods without eating if no intervention is exerted. B: Does not address the problem created by the continuous activity. D: Client is not amenable to teaching while in manic state.

2. **Correct Answer: A,** Client is displaying excessive happiness or elation and laughing which would be appropriate response to the euphoric mood. B: Client with dysthymia does not exhibit manic symptoms. C: Does not describe a manic presentation. D: Person with a flat affect would not be laughing.

3. **Correct Answer: C,** Shows acceptance and genuine concern for the person—shows individual worth. A: Implies disapproval and

punishment for behavior of the client. B: Allowing continuance of delusional thought processes is nontherapeutic. D: Reprimanding is inappropriate—behavior will improve symptomatic treatment is effective.

4. **Correct Answer: B,** Needs to provide structured activities that offer opportunity for positive and encouraging experiences. A: Does not offer a structured approach for stimulation. C: Supports the client's feeling of worthlessness and withdrawal. D: May be too demanding for client or chance for regress.

5. **Correct Answer: C,** Therapeutic lithium serum levels are 0.6 to 1.2 mEq/L. Giving additional doses could push levels to a toxic level. A: Not indicated. B: Level indicates a reduction is needed rather than increase. D: Medication dosage adjustment may be all that is needed to maintain therapeutic response.

6. **Correct Answer: D,** Photosensitivity is a side effect of tricyclic antidepressant drug agents. A: Stimulants would counteract the effect of an antidepressant medication. B: Medication must be tapered and should not be discontinued unless supervised by the physician. C: Therapeutic levels of the chemical neurotransmitters must be maintained in order for effective response of the drug.

7. **Correct Answer: B,** These contain tyramine and should be avoided when taking an MAOI. A, C, D: No interactions with these foods.

8. **Correct Answer: A,** Anhedonia is a lack of pleasure in things the individual previously enjoyed. B: Anergia relates to a decrease in energy level. C: Euphoria is an excessive feeling of happiness. D: Negativism is a learned sense of helplessness or ongoing feeling that something considered essential for happiness is missing from their life.

9. **Correct Answer: D,** Validating the client's feelings of worthlessness and hopelessness begins to establish a trusting relationship with the client. A: Inappropriate questioning and nontherapeutic. B: Reassuring cliché that closes the interaction to further response. C: More therapeutic to access the client's feelings than reasoning behind the words.

10. **Correct Answer: B,** Client in state of depression may need assistance with hygiene, elimination, and nutrition needs. A, C, D: These will be addressed as treatment progresses.

Chapter 11
Fill in the Blank
1. Anticholinergic; extrapyramidal
2. AIMS Assessment Scale
3. Illusions
4. Water intoxication
5. Grandeur
6. Blunted or flat

Matching
1. **F**
2. **G**
3. **E**
4. **B**
5. **D**
6. **C**
7. **A**

Multiple Choice
1. **Correct Answer: B,** Having delusions of persecution. Client believes others are telling him to harm himself. A: Hallucinations are perceptual disturbances rather than disorganized thinking. C: Would indicate belief that external thoughts are being tranferred into one's mind. D: Loose associations are concepts that are unrelated to one another.

2. **Correct Answer: D,** Decrease in amount or speed with which a person talks. Poverty of speech indicates a decreasing quality of speaking in which the person may not answer questions or stop in the middle of thoughts. A: This would be described as word salad. B: Rhyming is referred to as clang associations. C: Describes thought insertion.

3. **Correct Answer: A,** "I know seeing the elf is frustrating to you, but no one else sees it." Acknowledges the feelings produced by the perceptual alteration, while reinforcing reality of it as nonexistent to others. B: Encourages the client to continue the perceptual alteration. C and D: Belittles the discomfort the client is feeling in response to distortion of reality.

4. **Correct Answer: A,** Signs of extrapyramidal side effects to the drug. Protrusion of the tongue and pill-rolling of the fingers are both late-appearing and irreversible movements indicating the extrapyramidal side effect of tardive dyskinesia. B: Tardive dyskinesia is common after long-term use but is not a normal response. C: These are definitely related to the medication and not part of the illness. D: Indication that reduced, not increased, dosage is needed or medication to counteract these effects.

5. **Correct Answer: C,** "I need to take the medication when I eat so it doesn't upset my stomach." Risperidone can cause the adverse effect of photosensitivity. The client should be advised to wear sunscreen and protective clothing to avoid any negative effect. A: Drug should be taken with food to avoid gastric irritation. B: Medication can actually take several days to weeks to achieve full benefit. D: Orthostatic hypotention can occur as a side effect of this drug.

6. **Correct Answer: D,** Protruding tongue movements. The drug Cogentin is an anticholinergic drug for counteracting the extrapyramidal side effects of tardive dyskinesia as a result on antipsychotic drugs. Protruding tongue movements would indicate symptoms of tardive dyskinesia. A: Antipsychotic agent should diminish the delusional thinking. B: Not an indication for Cogentin. C: These would be expected negative symptoms of schizophrenia.

7. **Correct Answer: C,** Having auditory hallucinations. Perceptual disturbances appear early in the disease and are considered positive symptoms. A, B, and D: All develop slowly over time and are reflected in person's inability to deal with the effect of the illness on their life.

8. **Correct Answer: B,** Offering sugar-free hard candy or frequent liquids. Dry mouth is one of the anticholinergic side effects of the antipsychotic agents. A: This is an intervention for clients taking lithium carbonate. C: Frequent oral hygiene is recommended to help moisten mouth. D: Unrelated to these drug agents.

9. **Correct Answer: D,** Client frequently misinterprets social and environmental stimuli. Clients with paranoia often misinterpret things and sounds in the environment as endangering them and will act in repsonse. A: Most clients with paranoia are very alert to environmental changes. B: Clients with schizophrenia have very little insight into the illogical nature of their symptoms. C: Recognition of the distortions in thinking is lacking in most cases of schizophrenia.

10. **Correct Answer: A,** Matter-of-factly reinforce the need to take the medication. A firm matter-of-fact approach reassures the client of reality and the need for medication to treat the illness. B and C: Reinforce the distorted thinking and paranoid delusion. D: Delay will cause an increase in symptoms.

Chapter 12
Fill in the Blank
1. Consistent; stable
2. Ambivalent
3. No-win
4. Entitlement
5. Self-mutilation
6. Antisocial

Matching
1. **F**
2. **E**
3. **I**
4. **G**
5. **A**
6. **D**
7. **H**
8. **B**
9. **C**

Multiple Choice
1. **Correct Answer: B,** Self-injury is an outward focus of control over inner pain and a chronic sense of emptiness and self-hate. A: Arrogance is not typical in the self-mutilator. C: Suspicion is more common in paranoid disorder. D: Not a component of self-mutilation.
2. **Correct Answer: D,** With little insight into their behavior, those with personality disorders need limits with consequences that require taking responsibility for the behavior. A: Puts client on the defensive and invokes negative response. B: Behavior modification is more effective in these disorders. C: This should be used only in the event the client poses an actual threat to self or others.
3. **Correct Answer: B,** The individual tends to be self-indulgent, arrogant, and demanding. Treatment is ineffective because of the person's denial or inability to identify the problem in their inflexible and maladaptive behavior. A: Most persons with these disorders are unable to identify the problem. C: Most are oblivious to the problem with change doubtful. D: They tend to be unaware of how their behavior is seen by others.
4. **Correct Answer: B,** Persons who become involved in repeated abusive or destructive relationships are actually reinforcing and feeding a type of self-hate and redirected self-injury. A: Characteristic of those who are secluded with emotional indifference toward social relationships. C: Would be seen as odd behavior but not self-destructive. D: Exactly the opposite—person sees him or herself as superior.
5. **Correct Answer: C,** Demonstrates a grandiose sense of self-importance and claim that others owe him because of this superiority. A: Blaming others for one's own problem. B: Seeing the world in "all or none" terms. D: Conflicting views of a situation.
6. **Correct Answer: D,** The client's behavior and interactions with others will indicate whether the individual has recognized the problem and its impact on subsequent behavior. A, B, C: Client can do all of these and cannot identify the problem in their own behavior.
7. **Correct Answer: C,** Those with antisocial personality disorder exhibit a persistent pattern of disregard and infringement on the rights of others by their defiance of moral law and order in a society. A: This describes self-mutilation. B: Related to insecurity and inability to see behavior as cause of failure. D: More common to obsessive-compulsive personality disorder.
8. **Correct Answer: B,** The person with a histrionic personality displays a pattern of egocentric and excessive emotion in a demanding manner to gain personal attention, and is uncomfortable in situations where center-stage is not afforded them. A, C, D: Do not exhibit this type of behavior.
9. **Correct Answer: D,** Narcissistic personality disorder indicates a continued need for self-indulgent attention and admiration with little regard for the feelings of others. A: Describes a dependent personality. B: Descriptive of an obsessive-compulsive personality. C: Commonly seen in schizotypal personality disorder.
10. **Correct Answer: A,** All personality disorders incorporate deeply ingrained, persistent, inflexible, and maladaptive patterns of behavior that are in conflict with a cultural norm. B, C, D: All descriptive of individual personality disorders.

Chapter 13
Fill in the Blank
1. Somatization
2. Secondary gain
3. Primary gain
4. "La belle"
5. Physician shopping

Matching
1. **E**
2. **D**
3. **A**
4. **B**
5. **C**

Multiple Choice
1. **Correct Answer: C,** Person with illness anxiety disorder has excessive fear they have a serious illness despite medical testing and reassurance the disease does not exist. A, B, D: Common complaints in somatization disorder.
2. **Correct Answer: B,** Focus on the symptoms provides attention and concern for the client by physicians and family. The primary gain is achieved as the anxiety is relieved by diverting the focus to a physical problem. A: Characteristic of somatoform disorders is there is no medical evidence to support the symptoms. C: Client is usually unaware of the psychological basis for the symptoms. D: In conversion disorder there is an attitude of indifference or little concern over the implication of the symptoms.
3. **Correct Answer: A,** Helps the client to focus on using energy for positive outcomes rather than the anxiety-driven somatic complaints. B: The focus should be on reducing the need for the perceived dependency which provides secondary gain. C: Since the client is unaware of the underlying psychological conflict, confrontation should be avoided. D: Clients are encouraged to express feelings of anxiety and recent emotional events.
4. **Correct Answer: D,** A common symptom of somatoform pain disorder is an unchanging description of the location and characteristics of the pain. A: Although repeated visits are common, there is no pattern of time lapse between them. B: Impairment is more likely to increase in interference with daily activity. C: Analgesia use tends to increase adding to the potential for substance dependence.
5. **Correct Answer: C,** As client becomes aware of relationship of feelings and symptoms, the focus should be on reducing the perceived loss of function toward performance of self-care needs independently and willingly. A, B, D: All encourage the continuation of the perceived dependency that feeds a secondary gain of attention while avoiding the underlying psychological issues.

6. **Correct Answer: C,** The somatic symptoms provide a psychological or primary gain as the anxiety is relieved and focus is diverted to the physical problem. A: The client using somatization is unaware of the psychological factors. D: In some instances, the person may acknowledge the disease does not exist, but the fear and distress over the symptoms continues. B: Using somatization relieves but does not effectively resolve the psychological discomfort.

7. **Correct Answer: B,** Social isolation and physical inactivity along with the continued perceived pain pose a significant risk for symptoms of depression and contemplated suicide. A: Sleep disturbances are common with chronic pain and may be a contributing factor. C: This occurs in conversion disorder where little concern is shown over the symptoms. D: The person with chronic pain is more likely to receive increased attention as primary and secondary gain is achieved.

8. **Correct Answer: A,** Inadvertent movement of the limb when attention is directed away can be a clue to the conversion nature of the symptoms. B: Concern of a spouse over his wife is not unusual. C: Functional use of unaffected limb expected. D: Visits unrelated to current complaint not at issue.

Chapter 14
Fill in the Blank
1. Dissociation
2. Repressed
3. Host
4. Switching
5. Depersonalization

Matching
1. D
2. A
3. E
4. B
5. C

Multiple Choice
1. **Correct Answer: C,** The person with dissociative fugue has an inability to recall some or all of his or her past identity and may be accompanied by a sudden and unexpected travel away from home where a new identity may be assumed. A: Feeling of detachment while illogical nature of the feelings is recognized. B: Intentional dissociation to avoid a legal, financial, or unwanted personal situation. C: Feeling of being detached from mental thoughts of body but disorientation does not occur.

2. **Correct Answer: B,** Focus on the primary personality with reassurance for positive outcome. A: Places focus on dissociated identity. C: Avoidance. D: Response should emphasize a trusting environment.

3. **Correct Answer: A,** Provides increased perception and insight into present symptoms and problems. B, C: Outcomes for dissociative identity disorder. D: Would not be an outcome for problem identified.

4. **Correct Answer: C,** Flooding the client with details of past traumatic events may cause the client to regress further into the dissociative state that is serving as protection from the emotional pain. A, B: Focus on current rather than underlying traumatic events. D: Introducing details on the first session will likely be too overwhelming for the client and cause further regression.

5. **Correct Answer: C,** Clarification of events the client is describing to the nurse. A: There is no indication from the client to convey a

message of anger. B: Minimizes the difficulty the client has in relating traumatizing events. D: Demeaning statement that will likely block communication efforts.

6. **Correct Answer: B,** Although she can remember portions of her life, the client does not remember the painful details of her child who died. A, B, D: All describe other types of amnesia.

7. **Correct Answer: D,** Host or primary personality usually is submissive, depressed, and the one that seeks treatment. A, B: True of alternate personality states that assume persona to deal with feelings and emotions that are overwhelming to the primary personality. C: Host personality is usually unaware of the other personality states.

8. **Correct Answer: B,** Clients with depersonalization disorder have persistent and repetitious feelings of being detached from their thoughts or body without the presence of disorientation. A, C, D: Descriptive of other dissociative disorders.

Chapter 15
Fill in the Blank
1. Substance
2. Enables
3. Addiction
4. Detoxification
5. Alcohol-induced delirium
6. Wernicke–Korsakoff syndrome

Matching
1. I
2. A
3. J
4. G
5. D
6. F
7. E
8. C
9. H
10. B

Multiple Choice
1. **Correct Answer: D,** It is important for the nurse to notify the physician of changes in vital signs that could indicate complications during withdrawal. A: Fluids are not increased during withdrawal—the client has been usually been drinking for a period of time. B: Fall precautions are not indicated with the symptoms identified in the question. C: Irrelevant to the situation.

2. **Correct Answer: A,** Blood alcohol level, slurred speech, and staggering gait are symptoms of alcohol intoxication. B, C, D: Symptoms listed do not define any of these situations.

3. **Correct Answer: A,** Client is denying responsibility for his actions by saying "I can handle it," and he is not an alcoholic, despite his drinking pattern. B: Blame to another is not indicated in these statements by the client. C: Client is not transferring feelings to another person. D: Client is not substituting false reasoning for his behavior.

4. **Correct Answer: D,** Acknowledges and demonstrates respect for the client as a person with a problem who needs treatment. A: Belittles the person as a problem. B: Puts client on the defensive—blocks communication. C: Categorizes the client and blocks further therapeutic communication.

5. **Correct Answer: B,** Agreeing accepts her excuses for the behavior and does not help her to take responsibility for her actions and

own problem. A, C, D: Each offers a support for assisting her in a therapeutic outcome.

6. **Correct Answer: D,** Other respiratory symptoms and watery eyes are symptoms of recent drug inhalation. A, B, C: Indicate symptoms of other types of drug intoxication.
7. **Correct Answer: C,** Chronic alcohol users are usually deficient in these vitamins. A: Methadone is not used for alcohol treatment. B: Stress management not a priority at this point in treatment. D: Suicide interventions not indicated at this time.
8. **Correct Answer: B,** Client must first acknowledge he has a problem in order to be committed toward abstinence. A, C, D: All may be necessary once he has taken the initial step toward recovery.
9. **Correct Answer: C,** Hallucinogenic drugs alter the perception causing distortions of reality, such as distance or height. A, B, D: Symptoms would not be defined in these terms.
10. **Correct Answer: A,** Cannabis or marijuana is detectable in a urine sample for a longer period of time than other drugs. B: Cannot be detected after a short period of time. C: Determined by blood levels, not urine samples. D: Drug not detected by this method.

Chapter 16
Fill in the Blank
1. Perception
2. Self-control; failure
3. Controlling or overprotective
4. Purging
5. Weight
6. 30 minutes

Matching
1. **C**
2. **E**
3. **B**
4. **A**
5. **D**

Multiple Choice
1. **Correct Answer: C,** Extreme weight loss from self-imposed restricted food and nutrient intake. Extreme weight loss from self-imposed restricted food and nutrient intake is characteristic of anorexia. A, D: Weight gain and overeating are not seen in the pattern of anorexia. B: Usually talks about and prepares food for others but does not consume any.
2. **Correct Answer: A,** Provide opportunities for independent decision making. Fosters a sense of control for the client. B: Further depletes the client's sense of value and self-worth. C: A firm supportive approach should be used rather than one of sympathy which enables behaviors to continue. D: Discussions that focus on food are avoided.
3. **Correct Answer: B,** Antidepressant. Antidepressant medications combined with psychotherapy have been used successfully to combat feelings of worthlessness. A, C, and D: Medications not used in treating the eating disorders.
4. **Correct Answer: C,** "Tell me about the last time you did binge eating and what you did afterward." Open-ended statement to encourage communication and acquire information. A: Puts client on defensive and minimizes her underlying psychological problem and feelings. B: Demeaning and critical of the client. D: Does not show understanding of the underlying issues in eating disorder.
5. **Correct Answer: A,** Purging behavior. Electrolyte imbalance, teeth enamel erosion, and calluses of the fingers and hands are

common signs of purging behaviors. B, C, and D: Symptoms in question not specific to these aspects of the disorder.
6. **Correct Answer: C,** Frequent mirror-viewing and measuring of body parts. Viewing oneself in the mirror and measuring of body parts are an attempt to reinforce their perceived self-image which is dependent on body shape and size.
7. **Correct Answer: B,** Anxiety, related to feelings of hopelessness and lack of control. Anxiety is demonstrated in self-imposed guilt and excessive self-criticism for failure to meet their unrealistic self-standards and perceived lack of control. A: Fluid volume deficit, rather than excess results from purging behaviors. C: Clients with eating disorders tend to deny the medical complications and potential loss of health related to their condition. D: Body image disturbance and powerlessness better address the lack of insight and irrational thinking problems related to these disorders.

Chapter 17
Fill in the Blank
1. Sexual dysfunction
2. Diabetes mellitus
3. Inhibition to arousal
4. Personality
5. Thinking

Matching
1. **E**
2. **G**
3. **D**
4. **A**
5. **B**
6. **C**
7. **F**

Multiple Choice
1. **Correct Answer: C,** "I know it must be difficult for you to talk with a stranger about such a private matter. We can discuss it at a later time." The nurse would use an empathetic approach that acknowledges the client's right to choose when to discuss sexual functioning, but also offers to listen when the client is ready to do so. A: Blocks further communication with the client on any problem. B: Sympathetic response that agrees with the client and closes communication. D: Attempts to force client to talk about an uncomfortable subject.
2. **Correct answer: B,** "Tell me more about what happens when you have sexual intercourse." Open-ended statement that encourages the client to continue talking about the problem. A: Client's statement does not mention abuse making response inappropriate. C: Delaying when client is ready to talk discourages communication. D: Statement makes judgmental assumption.
3. **Correct answer: A,** Using an empathetic and nonjudgmental approach. Nurse would appropriately use an empathetic approach that acknowledges the client has a substance problem but does not judge the client based on his sexual paraphilia. B: It is inappropriate to discuss one client with another. C: Judgmental action not warranted by behavior at this time. D: Client is being admitted for treatment of polysubstance abuse.
4. **Correct Answer: D,** Consents to expose the errors in his thinking. Acknowledgment of his problem with voluntary consent to treatment poses the best chance for success. A: Imposed consequence of his actions. B: Does not indicate readiness to accept treatment. C: Admitting the sexual pedophilia does not indicate willingness to alter his behavior.

5. **Correct Answer: C,** Fear and withdrawal when touched. Victim of sexual abuse is usually very guarded with any form of physical assessment. A: Openness and willingness to share about the experience is unlikely. B: It is unlikely that anger would be displayed at this point in the child's response to abuse. D: The child who has been abused will be unlikely to trust anyone at this point.

6. **Correct Answer: A,** "I really want to respond to my husband, but the feeling just isn't there." Client statement indicates a possible sexual desire or arousal disorder related to effects of antidepressant medication. Most clients with depression experience some decrease in libido. B, C, and D: Usual symptoms of a depressive state.

Chapter 18
Fill in the Blank
1. Genetics
2. Dyslexia
3. Sixth grade
4. Stuttering
5. Attention
6. Echopraxia

Matching
1. **F**
2. **E**
3. **D**
4. **A**
5. **B**
6. **G**
7. **I**
8. **H**
9. **C**

Multiple Choice
1. **Correct Answer: C,** Feeling and content response invites the mother to continue expressing her feelings without judgment or comment. A: Judgmental question placing mother on the defense about her comments. B: Seemingly infers child is responsible for the problem. D: Takes focus off the child.

2. **Correct Answer: B,** The child with dyslexia has difficulty in the reading and spelling domains of cognitive skills. A, C, D: These disorders do not affect the cognitive areas of reading and writing.

3. **Correct Answer: B,** The child with separation anxiety experiences excessive anxiety related to separation from home or attachment figures. A, C, D: Not applicable to the symptoms in the question.

4. **Correct Answer: A,** Client's history shows a pattern of violent and aggressive behaviors that have resulted in or threatened harm to other people. The potential for serious injury to other clients or personnel would receive a priority. B, C, D: All may be applicable at some point in the treatment plan.

5. **Correct Answer: D,** Giving away prized possessions is a warning sign for suicide risk. A, B, C: Not indicative of suicidal behavior.

6. **Correct Answer: A,** The child with expressive language disorder has difficulty understanding words and sentences or associating and organizing incoming information. This would make it difficult for the child to follow rules of a game. B: More common in autistic disorder. C: Indicative of separation anxiety disorder. D: Symptom of behavioral disorder.

7. **Correct Answer: C,** Repetitive or prolonged sounds separated by pauses describes a stuttering disorder. A: Structural area of language. B: Sudden tic-like obscene gesture. D: Repetitive movements

8. **Correct Answer: C,** Child with IQ of 54 could work at simple jobs and have independent supervised living. A: Institutional care not indicated at this intelligence level. B: Would not be capable of independent living or providing own income. D: Would function at higher level than activities of daily living only.

9. **Correct Answer: A,** Turning up the volume indicates child may have a hearing problem that would contribute to the learning disorder. B, C, D: Irrelevant in evaluating for learning disorder.

10. **Correct Answer: B,** Child with oppositional-defiant disorder has a repetitive pattern of negative, defiant, disobedient, and hostile behavior toward authority figures. A, C, D: Not relevant to the behavior described.

Chapter 19
Fill in the Blank
1. Delirium; dementia; amnestic disorders
2. Consciousness; short
3. Metabolize and excrete the drug
4. Irreversible; progressive
5. Pneumonia; urinary tract infections; infected decubitus ulcers
6. Catastrophic events

Matching
1. **D**
2. **B**
3. **E**
4. **F**
5. **A**
6. **H**
7. **G**
8. **C**

Multiple Choice
1. **Correct Answer: C,** Inability to recognize himself in the mirror is symptomatic of agnosia, or loss of comprehensive ability to recognize objects or individuals. A, B, and D: Do not apply to this example of loss.

2. **Correct Answer: A,** Because of the inability to recognize himself in the mirror, he believes someone else is in the bathroom. This triggers anxiety that there is something wrong and retreat to another location to eliminate is likely. B: He seemingly knows he needs to eliminate in the bathroom. C and D: Not indicated by his behavior.

3. **Correct Answer: C,** The symptoms can usually be reversed once the cause is determined. A, B, and D: Do not apply to course of delirium.

4. **Correct Answer: B,** Filling in the gaps when memory falters is common in the early stages of dementia. A, C, and D: Do not describe the example in the question.

5. **Correct Answer: D,** Repeating words or sentences correctly describes echolalia. A: Babbling would be unintelligible sounds. B: Repetition of one word. C: Repeating one syllable.

6. **Correct Answer: B,** Clients with AD may misinterpret the nurse's action, and trying again later will usually allow the client to forget the issue. A: Client unable to encode and comprehend the explanation. C: Client is not cognitively able to refuse the medication. D: Only if repeated efforts to give the medication are unsuccessful.

7. **Correct Answer: C,** Client is unable to encode and interpret the spoken verbal message. Cueing will assist the client to follow through with the requested action. A: Saying the words another

way adds another challenge. B: Client unable to comprehend or reason. C: It would be unsafe for client to continue ambulating with loose shoestrings.

8. **Correct Answer: A,** Placing her on a lower bed would provide the safest means of avoiding a fall. B: Bedside commode may not be understood as appropriate by the client and would add clutter to the environment. C: The client will attempt to get out, over, or through side rails and poses a safety hazard. D: A sedative increases the likelihood of the client falling and poses a safety threat.

9. **Correct Answer: B,** Client is most likely overwhelmed and confused by the variety of items on the tray. Reduce choices by setting one item or bowl of food in front of the client at a time.

A: Keeping a regular schedule adds structure and reduces confusion about mealtime and sleep–wake cycles. C: Actions demonstrate confusion, not lack of appetite. D: Client most likely unable to interpret verbal command.

10. **Correct Answer: D,** The person with AD loses the ability to recognize the present and will remember grown children as youngsters, and often will think grandkids are their own children. Helping family members to understand this and encouraging reminisce about the past will help the client with the confusion. A: Arguing or correcting her may induce negative behavior in response. B: Pictures from the past are a better approach for reminiscence since current is not understood. C: Asking for information reminds client of their losses and feelings of loss.

Glossary

A

acceptance: ability to see the client as a person with worth and dignity who is not judged or labeled by the standards of another.

acceptance: final stage of grief when a person begins to experience peace and allows life to provide new experiences and relationships.

accommodation: process of responding to cognitively unbalancing information about the environment by modifying relevant schemas, thereby adapting the schemas to fit the new information and reestablishing cognitive balance.

acetylcholine: neurotransmitter found in various organs and tissues of the body, thought to play an important role in the transmission of nerve impulses at synapses and myoneural junctions. It is quickly destroyed by an enzyme, cholinesterase.

active listening: giving critical attention to verbal comments and observing nonverbal behaviors for content and inconsistencies while attempting to understand the client's view of a situation.

adaptation: manner in which individuals manage their anxiety.

adaptive coping: rational and productive way of resolving a problem to reduce anxiety.

addiction: physiological and psychological dependence upon alcohol or certain drugs of abuse noted for their effects on the central nervous system that is characterized by withdrawal symptoms when the substance is discontinued.

affect: describes facial expression that is displayed in association with the mood.

ageism: discrimination against aged persons.

aggression: behavior that may result in both physical and psychological harm to oneself or another verbally or nonverbally.

aging: manifestations of changes that advance in a continuous and progressive manner during the adult years.

agnosia: loss of comprehension of auditory, visual, or other sensations although the sensory sphere is intact.

agoraphobia: fear of being in a place from which escape might be difficult or embarrassing.

akathisia: motor restlessness, inability to sit still.

alogia: decrease in amount or speed of speech where person may not answer questions or stop talking in the middle of a thought (see also, poverty of speech).

Alzheimer's disease (AD): chronic, organic mental disorder or dementia due to atrophy of frontal and occipital lobes that involves a progressive, irreversible loss of memory, deterioration of intellectual functions, apathy, speech and gait disturbances, and disorientation.

American's with Disabilities Act (ADA): first federal civil rights law to prohibit discrimination against individuals with mental and physical disabilities.

amnesia: loss of memory applied to episodes during which individuals forget their identity, though they conduct themselves properly and following which no memory of the period exists.

anal stage: Freudian stage from 2 to 4 years during which pleasure is achieved from an awareness and control of urination and defecation.

anergia: marked decrease in energy level that may slow a person to a dependency on others for even basic needs.

anger: natural, adaptive emotion triggered in response to threats, insulting situations, or anything that seriously hampers the intended actions of an individual.

anhedonia: lack of interest in previously enjoyed activities.

anomia: inability to remember the names of objects.

anorexia nervosa: disorder characterized by extreme concern with body weight, an intense fear of becoming fat, and maintenance of body weight below expected levels for height and age. Individuals often perceive themselves as heavier than they are, or place unrealistic value on body weight and shape.

antianxiety agents (anxiolytics): drug agent used to counteract or diminish anxiety.

anticipatory anxiety: anxiety that is experienced for some time prior to an event or happening.

anticipatory grief: grief experienced before the impending death of a loved one.

antidepressants: central nervous system depressant that acts to prevent, cure, or alleviate mental depression.

antimanic: mood-stabilizing agent used to treat manic episodes associated with bipolar disorder or to diminish future episodes.

antipsychotic agents: drug agents, also referred to as neuroleptics, that are used to treat serious mental illness such as bipolar affective disorder, depressive and drug-induced psychosis, schizophrenia, and autism. They may be used in some cases of movement disorders (Tourette's syndrome) and nausea or intractable hiccups.

anxiety: built-in part of our basic instinct to respond in the event we are confronted with a threat to our well-being.

anxiolytic: drug agent used to counteract or diminish anxiety.

aphasia: absence or impairment of the ability to communicate through speech, writing, or signs, due to dysfunction of brain centers.

apraxia: inability to perform purposeful movements although there is no sensory or motor impairment.

assessment: first step of the nursing process in which subjective and objective data are collected.

assimilation: absorption of newly perceived information into the existing subjective conscious schema structure.

automatic relief behaviors: subtle unconscious behaviors that are aimed at relieving anxiety.

avolition: lack of motivation.

B

bargaining: step in grief process in which deals with God are attempted as a way to prolong the inevitable.

batterer: abusive partner who inflicts emotional and physical harm to another individual.

behavioral therapy: emphasizes the principles of learning with positive or negative reinforcement and observational modeling to incur behavioral change.

behaviorism: theory of conduct that regards normal and abnormal behaviors as the result of conditioned reflexes separate from the concept of will or choice.

bereavement: expected reactions of grief and sadness after learning of the loss of a loved one.

binge eating: recurrent eating of an amount in excess of 1,000 calories in a short period of time with a lack of control over eating during the episode.

biofeedback: training program designed to develop one's ability to control the autonomic or involuntary nervous system using monitoring devices, followed by an attempt by the individual to reproduce the conditions that caused the desired change.

biomedical therapy: application of biological and natural sciences to the study of medicine.

bipolar disorder: brain dysfunction that causes abnormal and erratic shifts in mood, energy, and functional ability.

blackout: sudden loss of consciousness; an episode of forgetting all or part of what occurred during or following a period of alcohol intake.

blocking: unconscious block that results in loss of thought process and person stops speaking.

bulimia nervosa: eating disorder characterized by periods of significant overeating (binge eating) and inappropriate methods of compensating for the overeating to prevent weight gain such as self-induced vomiting, use of laxatives or diuretics, and excessive exercise.

bullying: psychological harassment or physical confrontation used repeatedly to intentionally bring harm or humiliation to one seen as weak or different.

burnout: condition of mental, physical, and emotional exhaustion with a reduced sense of personal accomplishment and apathy toward one's work.

C

catastrophic events: overwhelming state of anxiety or panic experienced by a demented individual in response to any type of new situation related to an inability to process environmental observations accurately.

catalepsy: extreme form of posturing for extended periods of time.

catatonic behaviors: involve a decreased reaction to environmental surroundings.

central traits: general prominent features most often descriptive of a person, some of which are seen in behaviors.

chemical restraint: use of a drug to control behavior.

chronic sorrow: prolonged and intensified feelings of loss that render life as meaningless and a mere existence.

circumstantiality: cannot be selective when speaking and describes in lengthy, great detail.

clang associations: words strung together in rhyming phrases that have no connected meaning.

Client Bill of Rights: declared law by the Mental Health Systems Act passed in 1980, entitles all clients to receive care based on a current and individualized treatment plan with a description of services that are available and those offered upon discharge.

clinical psychologist: mental health professional who administers and interprets psychological testing used in the diagnostic process, and provides various types of therapy to assist in resolution of mental health issues.

codependent: tendency to feel a responsibility for drug user's problem while internalizing a form of guilt for the behavior of that person.

cognitive therapy: based on the cognitive model of how individuals respond in stressful situations to their subjective perception of the event. Therapy strives to assist the individual to reduce anxiety responses by altering the cognitive distortions.

compensatory methods: inappropriate and risky methods of preventing weight gain such as purging or induced vomiting and the use of laxatives, diuretics, or enemas.

compulsion: uncontrolled impulse to perform an action or ritual repeatedly to decrease anxiety.

concrete mental operations: stage of cognitive development in Piaget's theory of development, in which the individual engages in mental manipulations of internal images of tangible objects.

confabulation: behavioral reaction to memory loss in which the person fills in memory gaps with inappropriate words.

confidentiality: client's right to prevent written or verbal communications from being disclosed to outside parties without authorization.

conscious: being aware and having perception of the environment; having the ability to filter that information through the mind with the awareness of doing so.

continuous amnesia: encompasses a period up to and including the present that is lost from conscious recollection.

contracting: a behavioral technique in which the client and therapist draw up a contract to which both parties are obligated. The contract requires the client to demonstrate specific behaviors that are included in the therapy. In exchange, the therapist will give certain rewards that the client has requested.

conventional grief: feelings of sadness expected or experienced after a loss.

conventional level: stage in Kohlberg's theory of moral development in which decisions are based on the demands and pressures of society and the expectations of peers.

conversion disorder: symptoms are exhibited that indicate a sensory or neurological impairment that is not supported by results of diagnostic testing.

copropraxia: sudden tic-like obscene gesture.

craving: strong inner drive to use a substance.

cued: panic attack in which an identified trigger can be associated with the event.

cultural identity: binding force of a unique common heritage including beliefs, norms, values, and behaviors between members of a cultural group.

D

defense mechanism: methods for protecting the ego from anxiety associated with conflicting urges and restrictions of the id and superego.

delirium: state of mental confusion and excitement that happens in a short period of time and is characterized by disorientation for time and place, usually with illusions and hallucinations.

delirium tremens: alcohol-induced delirium lasting from 72 to 80 hours that produced a state of profound confusion and delusions along with other withdrawal symptoms.

delusion: fixed, false belief without appropriate external stimuli that is inconsistent with reality and the person's own knowledge or experience.

delusion of reference: false belief that the behavior of others in the environment refers to oneself.

dementia: broad impairment of intellectual function that usually is progressive and that interferes with normal social and occupational activities.

denial: stage of grief process in which there is shock and disbelief that the event is occurring, allowing time for adjustment and development of coping strategies.

depersonalization disorder: marked by a persistent and repetitious feeling of being detached from one's mental thoughts or body without the presence of disorientation.

depression: persistent and prolonged mood of sadness that extends beyond 2 weeks duration.

derailment: vague, unfocused, illogical, gradual, or sudden change in thought process without thought blocking (see also loose associations).

derealization: perception the external environment is unreal or changing.

detoxification: first phase of dependency treatment lasting from 3 to 5 days that consists of immediate withdrawal from the physical and psychological effects of the drug.

developmental crisis: occurs at a predictable time period in an individual's life related to maturational stages and changes.

disorientation: inability to be cognizant of time, direction or location, and person.

dissociation: mental mechanism that allows our mind to separate certain memories from conscious awareness and repress them into the unconscious level.

dissociative amnesia: characterized by an inability to remember important personal information that is usually of a traumatic or stressful nature.

dissociative fugue: inability to recall some or all of a person's past or identity, accompanied by the sudden and unexpected travel of the person away from home or place of employment.

dissociative identity disorder: two or more distinct identities or personalities present in the same person that alternate in assuming control of the person's behavior.

distress: negative stress in response to a threat or challenge that exhausts and drains energy from the individual.

domestic violence: pattern of behavior that is used by the perpetrator or batterer to gain power and control over another person through fear and intimidation.

dopamine: catecholamine neurotransmitter; a precursor in the synthesis of norepinephrine important in understanding the pathology of schizophrenia and parkinsonism.

drug-induced parkinsonism: symptoms that mimic parkinsonism such as tremors, rigidity, akinesia, or absence of movement with diminished mental state.

dysfunctional grief: prolonged and intensified reaction or failure to complete the grieving process and cope successfully with a loss.

dyslexia: learning disorder in the reading domain.

dystonia: muscle rigidity that affects posture, gait, eye movements.

E

echolalia: involuntary parrot-like repetition of words spoken by others, often accompanied by twitching of muscles.

echopraxia: repetitive tic-like movements.

eclectic: selecting from various sources what seems to be the best.

ego: in Freudian theory, one of the three major divisions in the model of the psychic apparatus that possesses consciousness and memory, and serves to mediate between the id and the superego or conscience.

electra conflict: psychosexual stage that Freud describes as a time in which a girl begins to feel romantic feelings for her father but fears the wrath of her mother.

electroconvulsive therapy (ECT): biomedical treatment using low-voltage electric shock waves to the brain along with general anesthesia and muscle relaxants that is usually administered two to three times weekly for 6 to 12 treatments. ECT is reserved for severe cases of mental illness that have not responded to medication and other therapeutic interventions.

emotional abuse: words or nonverbal language that is used to criticize, demean, or humiliate and inflict psychological trauma on another person.

emotional numbing: expression of little or no emotion soon after an event as an attempt to prevent future mental pain.

empathy: awareness of what another person is saying and feeling with a perception of the situation from that person's perspective.

enabling: pattern of either consciously or unconsciously helping the maladaptive behavior of a drug abuser to continue.

encopresis: involuntary passage of feces in inappropriate places after age of voluntary control has been established.

entitlement: narcissistic claim of being superior and owed by others.

enuresis: involuntary passage of urine after age of voluntary control has been established.

equilibration: process of cognitive development in which a person seeks to balance between information and experiences encountered in the environment with existing modes of thought and schemas.

ethics: a set of principles or values that provides dignity and respect to clients by protecting them from unreasonable treatment.

euphoria: excessive feeling of happiness or elation.

eustress: positive and motivating stress shown by one's confidence in the ability to master a challenge or stressor.

evaluation: step of nursing process which determines the success of nursing interventions in meeting the criteria outlined in the expected outcomes.

exhibitionism: tendency to attract attention to oneself by any means; psychosexual disorder manifesting an abnormal impulse that causes one to expose the genitals to a member of the opposite sex.

expected outcomes: planning measurable and realistic outcomes that anticipate the improvement or stabilization of the problem identified in the nursing diagnosis.

external stressors: aspects of the environment that may be adverse to one's well-being.

extrapyramidal side effects: effects produced by antipsychotic drugs that block dopamine causing irritation of the pyramidal tracts of the central nervous system that coordinate involuntary movements.

F

factitious disorder: falsification of medical or psychological signs and symptoms without obvious external benefits.

fight-or-flight response: reaction to an immediate threat in which there is a surge of adrenalin into the bloodstream.

flight of ideas: rapid shift between topics that are unrelated to each other.

focusing: communication technique that helps client concentrate on a specific issue.

formal operations: stage of cognitive development in Piaget's theory in which the individual can engage in mental manipulation of abstract ideas or symbols that may not have a specific concrete basis.

free-floating anxiety: occurs when a person is unable to connect the anxiety to a stimulus.

frotteurism: recurrent intense sexual urges and fantasies involving touching and rubbing against a nonconsenting person, usually in crowded places where arrest is unlikely.

G

generalized amnesia: inability to recall important personal information usually of a traumatic or stressful nature that is too extensive to be explained by ordinary forgetfulness.

generalized anxiety: person experiences an increased level of anxiety and worry about various situations on most days over a period of at least 6 months.

genital stage: Freudian psychosexual stage that occurs as the child enters puberty and adolescence.

genuineness: attribute of realness and concern that fosters an honest and caring foundation for trust.

grandiosity: unrealistic or exaggerated sense of self-worth, importance, wealth, or ability.

grief: emotional process of coping with a loss.

group therapy: process of helping clients to develop an understanding of and insight into their feelings, behaviors, and roles in relationships through involvement and interaction with others who have similar problems.

H

hallucination: false sensory perceptions unrelated to actual external stimuli.

hierarchy: ordering or classification of anything in descending order of importance or value.

holistic: philosophy that individuals are complete organisms and function as complete units that cannot be reduced to the sum of their parts.

hostility: anger-based aggression or an intense feeling of animosity toward someone or something.

humanistic: theoretical view of the developing person as a whole that includes the physical, emotional, spiritual, intellectual, and social aspects of life.

humanistic therapy: nondirective approach that centers on helping the client to explore his or her own view of feelings and choices with a focus on current problems.

hypomania: state of mild or moderate mania that lasts for a period of at least 4 days.

hysteria: nervous disorder marked by ineffective emotional control.

I

id: the obscure, inaccessible division of the psyche that serves as a collection of instinctual drives continually striving for satisfaction in accordance.

ideas of reference: belief that some events have a special personal meaning.

illness anxiety disorder: condition in which there are increased body sensations with extreme anxiety about the possibility of an existing serious undiagnosed illness that cannot be supported by medical testing.

illusions: mental misperception of actual sensory stimuli.

informed consent: explanation of client rights and institutional policies that give the client, or those who may have legal guardianship for the client, the ability to accept treatment, or refuse any aspect of treatment.

inhalants: volatile substances such as gasoline and paint if used for the purpose of intoxication.

intellectual disability: significant limitations in both intellectual functioning and adaptive behavior.

internal stressors: physical strain such as chronic or terminal condition, or psychological issue such as worry that affect the body response.

interpersonal: concerning the relations and interactions between persons.

involuntary commitment: person is admitted to a psychiatric unit against his or her will by order of a court official.

L

la belle indifference: attitude demonstrating little anxiety or concern over the implications of their symptoms.

latency stage: psychosexual theory stage during middle childhood in which the sexual desires and feelings remain subdued.

level of differentiation: degree to which a person's intellect or emotions control his or her functioning.

lewy body disease: progressive disease causing dementia similar to AD in which round deposits of protein called Lewy bodies develop in nerve cells throughout the brain. Visual hallucinations and intermittent mental alertness are distinguishing symptoms.

localized amnesia: usually occurs within a few hours following the event or traumatic event.

logoclonia: repetitious, continuous, and excessive monosyllabic utterances.

loose associations: vague, unfocused, illogical collection of thoughts seen in psychosis (see also, derailment).

loss: actual or perceived change in the status of one's relationship to a valued object or person.

M

magical thinking: belief that thoughts, words, and actions can cause or prevent an occurrence by extraordinary means.

maladaptive coping: unsuccessful attempts to decrease anxiety without attempting to solve the problem allowing anxiety to continue.

malingered fugue: dissociation in person trying to avoid a legal, financial, or unwanted personal situation.

mannerisms: repetitive, goal-directed movements.

mania: frenzied unstable mood in which the person may be out of touch with reality.

manipulation: conscious or unconscious process by which one person attempts to influence another person in order to get his or her own needs or desires met.

mental health: state of well-being in which an individual realizes his or her own abilities, copes with normal stressors of life, works productively, and is able to make a contribution to society.

Mental Health Act of 1983: addressed the rights of people regarding admission to a psychiatric hospital, the right to refuse admission against their will, rights while in treatment, and those following discharge.

Mental Health Parity and Addiction Equity Act of 2008: requires group insurance plans to cover mental illnesses the same way as physical ones, including no more higher copays, deductibles, and limits on hospital stays.

mental illness: clinically significant behavioral or psychological syndrome or pattern that occurs in an individual and is associated with distress or dysfunction.

milieu: environment or setting.

monoamine oxidase inhibitor (MAOI): group of drugs that inhibit monoamine oxidase; effective in treating depression.

mood: emotion that is prolonged to the point that it colors a person's entire psychological thinking.

mood disorder: refers to a condition in which the person experiences a prolonged alteration in mood.

mood-stabilizing agents: used to treat manic episodes associated with bipolar disorder or to diminish future episodes.

Munchausen syndrome: deliberate falsification of an illness in another for attention of assuming the sick role.

N

narcissism: derived from the Greek, meaning "excessive love and attention given to one's own self-image"; person has continued need for lavish attention and admiration with little regard for the feeling of others.

necrophilia: abnormal concern or sexual intercourse with a dead body.

negativism: learned sense of helplessness.

neologism: meaningless new word created to which the person gives a special significance as seen in psychosis.

neuroleptic malignant syndrome: potentially fatal reaction most often seen with high-potency antipsychotic drugs causing muscular rigidity, tremors, inability to speak, altered level of consciousness, hyperthermia, autonomic dysfunction, and elevated blood count.

neurotransmitter: substance released when the axon terminal of a presynaptic neuron is excited that travels across the synapse to act on the target cell to either inhibit or excite.

nursing diagnosis: identification of an actual or potential client problem based on conclusions about the collected data.

nursing interventions: actions taken by the nurse to assist the client in achieving the anticipated outcome.

nursing process: scientific and systematic method for providing effective individualized nursing care to resolve client problems.

O

objective data: information observed by the nurse or provided by others who are familiar with the client or additional members of the health care team.

objectivity: characteristic that allows the nurse to remain unbiased and open to what the client is saying about their problem and about themselves.

obsession: reoccurrence of persistent unwanted thoughts or images that cause a person intense anxiety.

oedipal conflict: psychosexual stage that Freud describes as a time in which a boy begins to feel romantic feelings for his mother but fears the wrath of his father.

Omnibus Budget Reform Act (OBRA): prevented the inappropriate placement of clients with mental illness into nursing homes.

oral stage: early stage during first 2 years when, according to Freudian theory, the child seeks pleasure from sucking and oral gratification of hunger.

orientation phase: introductory phase of the therapeutic relationship that involves getting to know the client, building trust, identifying problems and expectations, and establishing a baseline for the next step in the process.

P

palliative coping: coping strategy that temporarily relieves the anxiety but the problem still exists and must be dealt with at a later time.

panic attack: intense feeling of fear or terror that occurs suddenly and intermittently without warning.

paralalia: repetitious, sometimes continuous repetition of one word.

paraphilia: psychosexual disorder in which unusual or bizarre imagery or acts are necessary in order to achieve sexual excitement.

passive-aggressive: anger expressed in an indirect and subtle way that acts on hostile feelings.

pedophilia: unnatural desire for sexual relations with children.

persecution: false belief that one is being threatened or in danger of being harmed.

personality disorder: extreme pathological and maladaptive behavior patterns that are destructive to the person and others.

personality traits: defining characteristics that are unique to each individual.

phallic stage: psychosexual theory stage around the age of 4 years in which the child discovers pleasure in genital stimulation while also struggling to accept a sexual identity.

physical abuse: intentional acts of slapping, pinching, choking, scratching, stabbing, shooting, or homicide that are injurious to another person.

physical restraint: use of mechanical devices to provide limited movement by the client or to prevent harm to self or others.

postconventional: phase of moral development in which the individual recognizes the importance of societal rules as a basis for behavior but may also follow internal moral principles that supercede these rules.

postsynaptic receptor: cell component that is distal to the synapse that combines with a drug, hormone, or chemical to alter the function of the cell.

posturing: person in stupor assumes a rigid bizarre posture held against gravity, resisting efforts to be moved for extended periods of time.

poverty of speech: little or no verbal speech.

powerlessness: feeling of inability to control the outcome of one's actions or environmental situation.

preconscious: level of the mind not present in consciousness, but able to be recalled at will.

preconventional: phase of moral development in which moral reasoning is guided by punishments and rewards with a focus on avoiding punishment and obedience to authority without concern for the interests or feelings of others.

preoperational: second stage of cognitive development, according to Piaget, that is characterized by the development of internal mental representations (schema) and verbal communication.

presynaptic compartment: storage compartment for neurotransmitters located before the nerve synapse.

primary aging: changes that result from genetics or natural factors.

primary gain: relief that is felt when anxiety is converted into physical symptoms of a disorder.

prioritize: organizing nursing problems or diagnoses according to the intensity and immediate urgency of the problem.

prodromal phase: beginning of schizophrenia with insidious onset of symptoms of increasing anxiety, inability to concentrate, or complete goal-oriented tasks.

professional boundaries: gaps between the concern and perceived power of the nurse and the dependent nature of the client.

pseudoneurologic: symptoms that involve false voluntary motor or sensory functioning seen in conversion disorder.

pseudoself: the self a person presents to the world.

psychiatrist: physician who specializes in the study, treatment, and prevention of mental disorders.

psychodynamic therapy: based on Freudian psychoanalytic theory that assumes a person with insight into early relationships and experiences as a source of his or her problems can resolve these issues through analysis and insight.

psychogenic: psychological origin for conversion symptoms

psychological crisis: emotional response to a situation in which the person is totally overwhelmed and usual coping strategies fail or are not available.

psychopharmacology: study of the changes that occur as the drugs interact with the chemicals in the brain.

psychophysiological: symptoms that cannot be attributed to a medical condition.

psychosis: mental state in which there is mental disorganization and loss of contact with reality.

psychosocial: related to both psychological and social factors.

psychotherapy: method of treating disease by mental means rather than physical.

psychotropic agents: drugs that affect psychiatric function, behavior, or experience by exerting their primary effect on neurotransmitter systems of the body.

purging: evacuation of the digestive tract by means of self-induced vomiting, or by use of excessive diuretics, or laxatives.

R

rapid cycling: four or more mood shifts within 1 year.

reflection: communication technique that paraphrases the message client has conveyed to nurse.

reframing: way of restructuring our thinking about a stressful event into one that is less disturbing and over which we can have some control.

reinforcement: stimulus used in operant conditioning that increases the probability that a given behavior associated with the stimulus will be repeated.

relapse: recurrence of a disorder or symptoms after apparent recovery.

restating: repeats to client the content of interaction that serves to lead and encourage further discussion.

reuptake: deactivation of neurotransmitters by their entry into the presynaptic compartment from the synaptic cleft.

S

schizoaffective disorder: form of schizophrenia in which the person demonstrates symptoms of major depression or mania in addition to the primary symptoms of delusions, hallucinations, and disorganized behaviors of schizophrenia.

schizophrenia: form of psychosis characterized by disorganized thoughts, perceptual alterations, inappropriate affect, and decreased emotional response to reality.

seclusion: refers to the placement of a patient in a controlled environment in order to treat a clinical emergency.

secondary aging: changes that are influenced by environmental factors.

secondary gain: attention that is received from others as a result of physical symptoms.

secondary traits: personality traits that have some bearing on a person's behavior but that are not particularly central to what the person does.

selective amnesia: person retains memory of some portions of an event, but not all details surrounding the situation.

self-awareness: consciousness of one's own individuality and personality with an attitude of openness to make positive changes.

self-mutilation: intentional act of inflicting bodily injury to oneself without an intent to die as a result.

sensorimotor: first stage of cognitive development in Piaget's theory in which individuals largely develop in terms of sensory input and motor output abilities with reflexive responses and gradually expanding to schema and purposeful actions.

serotonin: potent vasoconstrictor thought to be involved in neural mechanisms related to arousal, sleep, dreams, mood, appetite, and sensitivity to pain.

serotonin-specific reuptake inhibitors (SSRIs): antidepressant drug agents used in the treatment of depression.

sexual abuse: any behavior using forced or unwanted sex that is inflicted on an unwilling participant.

sexual dysfunction: degree of persistent or recurrent symptoms, subjective distress, or decrease in the quality of sexual stimulation during any phase of the sexual response cycle.

sexuality: feelings and life of an individual as related to sex including the physical, chemical, and psychological functioning characterized by gender and sexual behavior.

sexual masochism: actual beating, binding, humiliating, or otherwise causing the victim to suffer.

sexual orientation: individual preference or sexual attraction.

sexual sadism: individual receives sexual excitement from observing psychological or physical suffering by the victim, while receiving additional satisfaction from the feelings of complete control over the victim.

situational crisis: unpredictable and sudden without warning such as natural disaster, fatal automobile accident, or sudden death.

social phobia: excessive and persistent irrational fear of specific objects or situations that actually pose little threat of danger.

solid self: self which includes the beliefs a person has about themselves and their environment as a result of life experiences.

soma: Greek word that refers to the body.

somatic symptom disorder: one or more somatic symptoms with accompanying abnormal thoughts, feelings or behavior disproportionate to the symptoms that cause disruption in the person's daily functioning.

somatization: predictable syndrome of physical complaints and symptoms that are expressed as a result of psychological stress.

specific phobia: characterized by an excessive and persistent irrational fear of specific objects or situations that actually pose little threat of danger.

splitting: extreme view of an all or none relationship with the world.

stress reaction: physical response to a stressor that is triggered by an arousal of the autonomic nervous system.

stress: condition that results when a threat or challenge to one's well-being requires a person to adjust or adapt to the environment.

stalking: harassing or threatening phone calls, e-mails, texts, mail, or unwanted appearances at victim's place of employment or home.

stupor: lack of awareness or orientation.

stuttering: repetitive or prolonged sounds or syllables with pauses and monosyllabic broken words.

subjective data: information provided by the client including history and perception of the present situation or problem.

substance: refers to any drug, medication, or toxins that share the potential for abuse.

substance abuse: maladaptive recurring use of a substance accompanied by repeated detrimental effects as a result of continued use.

substance intoxication: overindulgence or being poisoned by a drug or toxic substance.

suicidal erosion: long-term accumulation of negative experiences throughout a person's lifetime that leads to suicidal thoughts.

suicidal gesture: action that indicates a person may be about ready to carry out a plan for suicide.

suicidal ideation: verbalized thought or idea that indicates a person's desire to do self-harm or destruction.

suicidal threat: statement of intent accompanied by behavior changes that indicate a person has defined their plan to end their life.

suicide attempt: person carries out their plan with actions to end their life.

sundowning syndrome: increase in psychiatric symptoms of psychomotor restlessness and confusion at night or during evening hours.

superego: one of three psychodynamic concepts which includes all internal norms and values of society acquired during early development through interactions with parents as figures of societal authority.

switching process: changing of one personality to another that occurs very abruptly in dissociative identity disorder.

synaptic cleft: point of junction between two neurons in a neural pathway where neurotransmitters trigger receptor response.

T

tardive dyskinesia: extrapyramidal syndrome after long-term use of antipsychotic drugs with irreversible movements of the mouth and face that include grimacing, lip-smacking, grinding of teeth, and protruding tongue movements; cogwheel rigidity, pill-rolling, and tremors.

telemental health: use of electronic and telecommunication technology to deliver and manage long-distance mental health care to rural and underserved areas.

telephone scatologia: obscene phone calls that lead to sexual arousal.

temperament: individual differences in the intensity and duration of emotions including the characteristics of one's disposition.

termination phase: time of promoting the client independence in getting along with others, and depending on his or her own strengths through improved adaptive skills.

therapeutic milieu: a safe and secure structured setting that facilitates the therapeutic interaction between clients and members of the professional team amidst a supportive network in which there is a sense of common goals.

thought broadcasting: false belief that one's thoughts can be heard by others.

thought insertion: false belief that thoughts of others can be implanted in one's mind.

thought withdrawal: false belief that others can remove thoughts from one's mind.

tic: sudden, repetitive, arrhythmic, stereotyped motor movement or verbal speech.

tolerance: condition that develops through continued use of a substance as the brain adapts to repeated doses of the drug with a declining effect as it is taken repeatedly over time.

trait anger: a general biological leaning toward a volatile personality that reflects a quick response or irritation and fury or a quick temper.

transvestic fetishism: sexual arousal that results from cross-dressing by a man in women's clothing and fantasies of himself as a woman.

tricyclic agents (TCAs): drugs with three hydrocarbon rings that inhibit reuptake of norepinephrine and serotonin in the treatment of clinical depression.

U

unconscious: level of consciousness at which thoughts, wishes, and feelings are not retrievable to conscious awareness.

uncued: panic attack in which the person is unable to connect any particular stimulus with the panic attack.

unipolar: having depressive episodes but does not experience mania or hypomania.

unresolved grief: process of grieving becomes prolonged and may be considered abnormal or maladaptive when symptoms are still present 2 months after the loss.

V

validation: verify the nurse's perception of feeling conveyed by either verbal or nonverbal message of the client.

vascular disease (dementia): vascular disorder in which there are multiple large and small cerebral infarctions leading to a step-like pattern of dementia. Symptoms of dementia.

verbigeration: repeating of words, phrases, or sentences several time.

violence: an aggressive means to maintain power in a situation or relationship.

voluntary commitment: client is admitted for mental health treatment based on his or her chosen willingness to comply with the treatment program.

voyeurism: experiencing of sexual gratification by observing nude persons or the sexual activity of others.

W

water intoxication: condition in which an excessive amount of water is consumed, leading to abdominal cramps, dizziness, lethargy, nausea and vomiting, convulsions, and possible coma.

waxy flexibility: posturing in which a person's body part can be moved and it will remain in that position until moved by another person.

Wernicke–Korsakoff syndrome: mental disorder characterized by amnesia, clouding of consciousness, confabulation, memory loss, and peripheral neuropathy. The disorder is associated with thiamine and niacin vitamin deficiency seen in chronic alcoholism.

withdrawal: maladaptive change in behavior accompanied by physiological and psychological alterations that occur as the blood or tissue concentrations of a substance decline in a person who has engaged in heavy prolonged use of a substance.

word salad: meaningless and incoherent mixture of words or phrases.

working stage: phase in which outcomes and interventions toward behavior changes are planned and goals are developed to improve the client's well-being.

Z

zoophilia: sexual arousal by sexual contact with animals.

Index

Anxiety disorders, 302, 305
Anxiety scale (sample), 344
Anxiolytics, 130–131
Aphasia, 319
Appeals and complaints, 58
Appropriate care, 57
Apraxia, 319
APRN. *See* Advanced-practice nurses
Assertion, anger management, 24
Assessment, nursing process, 88–89
    components of, 89
Assimilation, 42
Attention deficit hyperactive disorder (ADHD), 77, 297–299
Autism Spectrum Disorder, 295–297
Automatic relief behaviors, 122
Autonomic nervous system, 5
Avoidant personality disorder, 195
    incidence and etiology, 195
    signs and symptoms, 195
Avolition, 168

B

Babies temperament
    difficult, 35
    easy, 35
    slow-to-warm-up, 35
Bailey, Harriet, Nursing Mental Diseases, 53
Bandura, Albert (Social Learning Theory), 46
Bargaining stage of grief, 12
Batterer, 21
Beck, Aaron Cognitive-Behavioral Theory, 46
Beck's Depression Scale, 345–346
Behavior alterations in psychosis, 164–165
Behavioral therapy, 77
Behaviorism, 46
Behavioristic Theory (Skinner), 45, 46
Benzodiazepine, 131
Bereavement, 11
Bethlehem Royal Hospital, 52
Binge-eating disorder, 267, 270
Binging, 267
Biofeedback, 79
Biomedical therapy, 78–79
Bipolar disorders (manic depression), 143–145
Blame and grief, 12
Blocking, 100
Blocks to therapeutic communication, 105
Body dysmorphic disorder, 129
Borderline personality disorder, 191–193
    incidence and etiology, 191, 193
    signs and symptoms, 191–192
Boston City Hospital Training School for Nurses, 53
Boundaries, professional, 112–113
Bowen, Murray (Family Systems Theory), 44–45
Bulimia nervosa, 268–270
Bullying, 20–21
Burnout, 8
Bush, George, Decade of the Brain, 54

C

Cannabis drugs, 246
Caregiver's role, 76
Care plan, 94–95
    sample, 94–95
Caring, 111
Case manager, 75
Catalepsy, 164
Catastrophic events, 319
Catatonic behaviors, 164
Catatonic schizophrenia, 169
CBT. *See* Cognitive behavioral therapy
Central traits, 34
Cerebral edema, 166
Characteristic behavior patterns, 64–65
Chemical restraint, 59
Chronic abuse, 49

Chronic sorrow, 13. *See also* Grief; Loss
Circumstantiality, 100
Clang associations, 144
Client advocate, 76
Client rights, 57–58
Clients
    ability to cope, 61, 62
    difficult behaviors of, 113–115
    dual diagnosis, 63
    independence, 112
    physical illnesses, 62
    psychological factors, 62
Clinical psychologists, 74
Clinton, Bill, 54
Cluster A personality disorders, 186–189
Cluster B personality disorders, 189–194
Cluster C personality disorders, 184–197
Cocaine, 249
Code of ethics, 113
Codependency, 235
Codependent, 235
Cognitive-Behavioral Theory (Beck), 46
Cognitive behavioral therapy (CBT), 77–78
Cognitive Development Related to Personality (Piaget), 42
Cognitive disorders, 315
Collaborative team approach, 73–75
Communication
    leading statements to client for providing information, 133
    in mental health nursing, 100
    nontherapeutic communication, 104–106
    response to difficult client behaviors, 113–115
        altered thought processes, 114–115
        manipulation, 114
        sexually inappropriate behaviors, 115
        violence/aggression, 114
    speech patterns of clients mental illness, 100–101
    therapeutic communication
        active listening, 103
        blocks to, 105
        nonverbal communication techniques, 102–103
        verbal communication techniques, 101–102
Community-based care, 53–54
Community Health Centers Amendment of 1975, 53
Community living centers, 57
Compassion, 111
Compensatory methods in bulimia, 269
Compulsions, 129
Concrete mental operations, 42
Conduct disorder, 302
Confabulation, 318
Confidentiality, 58
Conflict situation, 8
Conscious, 35
Continuous amnesia, 220
Contracting in therapy, 78
Control Theory (Glasser), 34–35
Conventional grief, 11. *See also* Grief; Loss
Conventional level, Moral Development Theory, 43
Conversion disorder, 208–209
Coping strategies (anxiety and stress)
    adaptive, 8
    dysfunctional, 8
    maladaptive, 8
    palliative, 8
Copropraxia, 303
Correctional facilities, 63–64
Counselor, 76
Countertransference, 36
Couples therapy, 78
Craving, 231
Creative art therapy, 79
Crisis. *See also* Anxiety; Stress
    intervention, 25–26
    psychological, 24–25
    types, 25
Cued panic attack, 123
Cultural identity, 3
Culture, 3
Cyclothymic disorder, 145

Family therapy, 78
Fight or flight response, 5
Flashbacks, 128
Flight of ideas, 101
Focusing, 102
Formal operations, 42
Free-floating anxiety, 122
Freud, Sigmund (Psychoanalytic Theory), 35–38

G

GABA, 131
Gender dysphoria disorder
  incidence and etiology, 285
  signs and symptoms, 284–285
Generalized amnesia, 219
Generalized anxiety disorder, 122–123
Genital stage, psychosexual development, 38
Genuineness, 110
Glasser, William (Reality Therapy and Control Theory), 34–35
Grandiosity, 144
Grief
  coping with, 13
  definition, 9
  dysfunctional, 13
  as process, 11
  reactions, 12
  stages of
    acceptance, 12
    anger, 12
    bargaining, 12
    denial, 12
    depression, 12
  types of, 10–11
Group therapy, 78

H

Haldol, 170
Hallucinations, 114, 115, 163
Health Insurance Portability and Accountability Act (HIPAA)
  of 1996, 58
Hepatitis B and C, 66
Heroin, 248
Hierarchy of needs (Maslow), 34
Histrionic personality disorder, 194
  incidence and etiology, 194
  signs and symptoms, 194
HIV, 66
Holistic concept of nursing, 61
Holistic view of human beings, 34
Homeless people, 166
Home milieu, 73
Hospital units, 57
Hostility, 20
Humanistic theories, personality, 34
Humanistic therapy, 77
Hydrocodone, 248
Hypomania, 144
Hysteria, 206

I

Id, 36
Ideas of reference, 188–189
Illness anxiety disorder, 208
Illusions, 114, 163
Independence of clients, 112
Individual psychotherapy, 77–78
Informed consent, 57–58
Inpatient psychiatric settings, 60–61
Inside the Criminal Mind (Samenow), 63
Institutionalized clients, 53
Intellectual Developmental Disability, 292–294
Interaction with society, 37
Intermittent explosive disorder, 300
Internal stressors, 6

Interpersonal Development Theory (Sullivan), 43
Interpersonal relationships, 43
Interventions, 25–26
  in nursing process, 92–93
Involuntary commitment, 60–61
Irrational thoughts, reframing, 9

J

JCAHO. *See* Joint Commission on Accreditation of Healthcare Organizations
Job-related burnout, 8
Joint Commission on Mental Illness and Health (1955), 53

K

Kinesics, 103
Kohlberg, Lawrence (Theory of Moral Development), 42–43
Kubler-Ross, Elisabeth, 12

L

La belle indifference, 209
Labile, 144
Latency stage, psychosexual development, 38
LCSW. *See* Licensed clinical social workers
Least restrictive environments, 57
Legal and ethical considerations in mental health care, 56–60
  client rights
    appeals and complaints, 58
    appropriate care, 57
    confidentiality, 58
    informed consent, 57–58
  ethics, 56
  nurse accountability, 59–60
  restraints
    chemical restraint, 59
    physical restraint, 59
  seclusion, 59
Level of differentiation, 44
Lewy body dementia, 322
Lewy Body Neurocognitive Disorder, 322
Licensed clinical social workers (LCSWs), 74
Licensed practical/vocational nurse (LPN/LVN), 74
Licensed professional counselors (LPCs), 74
Lipid solubility, 81
Lithium carbonate, 53, 81, 151
Lobotomies, 53
Localized amnesia, 219
Long term memory, 146
Long-term outcomes, 91
Loose associations, 101, 164
Loss
  age-related concepts of loss, 11
  coping with, 13
  definition, 10–11
LPC. *See* Licensed professional counselors
LPN/LVN. *See* Licensed practical/vocational nurse
LSD intoxication, 247

M

Magical thinking, 188
Major depressive disorder, 141–143, 145–150
Maladaptive coping, 8
Maladaptive defense mechanisms, 37–38
Malingered fugue, 220
Mania, 141
Manic depression (bipolar disorder), 143–145
Manipulation, 63
Mannerisms, 165
MAOI. *See* Monoamine oxidase inhibitors
Marijuana, 244
Maslow, Abraham, 34
Maslow's hierarchy of needs, 34, 91
Mellaril (Thioridazine), 170
Mental disorder. *See* Mental illness